Beyond Condoms

Beyond Condoms

Alternative Approaches to HIV Prevention

Edited by

Ann O'Leary

Centers for Disease Control and Prevention
Atlanta, Georgia

Springer Science+Business Media, LLC

Library of Congress Cataloging-in-Publication Data

Beyond condoms: alternative approaches to HIV prevention/edited by Ann O'Leary.
p. cm.
Includes bibliographical references and index.
ISBN 978-1-4757-7686-7 ISBN 978-0-306-47518-4 (eBook)
DOI 10.1007/978-0-306-47518-4
1. AIDS (Disease)—Prevention. I. O'Leary, Ann.

RA643.8 .B49 2002
616.97'9205—dc21

2001054193

ISBN 978-1-4757-7686-7

Originally published by Kluwer Academic / Plenum Publishers, New York in 2002
Softcover reprint of the hardcover 1st edition 2002

http://www.wkap.nl

10 9 8 7 6 5 4 3 2 1

A C.I.P. record for this book is available from the Library of Congress

Contributors

Andrea Allen • Department of Psychiatry, Mount Sinai School of Medicine, New York, New York

Sevgi O. Aral • Division of STD Prevention, National Center for HIV, STD and TB Prevention, Centers for Disease Control and Prevention, Atlanta Georgia

Bernard M. Branson • Division of HIV/AIDS Prevention, National Center for HIV, STD and TB Prevention, Centers for Disease Control and Prevention, Atlanta Georgia

Delia Easton • Division of HIV/AIDS Prevention, National Center for HIV, STD and TB Prevention, Centers for Disease Control and Prevention, Atlanta Georgia

Dana Fry • Center for Health Behavior and Communication Research, Annenberg School for Communication, University of Pennsylvania, Philadelphia, Pennsylvania

Eric Hollander • Department of Psychiatry, Mount Sinai School of Medicine, New York, New York

David R. Holtgrave • Division of HIV/AIDS Prevention, National Center for HIV, STD and TB Prevention, Centers for Disease Control and Prevention, Atlanta Georgia

Robert Janssen • Division of HIV/AIDS Prevention, National Center for HIV, STD and TB Prevention, Centers for Disease Control and Prevention, Atlanta Georgia

John B. Jemmott III • Center for Health Behavior and Communication Research, Annenberg School for Communication, University of Pennsylvania, Philadelphia, Pennsylvania

Charles Klein • City and County of San Francisco Department of Public Health, San Francisco, California

Susan Kippax • Mcquarie University, National Center in HIV Social Research, School of Behavioral Sciences, Sydney, Australia

Janet S. Moore • Division of HIV/AIDS Prevention, National Center for HIV, STD and TB Prevention, Centers for Disease Control and Prevention, Atlanta Georgia

Jon Morgenstern • Department of Psychiatry, Mount Sinai School of Medicine, New York, New York

Ann O'Leary • Division of HIV/AIDS Prevention, National Center for HIV, STD and TB Prevention, Centers for Disease Control and Prevention, Atlanta Georgia

Richard Parker • The Sociomedical Sciences Division, Joseph L. Mailman School of Public Health, Department of Health Policy and Institutions, Columbia University New York, New York

Lynn Paxton • Division of HIV/AIDS Prevention, National Center for HIV, STD and TB Prevention, Centers for Disease Control and Prevention, Atlanta Georgia

Thomas A. Peterman • Division of HIV/AIDS Prevention, Surveillance and Epidemology, National Center for HIV, STD and TB Prevention, Centers for Disease Control and Prevention, Atlanta Georgia

Steven D. Pinkerton • Center for AIDS Intervention Research, Department of Psychiatry and Behavioral Medicine, Medical College of Wisconsin, Milwaukee, Wisconsin

Martha Rogers • Division of HIV/AIDS Prevention, National Center for HIV, STD and TB Prevention, Centers for Disease Control and Prevention, Atlanta Georgia

Troy Suarez • Division of HIV/AIDS Prevention, National Center for HIV, STD and TB Prevention, Centers for Disease Control and Prevention, Atlanta Georgia

Richard J. Wolitski • Division of HIV/AIDS Prevention, National Center for HIV, STD and TB Prevention, Centers for Disease Control and Prevention, Atlanta Georgia

Foreword

Our contemporary division of the progress of time should be delineated as B.A.E. (Before the AIDS Epidemic, i.e., 1981) and P.A.E. Everyone keeps predicting the end of the epidemic, as *Newsweek* did in 1996 when combination therapy was introduced. But as far as we can tell from this vantage point, the virus continues, albeit a bit hobbled by a few drugs here and there, but moving forward nonetheless. Predictions are that over 100 million people will be infected with HIV by 2005. It is also clear that the number of people living with HIV in the US and other developed countries will continue to grow, as people with HIV live longer and better lives, but, paradoxically and perhaps as a result, the number of people acquiring HIV also continues to grow.

HIV vaccines are at least 20, and perhaps 40 years away. When they do come on board, they may not prevent infection but may, instead, change the course of illness in those infected and hopefully render them less infectious. Further, the first vaccines will, in all likelihood, be less than 100% effective. The next generation of prevention strategies need to combine the best of biomedical, social, and behavioral approaches in order to protect the population.

The male condom, along with reduction in the number of sexual partners or outright abstinence, have been the mainstay of HIV prevention. The male condom has its drawbacks and detractors, and abstinence until marriage and fidelity thereafter is an objective that few achieve. Hence, the need to promote alternatives in a serious way.

This welcome volume presents some of those alternatives—the female condom, social change, use of anti-depressant medications, treatment of sexually transmitted infections, treatment of HIV disease. These are beginnings and this book is a beginning. Let's hope that this book results in serious research on the efficacy of these approaches, alone and in combination, and the resulting addition of new tools to the HIV prevention armamentarium. Let us also hope that additional creative thinking goes forward and presents with even different options. We need as many as can be mustered. The P.A.E. era has just begun.

Thomas Coates

Preface

Since HIV was first identified and shown to be sexually transmitted, consistent use of latex condoms has been the standard prevention message given to individuals at risk of becoming infected with the virus or transmitting it to others. It is not surprising, given medicines past successes in identifying single "magic bullets" to solve health problems, and given the high level of prevention effectiveness demonstrated by consistent and correct use of condoms, that alternative strategies have seldom been sought. At the same time, consistent condom use is difficult for many individuals to achieve, and the prospect of a lifetime of this regimen is daunting to most of us. In the developing world, condom availability and affordability is often limited. Condoms prevent pregnancy, which is desired by many couples. Finally, while condoms, when properly used, are very effective in preventing HIV transmission, they are not 100% effective-they do sometimes break-and may not be available or accessible to everyone about to be engaged in sex.

Careful review of the HIV prevention literature suggests that, while behavioral intervention focusing on consistent condom use can produce significant behavior change, the majority of participants in these studies do not change their behavior completely, and many do not change at all. Specific difficulties exist for women at risk due to the behavior of primary male partners (see O'Leary, 2001); couples wishing to have children; persons with severe sexual self-control deficits; and individuals in impoverished countries who cannot obtain or afford condoms.

A growing view in HIV prevention is that the one-size-fits-all approach may not be the most effective public health strategy. Rather, different approaches or combinations of approaches may be optimal for particular individuals in diverse life circumstances. These approaches do not contradict condom use; most of them would be improved in effectiveness if combined with condom use. However, each has the potential, by itself, to produce a reduction in incident cases of HIV infection.

This volume brings together several alternative approaches, reviewing effectiveness and feasibility data and making specific suggestions for needed research. The amount of evidence for their public health impact varies across the strategies but is mostly inferential: few have yet been critically evaluated. In each case, research is greatly needed.

Chapter 1 by Susan Kippax describes research on "negotiated safety" agreements among men who have sex with men. In this approach, men who test HIV-seroconcordant (more advisable when both are negative) agree to abandon use of condoms with each other but to avoid risk behavior with others, thus protecting the dyad. While this chapter focuses on gay men, the approach may also be effective for some heterosexual couples (see O'Leary, in press for a review), particularly those who wish to conceive children. HIV antibody testing is an important, and until recently, underestimated tool in the prevention armamentarium. While individuals testing negative do not reliably reduce their behavioral risk, a number of reviews and metaanalyses have indicated that those who test positive, including serodiscordant couples, do (Weinhardt, Carey, Johnson, & Bickham, 1999). Indeed, a recent randomized comparison of HIV testing and health education yielded just these findings for the tested group in a three-country trial (The Voluntary HIVl Counseling and Testing Efficacy Study Group, 2000).

Many health-related behaviors are affected by elements of the environment, such as Policy and structural factors. Further, changes in policy and other environmental factors have been shown to change behavior. Examples from other domains include excise taxation, which has been shown to reduce consumption of tobacco and alcohol, and seat belt and motorcycle helmet laws. In HIV, structural factors have contributed enormously to the spread of the epidemic. To give one example, roads built to facilitate the transportation of cargo combined with trucking and roadside sex work to disseminate the epidemic in Africa and Asia. Klein, Easton, and Parker review structural interventions and their potential to reduce the HIV epidemic (Chapter 2) in primarily an international context where the work has been done. The need to identify structural and policy interventions to reduce the spread of HIV in the U. S. is pressing.

It can be particularly difficult for women to persuade their primary partners to use condoms. Some evidence suggests that violence-prone men may react violently to condom requests, possibly attributing the requests to female infidelity. In most cultures, women are relatively disempowered in sexual situations and do not make sexual decisions. Because some women are unable convince their male partners to use condoms, research and advocacy efforts have centered on the development and deployment of prevention technologies that are under the control of women themselves. At this time, we have two types of female-controlled technology: female condoms and vaginal microbicides. Unfortunately, while several microbicide candidates are under study, we do not yet have an agent that is effective against HIV in vivo. Moore and review and present the state of the science regarding these technologies.

Engaging consistently in safe sexual behavior is also difficult for those who suffer from sexual self-control deficits. Indeed, many individuals seek help in the form of psychotherapy or twelve-step groups. Gay men in HIV epicenters are especially likely to be concerned about this problem because it may be associated with heightened risk of infection or transmission of the virus. Chapter 9 by O'Leary, Suarez, and Morgenstem examines the potential role of specific serotonin reuptake inhibitors to increase control over sexual behavior. Recent research with male paraphilics and sex offenders suggests the efficacy of pharmacologic treatment of these conditions using these drugs. Possible mediating processes include reductions in anxiety, lowered depression and/or sexual side effects of reduced libido and sexual function. While to date there have been no studies of the effectiveness of this approach for HIV the chapter articulates a rationale for testing it, and describes an ongoing study that is doing just that. STDs are important cofactors in HIV transmission. Having STDs and their associated lesions potentiates the chance both of becoming HIV-infected if exposed, and of transmitting the virus if infected. In much of the developing world where condoms are less available, STD treatment has long been seen as an important component of HIV prevention. STD epidemics in the U. S. are also significant, particularly in communities most affected by HIV/AIDS, and STD control is just as important here. Chapter 5 reviews the evidence for the effectiveness of STD treatment as a prevention strategy in developing countries. Of particular interest are two large-scale trials, both conducted in Africa, in which STD control was evaluated for its effect on HIV incidence. These trials obtained different results; reasons for this difference are reviewed.

Wolitski and Branson review the understudied phenomenon of "gray area" behaviors-behaviors other than condom use that are performed in order to reduce the risk of HIV transmission. Partner selection strategies, oral sex, withdrawal prior to ejaculation, and using serostatus to make decisions about the "directionality" of behavior (e. g., a seropositive man engaging in receptive, but not insertive, anal sex) are discussed. There is evidence that use of these prevention measures is widespread, yet, their levels of risk reduction effectiveness is not known. This is an unfortunate gap in our knowledge base, and represents a failure of communication between behavioral scientists who observe these behaviors and the epidemiologists and bench scientists who are equipped to study their riskiness.

Sexual abstinence and delay of onset of sexual activity to prevent HIV may be an important prevention tool, particularly for young people. However, while abstinence messages have been the subject of much debate, the scientific knowledge base concerning their efficacy is inadequate. Nevertheless, Jemmott and Fry review this literature in Chapter 6 and conclude that, while no credible support exists for the effectiveness of the abstinence interventions that have been tested to date, researchers should continue to evaluate different ways of promoting abstinence and delaying sex among adolescents.

One of the more exciting developments in HIV care and prevention has been the arrival in 1996 of highly active antiretroviral therapies, or HAART. These medications and medication cocktails have prolonged the lives of thousands of infected individuals in the developed world (although they are not yet widely available in the developing world). Many of those on HAART regimens have serum levels of virus that are very low, and often even undetectable. An interesting effect of this is that when viral levels are low in the blood, they are also low in semen. This means that transmission risk is probably lower, possibly markedly so, according to the evidence that exists to date. Unfortunately, this silver lining has a dark cloud: HIV is developing resistance to these medications--partly but not entirely due to nonadherence-and new infections of drug resistant virus are occurring. If individuals use beliefs about their infectiousness based on their viral load in their sexual decision-making -- for example, assuming that if it was undetectable at last physician visit it is not necessary to use condoms with seronegative partners – but in the meantime resistance has developed and their viral load rebounded – the partner could become infected and not be helped by the new medications. Chapter 5 reviews the literature on prevention, including a discussion of post-exposure prophylaxis.

Evaluating the comparative cost effectiveness of alternative strategies will be an important priority, as discussed by Pinkerton and Holtgrave in Chapter 7. Public health dollars are limited and the HIV epidemic continues to grow, so it will be very important to spend those dollars in ways that maximize the number of HIV infections averted. Indeed, spending HIV prevention dollars in a cost-effective manner was a key recommendation in a recent Institute of Medicine report (IOM, 2000). What makes cost-effectiveness analyses particularly challenging in the face of multiple approaches will be the importance of matching at-risk individual, community or country to the most cost-effective prevention strategies for that entity. For example, sexual compulsivity affects a relatively small number of individuals, but those individuals may be "core transmitters" or highly at risk for infection. Cost-effective use of pharmacologic treatments (should they prove effective) must be matched to those few who would benefit from them, and it may be worth spending considerable resources to achieve this matching.

This point will be addressed in the final chapter, by O 'Leary, Aral and Peterman. We use the term "Prevention Triage" to describe this matching process, and discuss the complexities involved in the delivery of multicomponent public health strategies.

The HIV epidemic has ravaged the human race in the last twenty years. Our best efforts to date have not been sufficient even to contain, let alone reduce it. The pace at which we are gaining knowledge is inadequate under conditions of rapid changes in the biology of the virus and its treatment, social phenomena influencing behavior, and innovative thinking on the part of those at risk and infected (evidenced, for example in "gray area" behaviors). We researchers must be equally innovative and swift to respond to these changes if we are to make a difference in the HIV pandemic. It is my hope that each of these chapters will stimulate research leading to a better understanding of our prevention technologies and options, and a more effective prevention response.

Ann O'Leary

REFERENCES

Institute of Medicine (2000). No Time to Lose: Getting More from HIV Prevention. Monica S. Ruiz, Alicia R. Gable, Edward H. Kaplan, Michael A. Stoto, Harvey Fineberg, and James Trussell, Editors. Washington, D. C.: National Academy Press.

O'Leary, A. (2001). Women at Risk for HIV from a Primary Partner: Balancing Risk and Intimacy. *Annual Review of Sex Research*:2000. Society for the Scientific Study of Sex, 191-234.

The Voluntary HIV-1 Counseling and Testing Efficacy Study Group (2000). Efficacy of voluntary HIV-1 counseling and testing in individuals and couples in Kenya, Tanzania, and Trinidad: a randomised trial. *Lancet*, 356, 86-7.

Weinhardt, L. S., Carey, M. P., Johnson, B. T., &Bickham, N. L. (1999). Effects of HIV counseling and testing on sexual risk behavior: A meta-analytic review of published research, 9851997. *American Journal of Public Health*, 89, 1397-1405.

ACKNOWLEDGEMENTS

The editor would like to express her deepest appreciation to Daphne Cobb, Pat Thomas, and Laura Whelan for considerable technical assistance.

This book is dedicated to the memory of Kermit Graf.

Contents

Chapter 1

Negotiated Safety Agreements Among Gay Men

Susan Kippax
Mcquarie University
National Center in HIV Social Research
School of Behavioral Sciences
Sydney, Australia

1. NEGOTIATED SAFETY STRATEGY

HIV-seronegative people who engage in unprotected sexual intercourse cannot transmit HIV: they cannot infect another whether condoms are used or not. This premise underpins an HIV-prevention strategy adopted by gay men, a strategy in which anal intercourse is practised without the use of condoms. Under some conditions – when negotiated safety agreements are in place and adhered to – this strategy is an effective HIV-prevention strategy. The focus of this chapter is this HIV-prevention strategy, the 'negotiated safety' strategy.

As early as 1982 and before HIV was identified as the virus that caused AIDS (Callen 1983; Patton 1989), gay men had adopted condoms to protect themselves against AIDS. "Condoms every time" became the slogan underpinning an extremely successful health promotion strategy – at least in the industrialised world. In the late 1980s and early 1990s, however, a number of researchers documented the widespread practice of unprotected anal intercourse, anal intercourse without condoms, among gay men within regular relationships (Detels, English, Visscher, et al., 1989; Doll, Byers, Bolan, et al., 1991; Davies, 1992; Kippax, Crawford, Davis, et al., 1993; Dawson, Fitzpatrick, Reeves, et al., 1994; Bosga, de Wit, de Vroome, et al., 1995). Where such data were available, it was clear that unprotected anal intercourse was more likely with regular partners than with casual sexual partners.

While some researchers considered that the practice of unprotected anal intercourse signaled a waning of the 'safe sex' response of gay men, a 'relapse' (Stall, Ekstrand, Pollack et al., 1990; Ekstrand, Stall, Kegeles, et al., 1993), others were not so sure. A number of researchers (Davies, 1992; Davies, 1993; and Kippax, Crawford, Davis, et al., 1993) entertained the hypothesis that the practice adopted by men in relationships may be part of a deliberate 'safe sex' strategy. They argued that, under certain conditions, the practice of unprotected anal intercourse is safe with regard to HIV transmission and the strategy was named 'negotiated safety' (Kippax, Crawford, Davis, et al., 1993; Kippax 1996).

2. WHAT IS NEGOTIATED SAFETY?

The term 'negotiated safety' identifies the strategy, adopted by some gay and other homosexually active men, of negotiating and reaching agreement to dispense with condoms within an HIV-seronegative regular or committed relationship. It also refers to the patterns of sexual practice that conform to these negotiated agreements. For two men in a sexual partnership, dispensing with condoms for anal intercourse within the relationship is safe with respect to HIV transmission under certain conditions.

The conditions that apply are that:

- the sexual partners are in a regular relationship
- the sexual partners are HIV-antibody negative and are aware of each other's negative antibody status
- the sexual partners have reached a clear and unambiguous agreement about the nature of their sexual practice within and outside their relationship
- the agreement is that sexual practice outside their relationship is safe with regard to HIV transmission, and
- the agreement is kept.

These definitional conditions make 'negotiated safety' a complex strategy. Complexity is both a strength and a cause for concern. It is a strength because the very complexity of the strategy calls for clarification, and thus for communication and discussion between partners. It is a concern because the success of the simple slogan 'condoms every time' could be in danger of being undermined or overturned, since the negotiated safety strategy allows for the non-use of condoms under certain conditions.

The following section examines the complexity of the negotiated safety strategy by addressing each of the conditions in turn.

3. CONDITIONS OF NEGOTIATED SAFETY

3.1 Regular/casual distinction

Knowledge of one's sexual partner's serostatus is essential to negotiated safety agreements but such knowledge can never be completely relied upon. Within a regular or committed relationship however, there is a basis for trust. Hence the condition that negotiated safety should apply only to men in regular relationships.

Men within regular relationships can more reliably know their partner's serostatus and may use this knowledge as well as knowledge of their own serostatus in framing negotiated safety agreements regarding anal intercourse both inside and outside the relationship. Agreements to dispense with condoms within casual encounters or relationships do not fall within the ambit of 'negotiated safety' because of the absence of reliable knowledge about the serostatus of the casual sexual partner.

While most regular relationships are committed or 'primary' relationships, some men who regularly engage in sexual intercourse with one or two or occasionally more particular partners, or 'fuck buddies', might also identify these partners as regular. Relationships that are identified as either committed or 'fuck buddy' relationships are included within the notion of 'regular'. Most men can identify whether their relationship is a regular one or a casual one – except at the beginning of a relationship. As discussed below, the beginnings as well as the ends of relationships produce strains on negotiated safety.

3.2 HIV test status

As noted above, HIV testing is a necessary precondition of negotiated safety and both partners in the regular relationship need to be HIV-negative. The condition that those engaged in negotiated safety agreements be HIV-negative acknowledges the doubts that remain about superinfection Butto, Argentini, Mazzella et al. (1997).

The advent of reliable testing for HIV in the mid 1980s and the practice of gay men being tested regularly – in Australia (Grunseit, Rodden, Crawford et al. 1996; Kippax, Noble, Prestage et al. 1997), North America (Hoff, Stall, Paul et al. 1997; Myers, Godin, Lambert et al. 1996; Wagner, Remien and Carballo-Dieguez, 1998); the United Kingdom (Dawson, Fitzpatrick, Reeves et al. 1994; Elford, Bolding, Maguire et al.1999); and western European countries (Bochow 1997; Jeannin, Cohen and Bajos,

1998; Adam 1999; Davidovich, de Wit and Stroebe, 2000) – has made a negotiated safety strategy possible.

There are however large variations across the western world with regard to testing practice. In Australia approximately 85% of gay men recruited from gay venues in large cities reported having ever been tested (National Centre in HIV Social Research (a), 1999), with similar proportions reporting 'ever been tested' in a large New York City survey in 1999 (Gay Men's Health Crisis, 1999) and in France where gay men were recruited via readership of the French gay press (Adam 1999). Fifty seven percent of homosexually active men recruited from London Pride Festival reported having been tested (Hickson, Weatherburn, Reid et al., 1999), while 63% of gay men recruited through gay-identified venues in Canada (Meyers, Godin, Lambert et al., 1996) reported having done so. On the available data, in the countries under study, the smallest proportion of men reporting having ever been tested live in the Netherlands – between 40% and 49% of gay men, depending on how recruited (Davidovich, personal communication). In countries where HIV testing is not widespread, negotiated safety is likely to be an effective HIV-prevention strategy for only a small minority of men.

3.3 Talk and Communication

The requirement of knowing that one's own and one's partner's serostatus are concordant for HIV-negative antibodies necessitates talk about HIV serostatus. This necessity to talk has been captured by the education campaign designed by the AIDS Council of New South Wales (ACON), Australia, and known as the "Talk, Test, Test, Trust ...Together" campaign (Kinder 1996). The campaign was launched in May 1996 and run again in 1998. The decision to address unprotected anal intercourse within gay relationships was taken in order to provide realistic education material around the changing needs of gay men to the cumulative impact of the HIV epidemic (Kinder 1996).

The campaign specifically acknowledged and addressed concerns about men's ability to talk about intimate and emotional matters and the need for open communication. The "Test, Test" aspect of the slogan in the Negotiated Safety Poster campaign material contained the following advice to gay men: "Both of you need to get tested – be honest about your results. If both tests are negative then, ... Three months later, get tested again, before you stop using condoms. If you're both negative a second time...Reach a clear mutual agreement ... "(AIDS Council of New South Wales, 1998). The message on the poster was complemented by additional advice in a brochure suggesting a variety of ways to talk about getting tested and test results.

3.4 The negotiated agreement

Within negotiated safety there are agreements to be reached about sex *within* the regular relationship and agreements to be reached about sex *outside* the regular relationship. Sex within the regular relationship, by definition, includes unprotected anal intercourse. Sex outside the regular relationship may take a number of forms. There are a number of options and the three most common (Kippax, Noble, Prestage et al., 1997; Crawford, Rodden, Kippax et al., unpubl.paper; Davidovich, de Wit and Stroebe, 2000) may be described as follows:

1. the men opt for no sex outside the relationship at all; that is, they adopt mutual monogamy as a strategy.
2. the men opt for no anal intercourse outside the relationship and thus agree that any sex outside with casual partners is restricted to oral-genital sex, mutual masturbation or some other relatively safe sexual practice.
3. the men opt for anal intercourse outside the relationship, but agree that all such intercourse with casual partners is protected, that is that condoms are used 100% of the time.

Whatever the agreement reached about sex outside the regular relationship, the 'negotiated safety' agreement and the practices that conform to those agreements must be of the kind that, if adhered to, preclude the possibility of HIV transmission within the regular relationship.

Negotiated safety agreements should not be confused with monogamy. Monogamy is not the kind of agreement that necessarily precludes transmission and a simple-minded reliance on it without negotiation of a safety agreement is a truly dangerous strategy. It has been estimated, for example, that well over 50% of women infected with HIV in Africa and India have never had sex with anyone other than their husbands (Kippax, Crawford and Waldby, 1994; Piot, 1999). Agreed-upon mutual monogamy is an appropriate agreement but is only one of a number of possible 'negotiated safety' agreements.

Ensuring that the agreement is an appropriate one and that it is concise, clearly understood by both partners, and mutually agreed upon means there must be good communication. There must be "talk". As the Negotiated Safety Poster campaign put it: "Be honest with each other, and talk about all the issues. It is the talking that remains critical throughout.... Reach a clear, mutual agreement about sex inside and outside the relationship" (AIDS Council of New South Wales, 1998).

3.5 Trust together

Once embarked upon, the personal success of the negotiated safety strategy depends upon mutual trust and honesty. Trust and honesty go a long way to ensuring that the practice of unprotected anal intercourse within the relationship remains safe. It is safe only as long as both partners remain HIV seronegative.

As Davidovich, de Wit and Stroebe (in press) note trust, honesty, intimacy and love are subjective heuristics that do not necessarily guarantee safety. The agreement has to be kept – or if broken – acted upon. The Negotiated Safety Campaign Brochure illustrates this aspect: "... if you slip up it is important that as a couple you can talk about it without fear ... Honest communication is essential" (AIDS Council of New South Wales, 1998). The brochure also contained practical advice on what to do if a slip up occurred: "It means you will both have to go back to using condoms again. Agree to start the 'talk, test, test, trust process again ... together". In recognition of the same interpersonal issues, the strategy promotion material in the Netherlands contains a game for the partners in the regular relationship. The players, with the help of the cards, get to know intimate aspects of the sexual behaviour (in and outside of the relationship), and sexual desires and fantasies of their partners (Davidovich, personal communication).

4. IS NEGOTIATED SAFETY A SAFE OR RISKY PERSONAL STRATEGY?

Before turning to the very difficult task of assessing the long-term impact of the negotiated safety strategy on community HIV-prevention efforts and the related question of whether such a strategy might undermine the condom strategy, there is a prior question. Is it an effective personal risk-reduction strategy?

Given that the strategy was built on what was a pre-existing practice, the fact that gay men generally understood the message is not surprising. Process evaluation of the 1996 "Talk Test Test Trust ... Together" education campaign in Sydney revealed that recall of the campaign material was high. Most importantly no one understood the campaign as meaning that gay men could just give up condoms. The evaluators concluded that the campaign had been successful in that it "had added to gay men's understanding of how to negotiate unprotected sex within their relationships (Mackie 1996, p.36).

With regard to the question of effectiveness, the absence of HIV transmission within regular relationships in which negotiated safety has been adopted provides the ultimate test of negotiated safety as a personal risk-reduction strategy. There are no studies examining whether adopting negotiated safety agreements increases or decreases the risk of HIV transmission. Such studies – the most stringent test of the strategy – are needed. They would need to be longitudinal and track the sexual practice of men who remain in their HIV seroconcordant regular relationship over the duration of the study, and they would need to compare HIV transmission rates between those who have negotiated safety agreements in place and those who have not.

The next most stringent test of negotiated safety is a test of compliance with the negotiated safety agreement. Three studies have tested whether men who make negotiated safety agreements adhere to them. Two of these studies investigated negotiated safety among gay men in Sydney (Kippax, Noble, Prestage et al., 1997) and Australia (Crawford, Rodden, Kippax et al., unpubl.), the third examined negotiated safety and negotiated safety compliance among gay men in Amsterdam (Davidovich, de Wit and Stroebe, 2000). All three studies reported low levels of non-compliance with negotiated safety agreements, ranging from 10% in the Amsterdam study (Davidovich, de Wit and Stroebe, 2000), to 11% in the Sydney cohort study (Kippax, Noble, Prestage et al., 1997) and to 7% in the Australian sample (Crawford, Rodden, Kippax, et al., unpubl.). That is, all three studies indicated that the adoption of the strategy was successful in that around 90% of men in each study complied with their negotiated safety agreements and did not place their regular partners at risk of HIV infection. The last of these studies also found that although no class of agreement precludes risk behaviour, negotiated safety agreements were as effective in achieving low levels of risk as 'condoms always' agreements. While 7% of men who had a negotiated safety agreement engaged in risk practices, 9% of those who agreed to use condoms within their regular and/or casual relationships did so. These findings indicate that the negotiated safety agreements entered into by the men in this study were as effective in achieving low levels of risk practice as agreements to have only protected anal intercourse.

Some other studies, while examining the sexual risk behaviour of gay men in regular relationships, are unable to test the efficacy of the negotiated safety strategy directly, as they did not include any measure of agreements between men. Elford, Bolding, Maguire et al. (1999) report that while many gay men in central London engaged in unprotected anal intercourse only within their regular relationship, nearly half of these men were unaware of their own HIV status, their partner's or both. As Elford, Bolding, Maguire et al. (1999, pp1409-10) note: "under these circumstances, there is a risk of HIV transmission within the relationship. It appears that whereas gay men in a relationship have for the most part adopted the first principle of negotiated safety: to have UAI only with their main partner, not all have embraced the second principle: to establish that they are HIV seroconcordant."

Two recent studies in the United States also provide indirect evidence regarding some components of negotiated safety. Focusing on test status rather than relationship status, Ekstrand, Stall, Paul, et al. (1999) examined the risk behaviours of gay men recruited into the San Francisco Men's Health Study. The results indicated that a little over half the men reporting unprotected anal intercourse did so with partners whom they believed to be of the same serostatus, and classified these men as 'low transmission risk'. Eighty one percent of these 'low transmission risk' men were in a 'current relationship' and 91% had disclosed their HIV status to all their anal sex partners. These men are very different from men reporting unprotected anal intercourse with partners of unknown or different serostatus, 'high transmission risk' men: only 49% of these 'high transmission risk' men were in a current relationship and only 32% of them had disclosed their HIV status. While no information regarding agreements was available, the data suggest that the men in the 'low transmission risk' category may have been practising 'negotiated safety'.

Similar evidence comes from a study of gay men recruited in Portland and Tuscon. Hoff, Stall, Paul et al. (1997) concluded that the substantially lower rate of unprotected anal intercourse they found among men in discordant relationships compared with men in concordant relationships suggests that individuals and couples make judgments about sex and behaviour based on knowledge of one's own and one's partner's serostatus.

The findings from a study investigating gay men's seroconversions focuses our attention on those men for whom the strategy has failed (Kippax, Hendry, Kaldor, et al., 1996). This study analysed the stories that gay men gave of their recent seroconversion; a detailed narrative account of the occasion they believed led to their HIV infection. The men's retrospective accounts indicated that approximately half of the seroconversions occurred within a regular or primary relationship and that half again of these appeared to have been as a result of simple reliance on monogamy, implicit safety agreements, or some break down in a negotiated safety agreement. That is, in approximately 25% of the narrative accounts, an inability to talk openly, failures to negotiate and misplaced trust were cited alongside 'being in love' and 'passion' as reasons associated with HIV transmission.

> "...and after a number or couple of years of having protected sex with [my regular sexual partner], we stopped using protection last year because our understanding is that we are both monogamous and that's

still my understanding... But the upshot of it was that he'd had the virus for eight years and hadn't the courage to tell me."

The first three months of a relationship appeared to be particularly problematic, as was the end of a relationship.

"...it was a very very close, a very deep relationship... but it finished very quickly... He used to get very edgy around test time (every three months)... Basically with him I was receptive – prefer it ... I trusted him totally in all things, not just sexual."

While further research is needed, there are conclusions that can be drawn from these few studies. Negotiated safety is being practised in Australia and the Netherlands but by different numbers of men. The very different levels of testing in Australia and the Netherlands probably account for the different levels of uptake of the strategy – 29% in Australia (Crawford, Rodden, Kippax et al., unpubl.) compared with 12% in the Netherlands (Davidovich, de Wit, and Stroebe, 2000). The presence of a number of the elements of the negotiated safety strategy – disclosure of test status, seroconcordance, unprotected anal intercourse, and being in a regular relationship, also suggests that it is being practised by gay men in the United Kingdom, and in the United States.

Furthermore the indications are that the strategy is working in Australia and the Netherlands – at least in as much as the sexual partners within regular relationships adhere to their negotiated safety agreements. Whether this is because these two countries have advocated and promoted negotiated safety campaigns – in 1996 in Australia and 1998 in the Netherlands – awaits further confirmation.

The findings however also tell us that all men do not adhere to their agreements and/or that the negotiated safety agreements if made at all are not clear and /or mutually agreed. What these studies do not tell us – or only hint at – are the reasons for the non-compliance. For this, research is needed which gives us insight into the dynamics of partnerships, emotional and sexual relationships.

5. LOVE AND TRUST

While it is important that the men who adopt a negotiated safety strategy are in a regular relationship, the nature of regular relationships gives rise to the major problems associated with negotiated safety. These are human concerns; concerns about love, about intimacy and trust, and about open and honest communication.

McLean, Boulton, Brookes et al., (1994) reported that the emotional involvement inherent in regular relationships undermines safe sexual practice. While not focusing on negotiated safety, Flowers, Smith, Sheeran et al. (1997), using interpretive, phenomenological analysis of in-depth interviews of English gay men in relationships, found that within the context of romance men often privileged commitment, trust and love over health.

Ridge (1996) also using in-depth analytic techniques, interviewed a small number of Australian gay men, some of them more than once. The narratives he analysed suggested that honest two-way discussion based on equal relations around sexual issues was uncommon in these men's partnerships. Fear of rejection, fear of being perceived as vulnerable, anxiety about emotional intimacy, and imbalances of power were some of the reasons for this lack of good communication. Furthermore, like Flowers, Smith, Sheeran et al., (1997), Ridge also found that the emotions of love, romance and passion often over-rode health concerns. Fear of being HIV-positive, fear of one's partner discovering that the agreement had been broken, and fear of being found wanting, further complicate this already complex picture. Adam (1999) warns against a simplistic acceptance of negotiated safety. Negotiated safety agreements he argues are only as strong as the relationship within which the safety agreement is brokered.

The data reported above however indicate that the strategy does work for most men most of the time, at least insofar as we have been able to assess the strategy, that is, in terms of compliance with negotiated safety agreements. On the strength of the findings presented here, negotiated safety is a reasonably effective personal risk-reduction strategy.

The findings also point to sites of tension and to areas of strain – the interpersonal and partnership dynamics. These tensions are however the grounds on which relationships are built and do not provide good reason for eschewing negotiated safety. Negotiation, like relationships, needs nurturing and time should be allowed to develop the necessary skills. As the beginnings and likewise the ends of relationships are commonly fraught with difficulty, negotiated safety might be best left to calmer periods. However, as Adam and Sears (1996, pp75-76) concluded on the basis of their analysis of in-depth interview with people living with HIV: "Safer sex is not only a practical problem with a specific solution, but it is also a complex negotiation about love, trust, mutuality, and the erotic… This is not to argue that sexuality is not subject to conscious control, but rather that erotic and emotional relationships draw upon complex interweaving of social codes, practical negations, and layered meanings."

6. BROADER QUESTION OF SUCCESS OR FAILURE

Is it likely that the negotiated safety strategy will undermine the 'safe sex' culture? If nothing else, to advocate the use *and* non-use of condoms raises a range of significant educational issues.

Although there are is little evidence that bears on this question, two sources provide some data. The first concerns the proportion of men in regular relationships who continue to use condoms as their main risk-reduction strategy. Findings from six-monthly cross-sectional surveys of gay men recruited from sex clubs, saunas, social clubs and bars, and clinics in Sydney indicated that the proportion of gay men who had unprotected anal intercourse with their regular partner increased over time: from 23.4% in February 1996, three months prior to the "Talk Test Test Trust ... Together" campaign, to 34.0% in August 1999 (National Centre in HIV Social Research (b), 1999). These same surveys show that over the same time period the proportion of men using condoms always for anal intercourse with their regular partners decreased from 30.8% in February 1996 to 23.8% in August 1999. (The remainder of the men either did not engage in anal intercourse with their regular partner or had no regular partner at the time of interview.) Although it is likely that the increase in unprotected anal intercourse is in large part a result of the education campaign, Talk, Test, Test, Trust ... Together, these findings indicate that 'condoms always' is still a strategy that many men in regular relationships continue to employ. Similarly in the national survey of gay and other homosexually active men, Crawford, Rodden, Kippax et al. (unpubl.) found that of the men in regular relationships, while approximately one third had negotiated safety agreements, over one third continued to use condoms and engaged in protected anal intercourse only. The remaining 22% had either no agreement at all or some form of unsafe agreement.

It is also important to note that among the men practising negotiated safety, a sizeable proportion, around 41%, had an agreement with which they complied, to use condoms with their casual sexual partners (Kippax, Noble, Prestage et al., 1997).

Another concern regarding the undermining of the safe sex culture and 'condoms every time' is the leakage of negotiated safety to other forms of sexual practice. While it is true that a large proportion (68.5%) of HIV-positive gay men in Australia engage in unprotected anal intercourse with their HIV-positive partners, it remains unclear whether this is a risk practice (National Centre in HIV Social Research (a), 1999). While superinfection may be a problem, positive-positive sex does not transmit HIV. The more worrying trend has been an increase in unprotected anal intercourse with casual sexual partners amongst both HIV-positive and HIV-negative men. While there is some evidence that the increase is a response to treatment successes and availability (Van de Ven, Kippax, Knox et al., 1999), it is also possible that it is, at least in part, a function of negotiated safety.

The main point to make however is that since May 1996 when negotiated safety was promoted as a possible safe sexual strategy there has been no dramatic decrease in condom use – except within a negotiated safety agreement. Furthermore, for many men, the negotiated safety strategy means 'condoms every time' for casual sex. More importantly since May 1996 there has been no apparent increase in HIV transmission among gay men in Australia and the Netherlands. There is little if any evidence to indicate an undermining of the 'safe sex' message or, indeed, the 'safe sex' culture.

7. CONCLUSION

Negotiated safety, and the agreements that comprise it, is a complex HIV-prevention strategy. The debate about whether it is an effective personal and community strategy needs to continue and that debate needs to be positioned within the following framework:

- Unprotected anal intercourse commonly occurs between men in regular relationships. The question that must be addressed is whether to lower the risk of such behaviour or attempt to change it. The evidence that has been presented in this chapter indicates that the former move may be the most appropriate and sensible one. The available evidence also indicates that men need to be skilled in negotiating and warned of the dangers of negotiated safety at the beginnings of relationships.
- Whether negotiated safety undermines 'condoms always' in a manner that undermines safe sex culture remains to be demonstrated. Many men use condoms with their casual partners but not with their regular partners, other men continue to use condoms 'every time', while a small proportion of men never use them for anal intercourse. So providing a range of options for safe sex practice makes sense.

Education for health promotion that combines notions of personal freedom and personal choice with a practical response is more likely to be effective than education that inhibits desire and prohibits desired activity. Gay men are capable of developing their own risk avoidance and risk reduction strategies – indeed what researchers have called 'negotiated safety' was invented by them.

"... there is no truth, in that there is no single pre-determined method which all people can use to avoid further HIV transmission. Rather there are important problems which sexually active people need to face, and a range of possible solutions available to solve those problems. It is no mistake that some of the people whose lives are affected have worked out their own solutions to their own identified problems, using their own chosen processes to do so. The role of researchers, educators and policy makers should now be to help others do the same" Parnell (1996, p.105).

REFERENCES

Adam BD, Sears A: Negotiating sexual relationships after testing HIV-positive. *Medical Anthropology* 1996, 16: 63- 77.

Adam P: Unprotected sex with stable and casual partners among French gay men in a steady relationship, according to HIV status. Paper presented at the *10th Conference on Social Aspects of AIDS,* London; June 1999.

Butto S, Argentini C, Mazzella AM, Iannotti MP, Leone P, Leone P, Nicolosi A, Rezza G: Dual infection with different strains of the same HIV-1 subtype. *AIDS* 1997, 11: 694-696.

AIDS Council of New South Wales: Campaign Overview of 'Talk Test Test Trust ... Together" – 1998: Sydney 1998: 1-4.

Bochow M: Type of partnership as it affects the risk strategies of German gay men. Paper presented at *3rd AIDS Impact Conference,* Melbourne; June 1997.

Bosga MB, de Wit JBF, de Vroome EMM, Houweling H, Schop W, Sandfort TGM: Differences in perception of risk for HIV infection with steady and non-steady partners among homosexual men. *AIDS Educ Prev* 1995, 7: 103-115.

Callen M: *How to Have Sex in an Epidemic.* New York: News from the Front Publications; 1983.

Crawford J, Rodden P, Kippax S, Van de Ven P: Negotiated safety and other agreements between men in relationships: risk practice redefined. (under review)

Davidovich U, de Wit JBF, Stroebe W: Assessing sexual risk behaviour of young men in primary relationships – the incorporation of negotiated safety and negotiated safety compliance. (in press).

Davies PM, Project Sigma: On relapse: recidivism or rational response? In *AIDS: Rights, Risks and Reasons.* Edited by Aggleton P, Davies P, Hart G. London: Falmer Press; 1992: 133-141.

Davies PM: Safer sex maintenance among gay men: are we moving in the right direction? [letter]. *AIDS* 1993, 7: 2279-280.

Dawson JM, Fitzpatrick RM, Reeves G, Boulton M, McLean J, Hart GJ, Brookes M: Awareness of sexual partners' HIV status as an influence upon high-risk sexual behaviour among gay men. *AIDS* 1994, 8: 837-841.

Detels R, English P, Visscher BR, Jacobson L, Kingsley LA, Chmiel JS, Dudley JP, Eldred LJ, Ginzburg HM: Seroconversion, sexual activity and condom use among 2915 HIV seronegative men followed for up to two years. *J Acquir Immune Defic Syndr* 1989, 2: 77-83.

Doll LS, Byers RH, Bolan G, Douglas JM, Moss PM, Weller PD, Joy D, Bartholow BN, Harrison JS: Homosexual men who engage in high-risk sexual behavior: a multicenter comparison. *Sex Transm Dis* 1991, 18: 170-175.

Ekstrand ML, Stall RD, Kegeles S, Hays R, DeMayo M, Coates TJ: Safer sex among gay men: what is the ultimate goal? [letter]. *AIDS* 1993, 7: 281-281.

Ekstrand ML, Stall RD, Paul JP, Osmond DH, Coates TJ: Gay men report high rates of unprotected anal sex with partners of unknown or discordant HIV status. *AIDS* 1999, 13: 1525-1533.

Elford J, Bolding G, Maguire M, Sherr L: Sexual risk behaviour among gay men in a relationship. *AIDS* 1999, 13: 1407-1411.

Flowers P, Smith JA, Sheeran P, Beail N: Health and romance: understanding unprotected sex in relationships between gay men. *British J Health Psychol* 1997, 2: 73-86.

Gay Men's Health Crisis: GMHC releases largest survey since the start of AIDS on gay men's sexual practices in New York City. News Release, 1999, June 27:1-3.

Grunseit A, Rodden P, Crawford J, Kippax S: Patterns of serological testing in HIV-1 seronegative men. *Venereology* 1996, 9: 120-128.

Hickson F, Weatherburn P, Reid D, Henderson L, Stephens M: Evidence for Change: Findings from the National Gay Men's Sex Survey 1998. *Sigma Research Report;* November 1999: 1-77.

Hoff CC, Stall R, Paul J, Acree M, Daigle D, Phillips K, Kegeles S, Jinich S, Ekstrand M, Coates TJ: Differences in sexual behavior among HIV discordant and concordant gay men in primary relationships. *J Acquir Immune Defic Syndr and Human Retrovir* 1997, 14: 72-78.

Jeannin A, Cohen M, Bajos N: Voluntary HIV testing. In *Sexual Behaviour and HIV/AIDS in Europe.* Edited by Hubert M, Bajos N, Sandfort T. London: UCL Press; 1998: 287-302.

Kinder P: A new prevention education strategy for gay men: responding to the impact of AIDS on gay men's lives. Paper presented at the *Eleventh International Conference on AIDS,* Abstract We.C.442. Vancouver: July 1996.

Kippax S, Crawford J, Davis M, Rodden P, Dowsett G: Sustaining safe sex: a longitudinal study of a sample of homosexual men. *AIDS* 1993, 7: 257-263.

Kippax S, Crawford J, Waldby C: Heterosexuality, masculinity and HIV: barriers to safe heterosexual practice. *AIDS* 1994, 8 (suppl 1): S315-S323.

Kippax, S: A commentary on negotiated safety. *Venereology* 1996, 2: 96-97.

Kippax S, Hendry O, Kaldor J, Grulich A: Seroconversion in context. Paper presented at *8th Annual Conference of the Australian Society for HIV Medicine,* Sydney, November 1996.

Kippax S, Noble J, Prestage G, Crawford J, Campbell D, Baxter D, Cooper D: Sexual negotiation in the AIDS era: negotiated safety revisited. *AIDS* 1997, 11: 191-197.

Mackie B: Report & Process Evaluation of the 'Talk, Test, Test, Trust ... Together' HIV/AIDS Education Campaign. AIDS Council of New South Wales, October 1996: 1-36.

McLean J, Boulton M, Brookes M, Lakhani D, Fitzpatrick R, Dawson J, McKechnie R, Hart G: Regular partners and risky behaviour – why do gay men have unprotected anal intercourse? *AIDS Care* 1994, 6: 331-341.

Myers T, Godin G, Lambert J, Calzavara L, Locker D: Sexual risk and HIV-testing behaviour by gay and bisexual men in Canada. *AIDS Care* 1996, 8: 297-309.

National Centre in HIV Social Research (a): HIV/AIDS & Related Diseases in Australia: Annual Report of Behaviour 1999. Sydney, 1999:1-41.

National Centre in HIV Social Research (b): Sydney Gay Community Surveillance Report: Update to December 1999. Sydney, 1999, 9: 1-16.

Patton C: Resistance and the Erotic. In *AIDS: Social Representations, Social Practices.* Edited by Aggleton P, Hart G, Davies P. London: Falmer Press; 1989: 237-251.

Piot P: Action on AIDS in the new millennium: a critical time for Asia and the Pacific. Plenary address at 5th *International AIDS in Asia and the Pacific Conference: The Next Millennium: Taking Stock and Moving Forward,* Kuala Lumpur, October. 1999.

Parnell B: Unprotected sexual intercourse in 'safe' contexts: deciding what matters most. *Venereology* 1996, 2: 104-105.

Ridge D: Negotiated safety: not negotiable or safe? *Venereology* 1996, 2: 98-100.

Stall R, Ekstrand M, Pollack I, McKusick I, Coates TJ: Relapse from safer sex: the next challenge for AIDS prevention efforts. *J Acquir Immune Defic Syndr* 1990, 3: 1181-1187.

Van de Ven P, Kippax S, Knox S, Prestage G, Crawford J: HIV treatments optimism and sexual behaviour among gay men in Sydney and Melbourne. *AIDS* 1999, 13: 2289-2294.

Wagner GJ, Remien RH, Carballo-Dieguez A: "Extramarital" sex: Is there an increased risk for HIV transmission? A study of male couples of mixed HIV status. *AIDS Educ Prev* 1998, 10, 245-256.

Chapter 2

Structural Barriers and Facilitators in HIV Prevention: A Review of International Research

Charles Klein
City and County of San Francisco Department of Public Health

Delia Easton
Hartford Hispanic Health Council

And

Richard Parker
The Sociomedical Sciences Division
Joseph L. Mailman School of Public Health
Department of Health Policy and Institutions
Columbia University

1. INTRODUCTION

In this chapter we review the evolving history of international research on HIV prevention, with particular emphasis on work that has been carried out in the developing world. We begin with a brief analysis of the shifting paradigms that have guided HIV-related research and intervention over the course of the epidemic. We then provide an overview of a growing body of literature focusing on the structural and environmental factors that shape the spread of the HIV/AIDS epidemic and create barriers and facilitators in relation to HIV prevention programs. This discussion suggests that many issues identified through research in developing countries are equally pertinent in some parts of the so-called developed world, such as among inner city populations in the United States, where strikingly similar political and economic factors affect HIV infection patterns and prevention efforts. We conclude by identifying some of the key challenges confronting structural research and interventions in both developing and developed contexts.

2. SHIFTING PARADIGMS IN HIV/AIDS PREVENTION RESEARCH

The rapid spread of HIV infection and AIDS in societies around the world in the early-1980s quickly drew attention to the almost complete lack of scientific knowledge on the specific sexual and drug-using behaviors that appeared to be responsible for HIV transmission. As a result, much of the social and behavioral research that emerged in response to the epidemic in the mid-1980s focused on surveys of risk-related behavior and of the knowledge, attitudes and practices which might be associated with the risk of HIV infection (see, for example, Carballo *et al*, 1989; Chouinard and Albert, 1989; Cohen and Trussell, 1996; Turner, Miller, and Moses, 1989). Building on existing behavioral theories such as the Health Belief Model (Becker and Joseph, 1988), the Theory of Reasoned Action (Ajzen and Fishbein, 1980), and Social Learning Theory (Bandura, 1977), intervention research in the United States worked to promote behavioral change by providing members of target population groups adequate knowledge, information and awareness of risk, thereby stimulating rational decision-making processes that would lead to significant risk reduction (see Aggleton, 1996; Aggleton and Coates, 1995; Miller, Turner and Moses, 1990; Parker, 1996; Parker, Barbosa, and Aggleton, 2000; Sweat and Denison, 1995; Turner, Miller, and Moses, 1989). Similar initiatives were developed throughout the 1980s and early-1990s in many of the countries of the Anglo-European world, and, beginning in the late-1980s, in a number of developing countries in Africa, Asia and Latin America (see Carballo *et al*, 1989; Cleland and Ferry, 1995; Parker, Barbosa, and Aggleton, 2000).[1]

As behavioral research and interventions were developed in wide range of social and cultural settings in various parts of the world, it soon became

[1] Perhaps the clearest programmatic expression of this second research phase can be found in the large-scale "Partner Relations" and "KABP" surveys that were developed between 1988 and 1991 by the Social and Behavioral Research Unit of the Global Programme on AIDS at the World Health Organization (WHO/GPA/SBR) and were implemented with the collaboration of National AIDS Programmes in dozens of countries throughout the developing world (see, in particular, Carballo *et al*, 1989; Cleland and Ferry, 1995).

evident that these approaches were not easily implemented in the face of often radically different understandings of sexual expression and drug use in different societies and cultures, and even in different subcultures within the same society (see Aggleton, 1996; Parker, 1994; Parker, Barbosa, and Aggleton, 2000).[2] Moreover, as study after study found that information in and of itself is insufficient to produce risk-reducing behavioral change, the marked limitations of the information and reasoned persuasion based paradigm were made clear (see Aggleton, 1996; Cohen, 1991; Parker, 1994; Parker, Barbosa, and Aggleton, 2000). By the end of the 1980s, research findings and practical experience in countries around the world had demonstrated that a far more complex set of social and cultural factors inevitably mediate the structure of behavioral risk in all population groups and that the dynamics of individual psychology could never be expected to explain (or stimulate) behavioral change without taking these broader issues into account (see Aggleton, 1996; Aggleton and Coates, 1995; Parker, 1994; Parker, Barbosa, and Aggleton, 2000; Sweat and Denison, 1995).

Facing these challenges, researchers turned their attention to the social and cultural structures and meanings that shape and construct sexual experience and drug use in different settings. In these endeavors, the focus moved from behavioral frequencies and the subjective experience of individual psychology to the inter-subjective nature of cultural meanings related to sexuality and drug use—their shared, collective quality, not as the property of atomized or isolated individuals, but of social persons integrated within the context of distinct and diverse cultural settings (see Aggleton, 1996; Herdt and Lindenbaum, 1992; Kippax and Crawford, 1993; Parker, 1994; Parker and Aggleton, 1999; Parker, Herdt and Carballo, 1991; Parker, Barbosa and Aggleton, 2000; ten Brummelhuis and Herdt, 1995). Utilizing "insider"/"experience-near" approaches (see Geertz, 1983; Parker, 1989, 1991, 1994; Parker and Aggleton, 1999; Parker, Barbosa and Aggleton, 2000), researchers documented the significant variability in indigenous cultural categories and classification systems which organize sexual experience and injecting drug use, and in the process, repeatedly showed that many of the key categories used to describe HIV risk behavior in Western medicine and public health epidemiology (e.g. "homosexuality" and "prostitution") are neither present in all cultural settings nor unchanging in

[2] It is perhaps not surprising that much of this work first emerged in research in non-Western settings where the biomedical categories of epidemiological analysis failed to be fully applicable. Increasingly, however, cultural analysis has also been developed in specific sexual and drug cultures or subcultures in the industrialized West, offering important new insights even in settings where extensive behavioral research had already been carried out (see, for example, Clatts, 1995, 1999; Kane, 1991).

their meaning where they do in fact exist (see Gillies and Parker, 1994; Parker, 1994; Parker, Herdt and Carballo, 1991; de Zalduondo, 1991). This emphasis on the cultural meanings, identities, and communities which structure sexual practice and injecting drug use has led to a reformulation of the idea of HIV/AIDS-related interventions, one in which the emphasis has shifted from individual behavioral change to community-based efforts aimed at the transformation of norms and values and the constitution of collective meanings in ways that will effectively promote safer sexual and injecting practices (see Kippax and Crawford, 1993; Kippax *et al*, 1993; Parker, 1994, 1995; Parker, Barbosa, and Aggleton, 2000).[3]

Although the cultural contexts and meaning paradigm has generated new insights on the factors shaping HIV/AIDS epidemics and has promoted the development of culturally-sensitive, community-based prevention programs and interventions, as time has passed it has become increasingly apparent that political and economic factors have played a central role in defining the patterns and spread of the epidemic, and that these same factors have been responsible for many of the most complex barriers to effective AIDS prevention programs. By the early to mid-1990s, much as social and cultural analysis reacted to the perceived short-comings of earlier behavioral approaches, a new focus on the structural and environmental factors associated with the increased risk of HIV responded to the perceived limitations of both behavioral and cultural approaches (e.g. Aggleton and Coates, 1995; Friedman, 1998a; Parker, Barbosa, and Aggleton, 2000; Parker and Gagnon, 1995; Sweat and Denison, 1996).[4] Uniting what is an

[3] Again, work carried out through the World Health Organization's Global Programme on AIDS (GPA) provides a striking example of this shift in research paradigms. With the reorganization of GPA and the establishment of a Social and Behavioral Research and Support Unit (WHO/GPA/SSB), a program of research focusing on sexual cultures and contexts was developed from 1992 to 1995 that contrasts sharply with the previous, population-based survey research. Important aspects of this work have been extended, as well, by the Joint United Nations Programme on HIV/AIDS (UNAIDS) from 1996 to the present. For an overview of this work and the findings that it produced, see, in particular, Aggleton and Mane, 1998.

[4] Depending on the disciplinary frameworks and traditions within which research has been carried out, the categories and terminology employed in examining these issues have varied. Researchers working within the context of social sciences such as anthropology, sociology or political science, for example, have largely framed their analyses within the context of political economy (see, for example, Farmer, 1996; Singer, 1998). Researchers working within a more behavioral framework in psychology and, particularly, the behavioral sciences within public health, have generally been less explicit in linking their approach to political economy – and its apparently Marxist overtones – and have preferred to speak of structural and environmental forces. This lack of specificity in terminology has led to a good deal of definitional confusion and has highlighted the need for greater

extremely diverse structural and environmental factors literature is a rejection of strictly behavioral models and interventions and an overarching goal of providing a more dynamic and realistic understanding of the relationship between individual agency and socio-cultural and political economic structures. But exactly how structural intervention researchers should study and explain the multi-leveled processes involved in HIV/AIDS epidemics is not clear in this literature, since most writings have concentrated more on general descriptions of the structural forces driving HIV/AIDS epidemics than on fully articulated theories and methodologies. However, several promising theoretical frameworks can be found in this body of work, including political economy/critical medical anthropology (Farmer, Lindenbaum, and Delvecchio-Good, 1993; Lindenbaum, 1998; Parker, 1994, 1996; Schoepf, 1992a, 1992b; Singer, 1998), structuration theory (Webb, 1997), political ecology (Turshen, 1998), and multi-level causation models (for example, Sweat and Denison, 1995; Decosas, 1996).

What is perhaps most important to emphasize is the extent to which structural and environmental factors approaches have reframed the whole notion of behavioral risk within the more complex conception of social vulnerability (see, in particular, Mann, Tarantola and Netter 1992; Mann and Tarantola 1996). This distinction is much more than a change in terminology and implies a radical movement in the scientific paradigms that have thus far largely organized and guided HIV/AIDS research. By shifting the focus from the investigation of risk, perceived typically in individualistic and behavioristic terms, to the analysis of vulnerability, understood as socially structured and conditioned, this recent work has opened the way for a fundamental rethinking of the most basic problems confronting social research on HIV/AIDS. Equally important, by linking the analysis of societal or collective vulnerability to the question of discrimination and the violation of basic human rights, as well as the structures that maintain and perpetuate them, this paradigm has raised the possibility of a radically transformed public health practice in response to HIV/AIDS—a shift from the technical (or technocratic) management of the epidemic to one that confronts the underlying politics of the epidemic and that can transform the broader forces structuring HIV/AIDS vulnerability and enable members of affected communities to response more adequately to them (see Aggleton and Coates, 1995; Farmer, Connors and Simmons, 1996; Freidman, 1998b; Mann 1995; Mann and Tarantola 1996; Mann, Tarantola and Netter 1992;

---

conceptual reflection and clarity concerning both levels of analyzable phenomena as well as the productive relations of social organization and social change (see Friedman and O'Reilly, 1997; Friedman, Des Jarlais and Ward, 1994; Sweat and Dennison, 1995; Tawil, Vertser and O'Reilly, 1995).

Parker, 1996; Parker, Barbosa, and Aggleton, 2000; Singer, 1998; Sweat and Denison, 1995; Tawil, Vertser and O'Reilly, 1995). In the following sections of this article, we provide an overview of this structural and environmental factors literature, focusing first on the structural forces that have been identified as shaping the course of the HIV/AIDS epidemic internationally, then on the political context and policy processes through which different societies have responded to the epidemic, and, finally, on targeted interventions that have been designed to prevent the further spread of HIV within specific populations and communities.

3. OVERVIEW OF RESEARCH ON STRUCTURAL FORCES SHAPING THE EPIDEMIC

During the past decade, researchers have documented a number of structural factors that facilitate HIV transmission and its concentration within particular geographic areas and populations (Aggleton, 1996; Caraël, Buvé, and Awusabo-Asare, 1997; Singer, 1998; Sweat and Denison, 1995; Tawil, Vertser and O'Reilly, 1995; Turshen, 1995). These factors can be grouped into three analytically distinct but interconnected categories: (1) economic (under)-development and poverty; (2) mobility, including migration, seasonal work, and social disruption due to war and political instability; and (3) gender inequalities. This research reveals that despite the uniqueness of each local HIV/AIDS epidemic, the same general structures and processes are at work in Africa (Akeroyd, 1994; Anarfi, 1993; Bassett, 1993; Bond and Vincent, 1991; Decosas, 1995, 1996; Jochelson, Mothibeli and Leger, 1994, Romero-Daza and Himmelgreen, 1998; Schoepf, 1988, 1992a, 1992b, 1993; Schoepf *et al*, 1991; Turshen, 1998; Webb, 1997; Wilson *et al*), Asia (Archavanitkul and Guest, 1994; Brown and Xenos, 1994; Kammerer *et al*, 1995; Symonds, 1998; Tan, 1993), Latin America and the Caribbean (Daniel and Parker, 1993; Farmer, 1992, 1995; Farmer, Lindenbaum, and Delvecchio-Good, 1993; Kreniske, 1991; Lurie *et al*, 1995; Susser and Kreniske, 1997), and certain groups and communities in North America and Europe (Singer, 1998; Des Jarlais *et al*, 1992a; Friedman, 1998a, 1998b; Lindenbaum, 1998).

3.1 Economic Development

One of the key themes examined in the structural and environmental factors literature is the connection between economic development and

HIV/AIDS vulnerability. An excellent example showing the richness of this approach is Decosas's historical analysis (Decosas, 1996) of how the Akosombo dam project in Ghana in the 1960s contributed to the HIV/AIDS epidemic among the Krobo in the 1980s and 1990s. During the building of the dam, many Krobo men went downstream to work on the project, while many Krobo women provided services, including sexual-economic exchanges, for men in the construction area. When the creation of Lake Volta destroyed the Krobo's agricultural base, a sizable number of these women, and later on, their daughters, went abroad to work as prostitutes, and remittances from sex work became an important source of development in the region. Both these generations of women have high HIV incidence. Today, with the economic future of Ghana looking brighter, remittances from women working abroad are becoming scarce, fewer young girls are entering sex work, and HIV incidence among younger Krobo women is approaching the lower rates seen in the rest of Ghana. Decosas's analysis demonstrates the difficulties in establishing the mechanism of association between economic development and HIV, since causes and effects, as well as costs and benefits, are dynamic and play out over decades.

Farmer's work on Haiti similarly documents how displacements caused by large-scale development initiatives can propel the spread of HIV infection (Farmer, 1992). More broadly, and as will be discussed further below, international and intergovernmental development policies have been linked to the disintegration of traditional socio-economic structures and the accentuation of socio-economic inequalities, which in turn have contributed significantly to the severity of the epidemic in sub-Saharan Africa and other parts of the developing world.[5] Indeed, poverty itself has been identified as perhaps the key socio-economic force behind the epidemic, and virtually all of the structural and environmental literature has highlighted the synergistic effects of poverty, when linked to other forms of social inequality, instability and discrimination, in promoting the spread of HIV (Farmer, Connors, and Simmons, 1996; Friedman 1998a, 1998b; Singer, 1998).

3.2 Migration, Population Movement and Political Instability

In addition to the general conditions of poverty, research has linked migration/mobility to increased HIV incidence and vulnerability in a variety of contexts and places, including seasonal laborers in southern Africa (Jochelson, Mothibeli, and Leger, 1994; Romero-Daza and Himmelgreen,

[5] Similar processes of social disintegration have been identified as playing a key role in HIV/AIDS epidemics in US inner cities (Wallace, 1998; Wallace *et al*, 1992).

1998) and West Africa (Decosas); Dominican migrants to the United States (Kreniske, 1991); rural to urban migrants in Haiti (Farmer, 1992, 1995) and Zaire (Schoepf, 1988, 1992a); Filipino overseas contract workers (Tan, 1993); female sex workers in Thailand (Archavanitkul and Guest, 1994), Ghana (Anarfi, 1993), Zimbabwe (Wilson *et al*, 1990) and the Philippines (Tan, 1993), and male sex workers and other men who have sex with men in Brazil (Larvie, 1997; Parker, 1993, 1997). The causation patterns behind this mobility/HIV connection are complex. Male migrant laborers, for example, regularly frequent female sex workers (themselves often migrants) and/or establish secondary households in the field, leading to increased incidence of STDs and HIV in locations that usually lack adequate health-care services. Back in the communities of origin, women face severe economic and emotional demands, which they attempt to meet through agricultural and sometimes sex work. Finally, since male and female migrant workers move back and forth between two or more locations, HIV may spread from higher to lower incidence areas. As is discussed in greater detail in the following section, this migration-related vulnerability to HIV/AIDS can be further exacerbated by the introduction of "economic reforms" such as structural adjustment programs (SAPS). Bassett, for example, describes how Zimbabwe's structural adjustment in the 1990s reduced social expenditures and condom availability (Bassett, 1993), while Turshen outlines the negative health consequences that resulted throughout Africa after the World Bank imposed SAPS of the late 1980s and 1990s (Turshen, 1998). Equally if not more devastating in terms of increasing HIV/AIDS vulnerability have been the social and economic dislocations caused by war and political conflict (Turshen, 1995; Bond and Vincent, 1991; Webb, 1997). And even absent on-going armed conflict, political instability has been shown to exacerbate poverty and to stimulate migration to urban areas, where a series of factors, including sexism, sexual union patterns, STD prevalence, and governmental inattention to AIDS, all facilitate HIV transmission (Farmer, 1995).

3.3 Gender Inequality

These examples of the relationship between poverty, migration/mobility and HIV effectively demonstrate that the political economic factors driving the HIV/AIDS epidemic are closely intertwined with existing gender and sexuality structures, whose hierarchies make women, and especially low-income women, extremely vulnerable to HIV infection. Nonetheless, there have been few in-depth studies of gender and sexuality as structural, rather than simply behavioral, factors shaping HIV transmission. Farmer,

Lindenbaum and Delvecchio-Good (1993) attribute this neglect to the initial predominance of AIDS cases among gay men, the fact that social scientists only poorly understand sexuality, and the frequent reliance of AIDS intervention programs on superficial "rapid ethnographic assessments." The resulting inadequacies of AIDS research and interventions directed toward women has led some scholars to look more closely at gender and sexuality systems in order to develop more realistic and effective HIV risk reduction options for women (Elias and Heise, 1994; Gupta and Weiss, 1993; Heise and Elias, 1995; Kammerer *et al*, 1995; Michal-Johnson, 1994; Schoepf, 1992a, 1992b; Schoepf *et al*, 1991; Symonds, 1998; Zoysa, Sweat, and Denison, 1996). Heise and Elias (1995), for example, argue that the three pronged approach of most global AIDS prevention programs (i.e., partner reduction, condom promotion, and STD treatment) are inadequate to protect most of the world's women, who are poor and lack the power to negotiate the terms of sexual encounters. Moreover, the association of condoms with distrust, communication failures between men and women regarding sexual and reproductive health matters, and a lack of perception of HIV vulnerability, further limit many women's ability to practice safer sex (Heise and Elias, 1995; Michal-Johnson, 1994; Zoysa, Sweat, and Denison, 1996), a situation compounded by the lack of female-controlled HIV prevention technologies (Elias and Heise, 1994; Stein, 1990).

The gender and sexuality literature offers several impressive ethnographic analyses that illuminate the cultural and political economic factors behind HIV vulnerability. Kammerer *et al*'s work, for example, describes how state and capitalist penetration has produced a breakdown in the economy of the mountain tribes in the northern Thailand periphery (Kammerer *et al*, 1995). As a result, young people have migrated to valley towns to work, sometimes in prostitution, while at the same time traditional hillside sexuality and its core values of "shame, name and blame" present significant obstacles to taking precautions against HIV. Symonds (1998), also writing on Northern Thailand, likewise explains HIV vulnerability among the Hmong to be the product of a combination of political economic and cultural factors, including the entry of the highland Hmong into lowland markets, the growth of the commercial sex industry, injection drug use, racism and discrimination against the Hmong by the Thai majority, and sexual double standards. Schoepf's analysis of life histories of women in Zaire further shows that HIV is spread not through exotic cultural practices but because of normal responses to everyday problems such as substantial economic hardship and uncertainty (Schoepf, 1992b). In response to these dynamics, all three writers promote participatory and collaborative forms of action research with vulnerable women as a means to redefine the gendered social roles and socioeconomic conditions which contribute to the spread of

HIV (Schoepf, 1992a, 1992b, Schoepf *et al*, 1991; Kammerer *et al*, 1995; Symonds, 1998)

Finally, although considerably less research has been carried out on men who have sex with men in developing countries, findings show that HIV vulnerability related to gender inequality and sexism is also almost universally present in same-sex relationships (McKenna, 1996). In this context, the structures of gender inequality are typically replicated through the stigmatization of particularly effeminate homosexual men and transgendered persons, who often have few employment options outside of sex work and who frequently are subject to socially sanctioned physical violence (Parker, 1993). These studies suggest that men who have sex with men are present in nearly all societies and that multiple oppressions (e.g. homophobia, poverty, racism, and gender equality) syngeristically place such men at markedly increased vulnerability to HIV infection (Parker, Kahn, and Aggleton, 1998).

4. RESEARCH ON THE POLITICS OF AIDS-RELATED POLICY

A second major area of international and cross-cultural research on structural and environmental factors has centered on the politics of AIDS-related policy making and the impact of development and public health policies on the epidemic. This literature can be grouped into four categories. First, extensive debate has developed surrounding the link between policy, including structural adjustment programs, and the socio-economic instabilities that foster HIV transmission (Bloom and Glied, 1993; Elmendorf and Roseberry, 1993; Lurie, Hintzen, and Lowe, 1995; Sweat and Denison, 1995; Turshen, 1998; Quam, 1994). A second category has analyzed national HIV/AIDS policies (Brown and Xenos, 1994; Daniel and Parker, 1993; Feldman, 1994; Gil, 1994; Kirp and Bayer, 1992; Packard and Epstein, 1991; Parker, 1994, 1997; Quam, 1994; 54-61, Santana, 1997; Santana, Fass, and Wald, 1991; Scheper-Hughes, 1993; Shuey and Bagarukayo, 1995). Third, a number of writings have examined international injecting drug-related policies and programs (Bastos, 1995; Des Jarlais *et al*, 1992a; Drucker *et al*, 1998; Lurie, Reingold and Bowser, 1993; Stimson, 1994; Strathdee *et al*, 1998; Wodak *et al*, 1998). Finally, interwoven through each of these categories are examinations of the ethical and human rights issues raised by AIDS-related policies (Daniel and Parker, 1993; Friedman, 1998b; Mann and Tarantola, 1996; Mann, Tarantola, and

Netter, 1992; McKenna, 1996; Panos Institute, 1990; Parker, 1994; Santana, Fass, and Wald 1991; Santana, 1997; Scheper-Hughes, 1993).

4.1 Structural Policies and Social and Economic Devastation

As has been discussed in the previous section, cultural, political and economic upheaval, have, all been identified as critical structural factors fostering HIV transmission. Ironically, the very policies directed toward alleviating such conditions during the 1980s—e.g. international aid and structural adjustment programs (SAPS)—in fact exacerbated economic hardship and contributed to the explosion of HIV incidence in Asia and Africa during the late 1980s and early 1990s. Lurie *et al.* (1995), for example, describe how the decreasing demand for oil exportation following the 1970s oil embargo caused many developing countries to seek out international loans, whose availability was conditioned on the adoption of SAPS. In practice, the SAPS produced lower government spending, the decline of rural economics, and substantial rural to urban migration. As a result, many couples were separated, thereby multiplying the number of sexual contacts and intensifying the spread of HIV. Turshen (1992) similarly criticizes USAID AIDS interventions for supporting such adverse social and health outcomes of SAPS and failing to address the socio-economic determinants of HIV transmission. In contrast, Elmendorf and Roseberry (1993), representing the World Bank, defend the utility of SAPS and argue that economic decline, rather than decreases in central government health spending associated with SAPS, may be responsible for the high levels of HIV incidence in parts of sub-Saharan Africa.

4.2 National Policies Facilitating or Slowing HIV Transmission

Like the work on international development policies, studies of national HIV/AIDS policy-making and impact have been carried out in a number of different developing countries. Perhaps the most extensive discussion of national HIV/AIDS policies centers on Cuba, where the state has provided free food, shelter and treatment for people living with HIV/AIDS in sanitaria isolated from the rest of the Cuban populace (Santana, Fass, and Wald, 1991; Santana, 1997; Scheper-Hughes, 1993). Scheper-Hughes (1993) has argued that Cuban AIDS policy is worth examining because of the country's extraordinarily low HIV incidence although she recognizes that sexual puritanism and infrequent injecting drug use may also have contributed to these rates. Nonetheless, Scheper-Hughes cautions that this approach may not be applicable in other locations because of the ethical issues inherent in enforcing isolation. Somewhat differently, Santana explains that the sanitarium system is effective in Cuba because Cubans are used to sacrificing personal desires for the greater good (Santana, Fass, and Wald, 1991; Santana, 1997). Gil (1994) describes a similar dynamic in China, where national HIV prevention policies have been framed in terms of socialist cultural and moral values, and suggests that while these policies may be appropriate for rural populations who still conform to socialist ideology, they are less likely to be effective for urban dwellers, particularly since they do not acknowledge the gap between ideals of traditional sexuality and actual practices.

In Brazil, Parker has examined how the cultural, economic and political changes associated with that country's redemocratization in the 1980s affected the development of the Brazilian AIDS epidemic (Daniel and Parker, 1993; Parker, 1994, 1996). During the early and mid 1980s, Brazilian federal government officials largely ignored AIDS because they viewed it as a problem of homosexual men rather than the general populace. In response, non-governmental organizations filled the AIDS education void and played a key role in campaigning for and shaping more effective governmental AIDS policies (Parker, 1994, 1997). This link between governmental acknowledgment of the gravity of AIDS and the development of successful governmental interventions has been further highlighted in studies of Thailand's five year national AIDS program (Brown and Xenos, 1994) and Uganda's multi-sectoral approach to AIDS prevention and services (Shuey and Bagarukayo, 1996).

While national case studies provide important insights, there has unfortunately been little comparative research on the historical development of AIDS policies in developing countries (in spite of the fact that by far the greatest burden of the global pandemic has been concentrated in the developing world), or on how these policies have affected the epidemic, perhaps in part because funding for international, HIV-related policy research has been extremely limited. At least one long-term study of the history and consequences of national AIDS policy is currently underway in Brazil (Parker, 1997; Parker and Galvão, 1998; Parker, Galvão and Bessa, 1999), but such relatively large-scale undertakings are exceptional. Moreover, virtually no work has compared the development of AIDS policies in different developing countries, as Kirp and Bayer and their collaborators have carried out for the industrialized democracies of the Anglo-European world (Kirp and Bayer, 1992), making it especially difficult to assess the relative impact of different policy initiatives.

4.3 Drug Legislation, HIV Transmission and Prevention

Most international policy research on injecting drug use focused on two central themes: (1) the epidemiology of injecting drug use worldwide (Des Jarlais *et al*, 1992a, Des Jarlais *et al*, 1992b; Friedman, 1998b; Libonatti *et al*, 1993; Panda *et al*, 1997; Stimson, 1992, 1994; Stimson and Choopanya, 1998; Wodak *et al*, 1998); and (2) the development and implementation of harm reduction policies in particular national and local contexts (Bastos, 1995; Des Jarlais *et al*, 1992a, Des Jarlais *et al*, 1995, Choopanya *et al*, 1991; Des Jarlais *et al*, 1992a; Des Jarlais *et al*, 1992b; Drucker *et al*, 1998; Lurie, Reingold and Bowser, 1993; Stimson, 1994; Strathdee *et al*, 1998; Wodak *et al*, 1998). These writings indicate that those countries and localities which have focused on needle exchange, treatment availability, and other pragmatic approaches (e.g. Australia; the Netherlands; Glascow, Scotland; Lund, Sweden) have had more success in averting and/or containing HIV epidemics among injecting drug users than those settings where law enforcement and drug eradication approaches are emphasized (e.g. the United States, Malaysia, France; see Des Jarlais *et al*, 1995a; Des Jarlais *et al*, 1995b; Lurie, Reingold and Bowser, 1993; Starthdee, *et al*, 19978; Stimson and Choopanya, 1998; Wodak *et al*, 1998). In fact, comparative analyses of the epidemiology of injecting drug related HIV infection have highlighted how drug trafficking and law enforcement practices have led to the increased consumption of injecting drugs that can be efficiently transported and distributed (Des Jarlais *et al*, 1992a, Des Jarlais *et al*, 1992; Friedman, 1998b; Stimson, 1992, 1994). And as will be discussed in more detail below, studies of injecting drug use in both developed and developing countries demonstrate that many of the social processes associated with drug injecting are remarkably similar across place, suggesting that the elements needed for effective prevention policies and programs in sites as different as Bangkok, Glasgow, New York City and Rio de Janeiro are in many ways the same (Des Jarlais *et al*., 1992b; Des Jarlais *et al*, 1995a; Dolan, Stimson, and Donoghoe, 1993).

4.4 AIDS Policies and Ethics

Despite the far-reaching ethical implications of AIDS-related policy and programs, most of the structural and environment factors literature has limited its consideration of such questions to sweeping condemnations of the detrimental effects of structural adjustment policies and global economic inequalities. Exceptions to this trend include Sweat and Denison's review article on structural interventions, which discusses several well-known AIDS policies (e.g. the closing of the gay bath houses in San Francisco, Cuba's AIDS sanitaria, Thailand's 100% condom program) to highlight the potential for AIDS interventions to violate individual civil rights (Sweat and Denison, 1995), and Altman's comparative analysis of community-based AIDS advocacy organizations (Altman, 1994) and Parker's work on Brazilian AIDS activism (Daniel and Parker, 1993, Parker, 1994), both of which describe how nongovernmental organizations have successfully fought for the civil rights of people living with AIDS.

5. RESEARCH ON SPECIFIC STRUCTURAL AND ENVIRONMENTAL INTERVENTIONS

In comparison with the relatively large and compelling literature on the structural and environmental factors shaping the spread of the epidemic and the somewhat smaller but nonetheless important literature on the politics of AIDS-related policy making, the number of published studies that describe and/or evaluate specific structural interventions in detail is unfortunately rather restricted. More extensive references on these topics can be found in the abstracts of recent International AIDS Conferences, but the information provided here is almost always too limited to be of much use. Even more unfortunate is the fact that only a very small percentage of what is presented at the International AIDS Conferences goes on to be published in scientific journals or other formats—perhaps as little as about 5% according to one review of HIV/AIDS research conducted in Brazil (Bastos *et al*, 1998)—making it difficult to assess these findings. Based primarily on those studies that are published, however, it is nonetheless possible to identify at least some of the approaches that have received significant international attention, including targeted interventions that have been developed for injecting drug users, heterosexual women, female commercial sex workers, male truck drivers, and men who have sex with men, which we will describe in greater detail below. [6]

[6] It is worth noting the existence of a much larger "gray" literature of project reports, manuals, and popular media reporting, although in general most research scientists in the developing world lack the necessary infrastructure and financial support to analyze and disseminate their results adequately.

5.1 Injecting Drug Users

Injecting drug users have been the focus of some of the most extensive and discussed structural and environmental level interventions developed in response to the HIV/AIDS epidemic. Most of these interventions has followed harm reduction approaches, which were first developed in the Netherlands in the early 1980s and premised on the idea that although it was not possible for all injecting drug users to stop or diminish their injecting, it was nonetheless possible to reduce many of the harms associated with injection (Brettle, 1991; Des Jarlais, Friedman, and Ward, 1993; Friedman, de Jong, and Wodak, 1993; Heather *et al*, 1993; Hartgers *et al*, 1989; Wodak *et al*, 1998). Perhaps the best-known HIV-related harm reduction strategy is needle and syringe exchange. First used in the Netherlands, needle/syringe exchange programs quickly spread during the 1980s to Australia, the United Kingdom, Sweden, and the United States and other parts of the world where injecting drug use is practiced (Dolan, Stimson and Donoghoe, 1993; Drucker *et al*, 1998; Hartgers *et al*, 1989; Stimson and Choopanya, 1998; Strathdee *et al*, 1998). During the late 1980s and 1990s, needle/syringe program were implemented in many developing countries as well (Abdul-Quader *et al*, 1999;Wodak *et al*, 1998), including; Bueno *et al*, 1996; Conte *et al*, 1996; de Carvalho *et al*, 1996; Brazil (Loures *et al*, 1996), Thailand (Abdul-Quader *et al*, 1999), Vietnam (Abdul-Quader *et al*, 1999; Quan, Chung and Abdul-Quader, 1998), India (Abdul-Quader *et al*, 1999), and Nepal (Abdul-Quader *et al*, 1999; Peak *et al*, 1995). In many cases, these needle/syringe exchange programs have been complemented by street-based outreach, HIV risk reduction education, condom distribution, and other harm reduction strategies such as methadone treatment in Thailand (Des Jarlais *et al*, 1992b) and Nepal (Shreshtha *et al*, 1995); ready availability of needles and syringes at pharmacies in Thailand (Des Jarlais *et al*, 1992b); bleach distribution in India (Hangzo *et al*, 1997; Chatterjee *et al*, 1996), Nepal (Peak *et al*, 1995), and Malaysia (Palaniappan, 1996); and the substitution of less harmful means of ingesting drugs in India (i.e. buprenorphine tablets for buprenorphine injectors and/or heroin users, SHARAN, 1995). Although there are relatively few published studies on the efficacy of needle exchange and other harm reduction policies in the developing world, research suggests that many of these programs have resulted in significant reductions in drug-related HIV risk behaviors (Abdul-Quader *et al*, 1999; Chatterjee *et al*, 1996; Des Jarlais *et al*, 1992b; Kumar and Daniels, 1996; Peak *et al*, 1995).

Another common structural and environmental level intervention involving injecting drug users in many developed countries and a few developing countries is the establishment of drug-user organizations (Abdul-Quader *et al*, 1999; Friedman, 1996; Friedman *et al*, 1987; Friedman, Jong and Wodak, 1993; Jose *et al*, 1996). These organizations have served as a vehicle through which injecting drug users have come together, developed skills, implemented HIV risk reduction programs, conducted "community development," and advocated for themselves in political and social forums (Friedman, de Jong and Wodak, 1993). The particular forms and results of organizing and community building are context dependent; in general, these efforts have been more successful in countries that have implemented harm reduction policies (e.g. the Netherlands and Australia) rather than those which have emphasized law enforcement and repressive drug use policies (e.g. the United States, France, Malaysia). Nonetheless, even in more favorable environments, and it has been difficult for these organizations to develop a stable leadership core, and relatively few drug users have become involved in these organizations (Friedman, de Jong and Wodak, 1993).

Finally, one of the most innovative and controversial structural and environmental interventions directed toward injecting drug users is Needle Park, which existed as an open air drug scene from 1986 to February 1992 in Zurich, Switzerland (Huber, 1994). Building on a harm reduction approach (Ueberlebenshifle –"assistance to make survival possible"), more than twenty governmental and non-governmental organizations implemented a wide range of programs such as free condom and syringe distribution, medical help, resuscitation teams, mobile kitchens, and setting up showers and toilets at the Park. In practice, Needle Park generated several unforeseen consequences, including increases in drug-related deaths and the number of injections per user, low drug prices, and a migration of drug users to the Park from other parts of Switzerland and beyond (only 10% of the drug users were from Zurich). This transnational dimension of injecting drug use in Europe makes it is difficult to evaluate the evaluate Needle Park (e.g. given that Needle Park concentrated injection drug users from throughout Europe, what is the appropriate unit of analysis for measuring its effects?) and highlights the need for regional and international cooperation on structural and environmental level interventions directed toward injection drug users.

5.2 Heterosexual Women

Despite the impressive literature examining structural HIV vulnerability among heterosexual women (Farmer. Lindenbaum, and Delvecchio-Good, 1993; Farmer, Connors, and Simmons, 1996; Gupta and Weiss, 1993), it is striking how few projects have attempted to address this vulnerability through structural changes. Instead, the vast majority of prevention programs targeted toward women have concentrated on condom promotion and partner reduction strategies, even though it has been repeatedly shown that these behavioral approaches are inadequate given the realities of most women's lives (Heise and Elias, 1995; Goldstein, 1994; Parker and Galvão, 1996; Stein, 1990).

Most of the reported structural interventions with heterosexual women describe attempts to support safer sexual practices given the realities of gender and economic inequalities. Examples of such enabling approaches include testing and counseling programs that not only inform women of their serostatus and but also provide on-going psychosocial support for HIV decision making and risk reduction (Allen *et al*, 1993), and action research projects such as CONNAISSIDA in Zaire during the 1980s (Schoepf, 1988, 1992a, 199b, 1993; Schoepf *et al*, 1991). This strategy of promoting female economic empowerment as a means to avoid the risks of sex work and to promote greater autonomy in contraceptive use and sexual decision making has grown in importance as the fields of HIV/AIDS and reproductive health have become increasingly integrated in the 1990s (Schuler and Syed, 1994).

A related body of work on heterosexual women has focused on expanding the range of female-controlled HIV prevention methods (Elias and Heise, 1994; Rivers *et al*, 1998; Stein, 1990, 1995). For example, a recently completed cross-national study has provided comparative data on how the female condom, when added to the already existing prevention options available in developing country settings, can increase women's ability to protect themselves from HIV infection (Rivers *et al*, 1998). While the cost of most female-controlled or initiated methods still restricts their accessibility, various intervention studies currently underway seek to increase women's options through the elaboration of more complex dual protection prevention strategies within women's reproductive health services (Barbosa and Lego, 1997) and represent among the most important structural changes taking place in developing countries today.

5.3 Female Sex Workers

One of the most commonly targeted populations for structural and environmental level interventions in the developing world are female sex workers (Asamoah-Adu *et al*, 1994; Bhave *et al*, 1995; Gadgil, 1994; Kirubi *et al*, 1994 Lamptey, 1991; Rojanapithayakorn, 1994; Rojanapithayakorn and Hanenberg, 1996; Williams *et al*, 1992). Indeed, one of the most acclaimed structural interventions of any type is the One Hundred Percent Condom Program (Rojanapithayakorn, 1994; Rojanapithayakorn and Hanenberg, 1996), which seeks to prevent the sexual transmission of HIV through increasing condom utilization in Thai sex establishments to 100% and involves the active involvement of governmental authorities and owners of sex establishments. Condoms are supplied free of charge to all sex establishments, and if clients refuse to use them, sexual services are withheld; condom use is strictly enforced through provincial AIDS committees, local police, monitoring, and the imposition of sanctions on commercial sex establishments that fail to comply. Since its inception in 1989 and its expansion nationwide in 1991, condom use rates rose from under 50% in 1989 to 94% in 1993. However, despite the apparent success of the One Hundred Percent Condom Program, whether this approach is possible in other contexts is uncertain due to the particularities of Thai society (i.e. a hierarchical social structure, a very specific set of sexual values, a booming economy during the early 1990s, and a political system that combines a traditional monarchy with military authoritarian rule).

Whatever the transferability of the Thai One Hundred Percent Condom Program, the centrality of the cooperation of commercial sex establishments and governmental officials in promoting HIV risk reduction among female sex workers is nonetheless confirmed by the more mixed results of two projects in Bombay, India (Bhave *et al*, 1995; Gadgil, 1994). Bhave *et al.* (1995), describe a controlled study in which intervention group participants underwent a six month program of educational videos and small group discussions and were provided pictorial educational materials and free condoms. Women reported increased levels of condom use; however, and in stark contrast to the 100% Condom Use Program, both sex workers and madams were concerned about losing business if condom use was insisted upon. At the same time, levels of knowledge among control group women group remained low despite HIV testing and counseling, leading the authors to posit that high levels of illiteracy and isolation make it difficult for many women to understand even basic concepts about HIV transmission without intensive education.

Such structural obstacles to developing successful interventions were particularly evident in a peer education project among prostitutes and madams in the Kamathipua and Khetwadi areas of Bombay. The project sought to educate sex workers about their health problems, including HIV and STDs, and to create an on-going network of health educators among female sex workers in the two areas (Gadgil, 1994). Although women reported personal benefits from the training, most were not interested in attending follow-up meetings, nor did many women conduct education sessions among their peers, as madams did not allow them to leave their own brothels. This experience suggests, as Gadgil argues, that peer education and group empowerment models may not be successful in structural contexts where freedom of movement and camaraderie among sex workers are absent.

Finally, as in work focusing on women who are not commercial sex workers, a number of intervention projects have attempted to promote empowerment and personal autonomy through cultivating alternative employment opportunities for female sex workers. A project in Machakos Town and Nairobi, Kenya, for example, provided women with relevant HIV/AIDS, safer sex and fertility education, training in small business management, and start-up funds for their own businesses (mostly selling vegetables, fruits and grains or making handicrafts) (Kirubi *et al*, 1994). The authors report a decline in the number of the women's sexual partners, increased condom use, and the creation of an overall sense of well being and pride among the women as a result of not having to sell sex and expose themselves to HIV infection.

5.4 Truck Drivers

Interventions designed for male truck drivers and sex workers often overlap because of sex work is typically embedded within truck driver culture (e.g. truck drivers often provide transportation to women in exchange for sex; women offer truck drivers sex and/or a place to stay for a small fee) (Wilson *et al*, 1994). Mwizarubi *et al.* (1991), for example, describe an AIDS intervention in Tanzania which targeted truck drivers, their assistants, and their female sex partners at seven truck stops along the Dar es Salaam highway and sought to raise HIV and STD awareness, promote condom use and distribution, reduce the overall number of sexual partners, and encourage peer based STD/HIV education. During the project, AIDS awareness increased and condom distribution rose by 100,000; however, the authors report that women at truck stops remain in need of greater condom negotiation skills and empowerment more generally.

In Zimbabwe, Wilson *et al.* conducted semi-structured interviews, focus groups, and participant observation with 74 truckers. Baseline interviews revealed high levels of prior STD infection and low levels of knowledge of the efficacy of condoms as an HIV prevention strategy (Wilson *et al*, 1994). The truckers complained that the low wages and long hours they worked decreased their contact with wives and children and led them to seek companionship and sex while on the road. Based on these data, the authors suggest that structural interventions such as raising salaries and limiting overtime, providing nursery care so that wives could travel with their husbands, and providing truckers' better contact with their families through increasing telephone access, could all help reduce HIV transmission.

5.5 Men Who Have Sex With Men

In keeping with the small amount of research, intervention or otherwise, on men who have sex with men in the developing world, virtually no official governmental or intergovernmental programs have prioritized men who have sex with men, even in regions where homosexual transmission has been pronounced, as in Latin America and parts of Asia (McKenna, 1996; Parker, Kahn, and Aggleton, 1998). Nonetheless, in a number of regions, community-based organizations have developed groundbreaking prevention programs, particularly through strategies aimed at community mobilization (Parker, Kahn, and Aggleton, 1998), which in many cases overlap and complement structural interventions.

In Sri Lanka, a gay organization known as Companions on a Journey has combined outreach work with support networks and advocacy aimed at decriminalizing homosexual behavior (Parker, Kahn, and Aggleton, 1998). In Mexico, the Coletivo Sol, a community-based gay and AIDS-service organization, has worked with bathhouse managers and clients to provide information on safer sexual practices and to distribute condoms and water-based lubricants in these locations Asia (McKenna, 1996; Parker, Kahn, and Aggleton, 1998). In Brazil, a large-scale and long-term prevention program developed in Rio de Janeiro and São Paulo by the Associação Brasileira Interdisciplinar de AIDS (ABIA), the Grupo Pela Vidda-Rio de Janeiro, and the Grupo Pela Vidda-São Paulo combined intensive outreach work with safer sex workshops, cultural activities, collaboration with the owners and managers of commercial establishments, and the creation of special STD treatment and counseling programs for men who have sex with men in order to build social support networks and provide a safe environment capable of nurturing risk reduction (Parker, Kahn, and Aggleton, 1998; Parker, 1995).

This work among men who have sex with men in developing countries has rarely been systematically evaluated due to the lack of financial and technical resources, although novel forms of evaluation have been developed, such as the use of on-going ethnographic assessment to monitor and revise intervention activities in Brazil (Parker, Kahn, and Aggleton, 1998; Parker, 1999). These experiences suggest that community attachment strategies based not only on outreach work but also on the actual construction and/or reorganization of local environments may be particularly relevant today in many developed countries, where early prevention efforts designed for and by self-identified gay men have been redesigned and reinvented to reach men who have sex with men who do not necessarily share a defined gay identity or participate in organized gay communities. In such contexts, the perspectives of community mobilization and structural intervention may need to merge in order to construct safer environments and to sustain safer sex as a form of community practice (Watney, 1994).

6. KEY CHALLENGES FOR FUTURE RESEARCH

In conclusion, we would like to highlight the emergence of an important and growing body of international AIDS research that has moved beyond the more limited approaches of behavioral science to examine the structural and environmental forces and socio-cultural contexts which shape HIV vulnerability. Most of this work has remained relatively general in its analysis and can be criticized as being poorly operationalizable, since far-reaching dilemmas such as poverty, migration, and gender inequality are unlikely to be overcome in the short run or through the limited resources available for health-related interventions. Yet, contextual variables and AIDS-related policies must be seriously addressed if we are to bring about effective HIV risk reduction.

While the structural and environmental factors literature offers extremely important insights and reveals a number of productive intervention strategies that might be explored in both resource rich and poor settings, many importance challenges remain. Among these, a few are worth highlighting:

- How can we better document the effects of large-scale structural and environmental factors (e.g. poverty, the denial of humans rights) on the highly localized behavioral events (e.g. unprotected sex, needle sharing) that ultimately shape the course of HIV infection?

- How can we facilitate comparative analysis of policy processes which is attentive to local nuances and capable of systematically assessing how specific policies and programs affect transmission rates within particular population groups and communities?

- How can we design and implement focused structural interventions that address the consequences of large-scale factors such as economic justice and gender inequality and provide program clients options that produce meaningful reductions in behavioral risk, without presuming that such small-scale programs will end poverty or sexism?

- How can we develop rigorous methodologies to evaluate structural and environmental interventions, since by their very nature these interventions involve large-scale elements that cannot be controlled by experimental or quasi-experimental research designs?

- How can we adapt proven structural interventions to contexts in which some, but not necessarily all, of the same underlying structural factors are present or important?

The answers to these questions are not simple or straightforward and often take us far afield from the kinds of theoretical frameworks, methodologies and research designs that have been at the center of behavioral health research as a whole and HIV/AIDS research in particular. They push us, on the contrary, toward innovative approaches as well as new--and hopefully productive--dialogues with fields of work and disciplinary traditions that until recently have been at the margins of mainstream AIDS research. Yet the fact remains that despite recent advances in HIV treatment, in very few settings has AIDS prevention been able to declare victory over the epidemic. After nearly two decades, traditional behavioral intervention strategies have shown themselves to be incapable of slowing the spread of HIV infection, and only in contexts in which effective community mobilization and structural interventions have been implemented has HIV/AIDS prevention and control been truly realized. The time has come to move beyond the limitations of failed behavioral interventions and strike out in new directions aimed at achieving broad-based social and structural change.

REFERENCES

Aggleton, P. (1996). Global priorities for HIV/AIDS intervention research. *International Journal of STDs and AIDS*, 7 (suppl 2), 13-16.

Aggleton, P. & Coates, T. (1995). Social, cultural and political aspects. *AIDS*, 9 (suppl A), S237-238.

Aggleton, P. & Mane, P. (1998). Introduction to special HIV/AIDS symposium issue. Critical Public Health 8, 253-255.

Ajzen, I. & Fishbein, M. (1980). Understanding Attitudes and Predicting Behavior, Englewood Cliffs, NJ: Prentice Hall.

Akeroyd, A. (1994). HIV/AIDS in Eastern and Southern Africa. Review of African Political Economy, 60, 173-184.

Allen, S., Serufilira, A., Gruber, V., Kegeles, S., Van de Perre, P., Caraël, M., & Coates, T. (1993). Pregnancy and contraceptive use among urban Rwandan women after HIV testing and counseling. *American Journal of Public Health*, 83, 705-710.

Altman, D. (1994). Power and Community: Organizational and Cultural Responses to AIDS, London: Taylor & Francis.

Anarfi, J. (1993). Sexuality, migration and AIDS in Ghana: A sociobehavioral study. *Health Transition Review* 1993, 4 (suppl.), 273-295.

Archavanitkul, K. & Guest, P. (1994). Migration and the commercial sex sector in Thailand. *Health Transition Review*, 4 (suppl), 273-295.

Asamoah-Adu, A.S., Weir, M., *et al.* (1994). Evaluation of a targeted AIDS prevention intervention to increase condom use among prostitutes in Ghana. *AIDS*, 8, 239-246

Bandura, A. (1977). Social Learning Theory, Englewood Cliffs, NJ: Prentice-Hall.

Barbosa, R. & Lego, T. (1997). AIDS e direito reproductivo: Para além da transmissão vertical. In R.G. Parker (Ed.) Políticas, Instituições e AIDS: Enfrentando a Epidemia no Brazil, Rio de Janeiro: Jorge Zahar Editora/ABIA, 163-175.

Bassett, M. (1993). Social and economic determinants of vulnerability to HIV infection: The Zimbabwe experience. *AIDS Analysis Africa*, July/August, 9-11.

Bastos, F.I. (1995). Ruína e Reconstrução: AIDS e Drogas Injetáveis na Cena Contemporânea, Rio de Janeiro: Relume-Dumará Editora.

Bastos, F.I., Coutinho, K., Galvão, J., & Parker, R.G. (1998). Research on HIV/AIDS in Brazil—1983-1997: A comprehensive review. 12th World AIDS Conference Abstracts, Geneva, Switzerland, #43278.

Becker, M.H. & Joseph, J.K.. (1988). AIDS and behavioral change to reduce risk: A review. *American Journal of Public Health*, 78, 394-410.

Bhave, G.L., Lindan, C.P., Hudes, E., Desai, S., Wagle, U., Tripathi, S.P., & Mandel, J.S. (1995). Impact of an intervention on HIV, sexually transmitted diseases, and condom use among sex workers in Bombay, India. *AIDS* 1995, 9 (suppl 1), S21-S30.

Bloom, D.E. & Glied, S. (1993). Who is bearing the cost of the AIDS epidemic in Asia? In D.E. Bloom & J.V. Lyons (Eds.) Economic Implications of AIDS in Asia, New Delhi: UNDP.

Bond, G.C. & Vincent, C. (1991). Living on the edge: Changing social structures in the context of HIV. In H. Hansen & M. Twaddle (Eds.) Changing Uganda: The Dilemma of Structural Adjustment and Revolutionary Change, London: James Curry.

Brown, T. & Xenos, P. (1994). AIDS in Asia: The Gathering Storm, Asia Pacific Issues 16. Program on Population, Honolulu: East-West Center.

Brettle, R.P. (1991). HIV and harm reduction for injection drug users. *AIDS* 1991, 5, 125-136.

Bueno, R.C., Mesquita, F., Haiek, R., *et al.* (1996). Bleaching among IDUs in the city of Santos: Results on an intervention by an outreach team. XI International Conference on AIDS, Vancouver, Abstract No. Pub.C.1259.

Caraël , M., Buvé A., & Awusabo-Asare, K. (1997). The making of HIV epidemics: What are the driving forces? *AIDS*, 11 (suppl B), S23-S31.

Carballo, M., Cleland, J., Caraël, M., & Albrecht, G. (1989). A cross-national study of patterns of sexual behavior. *The Journal of Sex Research*, 26, 287-299.

Chatterjee, A., Hangzo, C.Z., Abdul-Quadar, A.S, *et al.* (1996). Evidence of effectiveness of street-based peer outreach intervention to change behavior among injecting drug users in Manipur, India. XI International Conference on AIDS, Vancouver, Abstract No. 4975.

Choopanya, K., Vanichseni, S., Des Jarlais, D.C. *et al.* (1991). Risk factors and HIV seropositivity among injection drug users in Bangkok. *AIDS*, 5, 1509-1513.

Chouinard, A. & Albert, J. (Eds.). (1989). Human Sexuality: Research Perspectives in a World Facing AIDS, Ottawa: International Development Research Centre.

Clatts, M.C. (1995). Hitting a Moving Target: The Use of Ethnographic Methods in the Development of Sampling Strategies for the Evaluation of AIDS Outreach Programs for Homeless Youth in New York City. NIDA Research Monograph, 157, 117-135.

Clatts, M.C. (1999). A demographic and behavioral profile of homeless youth in New York City: Implications for AIDS outreach and prevention. *Medical Anthropology Quarterly*, 13 (3), 365-374.

Cleland, J. & Ferry, B. (Eds.). (1995). Sexual Behaviour and AIDS in the Developing World, London: Taylor and Francis.

Cohen, M. (1991). Changing to safer sex: Personality, logic and habit. In P. Aggleton, G. Hart, & P. Davies (Eds) *AIDS:* Responses, Interventions and Care, London: The Falmer Press,19-42.

Cohen, B. & Trussell, J. (1996). Preventing and Mitigating AIDS in Sub-Saharan Africa: Research and Data Priorities for the Social and Behavioral Sciences, Washington, D.C.: National Academy Press.

Conte, M. Dávila, S., Mayer, R. *et al.* (1996). The syringe pass. AIDS stay: AIDS prevention for injection drug users. XI International Conference on AIDS, Vancouver, Abstract No. WeC.3567.

Daniel, H. & Parker, R.G. (1993). Sexuality, Politics and AIDS in Brazil, London: The Falmer Press.

De Carvalho, H.B., Mesquita, F., Massad, E., *et al.* (1996). HIV and infection of similar transmission patterns in a drug injectors community of Santos, Brazil. *Journal of Acquired Immune Deficiency Syndrome*, 12 (1), 84-92.

Decosas, J. (1996). HIV and development. *AIDS*, 10 (suppl 3), S69-S94.

Decosas, J., Kane, F., Anarfi, J., Sodii, K. & Wagner, H.U. (1995). Migration and AIDS. *Lancet*, 346, 826-828.

Des Jarlais, D.C., Friedman, S.R., Choopanya, K., Vanichseni, S., & Ward, T.P. (1992a). International epidemiology of HIV and AIDS among injecting drug users. *AIDS*, 6, 1053-68.

Des Jarlais, D.C., Choopanya, K, *et al.* (1992b). Risk reduction and stabilization of HIV seroprevalence among drug injectors in New York City and Bangkok, Thailand. In G.B. Rossi, E. Beth-Giraldo, L. Chieco-Bianchi, *et al* (Eds.) Science Challenging AIDS, Basel: Karger, 207-213.

Des Jarlais, D.C., Friedman, S.R., & Ward, T.P. (1993). Harm reduction: A public health response to the AIDS epidemic among injecting drug users. *Annual Review of Public Health*, 14, 413-450.

Des Jarlais, D.C., Friedman, S.R., Friedman, P., *et al.* (1995a). HIV/AIDS-related behavior change among injecting drug users in different national settings. *AIDS*, 9, 611-17.

Des Jarlais, D.C., Hagan, H.H. Friedman, S.R. *et al.* (1995b). Maintaining low HIV seroprevalence in populations of injecting drug users. *JAMA*, 274, 1226-1231.

De Zalduondo, B.O. (1991). Prostitution viewed cross-culturally: Toward recontextualizing sex work in AIDS research. *Journal of Sex Research*, 28 (2), 223-248.

Dolan, K.A., Stimson, G.V., & Donoghoe, M. (1993). Reductions in HIV risk behavior and stable HIV prevalence in syringe-exchange clients and other injectors in England. *Drug and Alcohol Review*, 12, 133-142.

Drucker, E., Lurie, P., Wodak, A., & Alcabes, P. (1998). Measuring harm reduction: The effects of needle and syringe exchange programs and methadone maintenance on the ecology of HIV. *AIDS* , 12 (suppl A), S217-S230.

Elias, C.J. & Heise, L.L. (1994). Challenges for the development of female-controlled vaginal microbicides. *AIDS*, 8, 1-9.

Elmendorf, A.E. & Roseberry, W. (1993). Structural adjustment: What effect on health? On vulnerability to HIV?. *AIDS Analysis Africa*, July/August, 4-7.

Farmer, P. (1992). AIDS and Accusation: Haiti and the Geography of Blame, Berkeley and Los Angeles: University of California Press.

Farmer, P. (1995). Culture, poverty, and the dynamics of HIV transmission in rural Haiti. In H. Brummelhuis & G. Herdt (Eds.) Culture and Sexual Risk: Anthropological Perspectives in AIDS, New York: Gordon and Breach, 3-28.

Farmer, P., Connors, M., & Simmons, J. (1996). Women, Poverty, and AIDS: Sex, drugs and structural violence, Monroe, ME: Common Courage Press.

Farmer, P., Lindenbaum, S., & Delvecchio-Good, M.J. (1993). Women, poverty and AIDS: An introduction. Culture, Medicine and Psychiatry, 17, 387-397.

Feldman, D. (Ed). (1994). Global AIDS Policy, Westport, CT: Bergin & Garvey.

Friedman, S.R. (1996). Theoretical bases for understanding drug user organizations. *The International Journal of Drug Policy* , 7, 212-219.

Friedman, S.R. (1998a). HIV-related politics in long-term perspective. AIDS Care, 10 (suppl 2), S93-103.

Friedman, S. R. (1998b). The political economy of drug-user scapegoating—and the philosophy and politics of resistance. Drugs: Education, Prevention and Policy, 5 (1),15-32.

Friedman, S.R. & O-Reilly, K. (1997). Sociocultural interventions at the community level. *AIDS*, 11 (suppl A), S201-S208.

Friedman, S.R., Des Jarlais, D.C., & Ward T.P. (1994). Social models for changing health-relevant behavior. In R.J. DiClemente & J.L. Peterson (Eds.) Preventing AIDS: Theories and Methods of Behavioral Interventions, New York: Plenum Press, 95-116.

Gadgil, A. (1994). Peer group education among prostitutes of Kamathipua and Khetwadi areas of Bombay. 10th International Conference on AIDS Abstracts, PD0457, Yokohama, Japan.

Geertz, C. (1983). Local Knowledge, New York: Basic Books.

Gil, V.E. (1994). Behind the wall of China: AIDS profile, AIDS policy. In D. Feldman (Ed.) Global AIDS Policy, Westport, Connecticut: Bergin and Garvey, 7-27.

Gillies, P. & Parker, R. (1994). Cross-cultural perspectives on sexual behaviour and prostitution. *Health Transition Review*, 4 (Suppl), 257-271.

Goldstein, D. (1994). Women and AIDS in Brazil: The emerging problem. *Social Science and Medicine*, 39, 319-329.

Gupta, G.R., Weiss, E. (1993). Women's lives and sex: Implications for AIDS prevention. *Culture, Medicine and Psychiatry*, 17, 399-412.

Hangzo, C., Chatterjee, A., Sarkar, S., *et al.* (1997). Reaching out beyond the hills: HIV prevention among injecting drug users in Manipur, India. *Addiction*, 92 (7), 813-820.

Hartgers, C., Buning, E.C., van Santen, G.W. *et al.* (1989). The impact of the needle and syringe-exchange program in Amsterdam on injecting risk behaviors. *AIDS*, 3, 571-576.

Heather, N., Wodak, A., Nadelmann, E., O'Hare, P. (Eds.). (1993). Psychoactive Drugs and Harm Reduction: From Faith to Science, Whurr Publishers, London.

Heise, L.L. & Elias, C. (1995). Transforming AIDS prevention to meet women's needs: A focus on developing countries. *Social Science and Medicine*, 40, 931-943.

Herdt, G. & Lindenbaum, S. (1992). The Time of AIDS: Social Analysis, Theory, and Method, Newbury Park and London: Sage Publications.

Jochelson, K., Mothibeli, M., & Leger, J.P. (1994). Human immunodeficiency virus and migrant labor in South Africa. In N. Krieger & M. Glenn (Eds.) AIDS: The Politics of Survival, Amityville, NY: Baywood Publishing Co, 141-160.

Jose, B., Friedman, S.R., Neaisgus, A., *et al.* (1996). Collective organization of injecting drug users and the struggle against AIDS. In T. Rhodes & R. Hartnoll (Eds.) AIDS, Drugs and Prevention, London: Routledge, 216-233.

Kammerer, C.A., Hutheesing, O.K., Maneeprasert, R., & Symonds, P.V. (1995). Vulnerability to HIV infection among three hilltribes in Northern Thailand. In H. Brummelhuis & G. Herdt (Eds.) Culture and Sexual Risk: Anthropological Perspectives in AIDS, New York: Gordon and Breach, 53-78.

Kane, S. 1991. HIV, heroin and heterosexual relations. *Social Science and Medicine*, 32 (9), 1037-1050.

Kippix, S., Connell, R.W., Dowsett, G.W., & Crawford, J. (1993). Sustaining Safe Sex: Gay Communities Respond to AIDS, London: Taylor and Francis.

Kippax, S. & Crawford, J. (1993). Flaws in the theory of reasoned action. In D.J. Terry, C. Gallois, & M.M. McCamish (Eds.) Theory of Reasoned Action: Its Applications to AIDS-Preventive Behaviour, London: Pergamon, 253-269.

Kirp, D.L. & Bayer, R. (1992). AIDS in the Industrialized Democracies: Passions, Politics, and Policies, New Brunswick, NJ: Rutgers University Press.

Kirubi, M., Ngugi, E.N., Kamau, P., Nyanbola, L., & Ronald, A. (1994). The impact of social economic and sexual empowerment: Commercial sex workers (CSWs). 10th International Conference on AIDS Abstracts, 447D, Yokohama, Japan.

Kreniske, J. (1991). AIDS in the Dominican Republic: Anthropological reflections on the social nature of disease. In G. Bond, J. Kreniske, I. Susser, & J. Vincent (Eds.) AIDS in Africa and the Caribbean, Boulder: Westview Press.

Kumar, S. & Daniels, D. (1996). Empirical evidence of behavior change. Paper presented at the Indo-US Workshop on Behavioral and Social Research on HIV Prevention, Bombay, India.

Lamptey, P. (1991). An overview of AIDS interventions in high-risk groups: Commercial sex workers and their clients. In AIDS and Women's Reproductive Health, New York: Plenum Press.

Larvie, P. (1997). Homophobia and the Ethnoscape of sex work in Rio de Janeiro. In G. Herdt (Ed.) Sexual Culture and Migration in the Era of AIDS: Anthropological and Demographic Perspectives, Oxford, Clarendon, 143-164.

Libonaati, O., Lima, E., Pergua, A., Gonzalez, R., Zacarais, F., & Weissenberg, M. (1993). Role of drug injection in the spread of HIV in Argentina and Brazil. *International Journal of STD & AIDS*, 4 (3), 135-141.

Lindenbaum, S. (1998). Images of catastrophe: The making of an epidemic. In M. Singer (Ed.) The Political Economy of AIDS, New York: Baywood Publishing Company, 33-58.

Loures, L.A., Bittencourt, L., Marques, F., *et al.* (1996). Dealing with a paradox: The national syringe exchange program in Brazil. XI International Conference on AIDS, Vancouver, Abstract No. We. C.3562.

Lurie, P., Fernandes, M.E., Hughes, V., Arevalo, E., Hudes, E., Reingold, A., & Hearst, N. (1995). Instituto Adolfo Lutz Study Group: Socioeconomic status and risk of HIV-1, syphilis and hepatitis B infection among sex workers in São Paulo State, Brazil. *AIDS*, 9, (suppl 1), S31-37.

Lurie, P., Hintzen, P., & Lowe, R.A. (1995). Socioeconomic obstacles to HIV prevention and treatment in developing countries: The roles of the International Monetary Fund and World Bank. *AIDS*, 9, 539-546.

Lurie, P., Reingold, A.L., Bowser, B. (Eds.) (1993). The Public Health Impact of Needle Exchange Programs in the United States and Abroad, Vol. 1, Atlanta, GA: Centers for Disease Control and Prevention.

Mann, J. Tarantola, D.J.M., & Netter, T.W. (Eds.) (1992). AIDS in the World, Cambridge, MA: Harvard University Press.

Mann, J. & Tarantola, D.J.M. (Eds.) (1996). AIDS in the World II, Oxford: Oxford University Press.

McKenna, N. (1996). On the Margins: Men who have Sex with Men and HIV in Developing Countries, London: Panos Institute.

Michal-Johnson, P. (1994). The dark side: Barriers to changing high-risk behaviors. *AIDS & Public Policy Journal*, 9, 18-19.

Miller, H.G., Turner, C.F, & Moses, L.E. (Eds). (1990). *AIDS:* The Second Decade, Washington, D.C.: National Academy Press.

Mwizarubi, B.K., Mwaijonga, C.L., Laukamm-Josten, U., Lwihula, G., Outwater, A. & Nyamwaya, D. (1991). HIV/AIDS Education and condom promotion for truck drivers, their assistants and sex partners in Tanzania. 7th International AIDS Conference on AIDS Abstracts, WD4017.

Packard, R. & Epstein, P. (1991). Epidemiologists, social scientists, and the structure of medical research on AIDS in Africa. *Social Science and Medicine*, 33, 771-794.

Palaniappan, N. (1996). Intervention among multiracial injecting drug users from different cultural and economic backgrounds. XI International Conference on AIDS, Vancouver, Abstract No. Mo.D. 1949.

Panda, S., Chatterjee, A., Sarkar, S., *et al.* (1997). Injection drug use in Calcutta: A potential focus for an explosive HIV epidemic. *Drug and Alcohol Review*, 16, 17-23.

Panos Institute (1990). The Third Epidemic: Repercussions of the Fear of AIDS, Budapest, London, Paris and Washington.

Parker, R.G. (1989). Youth, identity, and homosexuality: The changing shape of sexual life in Brazil. *Journal of Homosexuality* 17, 267-287.

Parker, R.G. (1991). Bodies, Pleasures and Passions: Sexual Culture in Contemporary Brazil, Boston: Beacon Press.

Parker, R.G. (1993). The negotiation of difference: Male prostitution, bisexual behavior and HIV transmission in Brazil. In H. Daniel & R.G. Parker Sexuality, Politics and AIDS in Brazil, London: The Falmer Press, 85-94.

Parker, R.G. (1994). Public policy, political activism, and AIDS in Brazil. In D. Feldman (Ed.) Global AIDS Policy, Westport, Connecticut: Bergin and Garvey, 28-46.

Parker, R.G. (1995). AIDS prevention and gay community mobilization in Brazil. *Development*, 2, 49-53.

Parker, R.G. (1996). Shifting paradigms in HIV/AIDS research and intervention: Behavior, culture and politics. In M. Poznansky, P.A. Gillies, & R. Coker (Eds.) Advancing a New Agenda for AIDS Research, London: Blackwell.

Parker, R.G. (1997). Migration, sexual subcultures, and HIV/AIDS in Brazil. In G. Herdt (Ed.) Sexual Culture and Migration in the Era of AIDS: Anthropological and Demographic Perspectives, Oxford, Clarendon, 55-69.

Parker, R.G. (1999). Beneath the Equator: Cultures of Desire, Male Homosexuality, and Emerging Gay Communities in Brazil, New York and London: Routledge.

Parker, R.G. & Aggleton, P. (1999). Culture, Society and Sexuality: A Reader, London and Philadelphia: UCL Press.

Parker, R.G., Barbosa, R., & Aggleton, P. (2000). Framing the Sexual Subject. In R.G. Parker, R. Barbosa, & P. Aggleton (Eds.) Framing the Sexual Subject: The Politics of Gender, Sexuality and Power, Berkeley and Los Angeles: University of California press, 1-25.

Parker, R.G. & Galvão, J. (Eds.) (1996). *Quebrando o Silêncio: Mulheres e AIDS no Brasil.* Rio de Janeiro: ABIA/IMS-UERJ/Relume-Dumará.

Parker, R.G. & Galvão, J. (1998). HIV/AIDS policy in Brazil. 12th World AIDS Conference Abstracts, Geneva, Switzerland, #355/43560.

Parker, R.G. , Galvão, J., & Bessa, M.S. (Eds.) (1999) *Saúde, Desenvolvimento e Política: Respostas frente à AIDS no Brasil.* São Paulo: ABIA/Editora 34.

Parker, R.G. & Gagnon, J. (Eds). (1995). Conceiving Sexuality: Approaches to Sex Research in a Postmodern World, New York and London: Routledge.

Parker R.G., Herdt, G., & Carballo, M. (1991). Sexual culture, HIV transmission, and AIDS research. *Journal of Sex Research*, 28, 77-98.

Parker, R.G., Kahn, S., & Aggleton, P. (1998). Conspicuous by their absence? Men who have sex with men (msm) in developing countries: Implications for HIV prevention. *Critical Public Health*, 8, 329-346.

Peak, A., Rana, S., Maharjan, S.H., *et al.* (1995). Declining risk for HIV among injecting drug users in Kathmundu, Nepal: The impact of a harm reduction programme. *AIDS* , 9, 1067-1070.

Quam, M. (1994). AIDS policy and the United States political economy. In D. Feldman (Ed.) Global AIDS Policy, Westport, CT: Bergin & Garvey, 142-159.

Quan, V.M., Chung, A., Abdul-Quader, A.S. (1998). Feasibility of a syringe-needle exchange program in Vietnam. *Substance Use and Misuse*, 33 (5), 1-14.

Rivers, K., Aggleton, P., Elizondo, J., Hernandez, G., Herrera, G., Mane, P., Niang, C.I., Scott, S., & Setiadi, B. (1998). Gender relations, sexual communication and the female condom. *Critical Public Health*, 8 (4), 273-290.

Romero-Daza, N. & Himmelgreen, D. (1998). More than money for your labor: Migration and the political economy of AIDS in Lesotho. In M. Singer (Ed.) The Political Economy of AIDS, New York: Baywood Publishing Company, 185-204.

Rojanapithayakakorn, W. (1994). The One Hundred Percent Condom Programme in Thailand, an update. 10th International Conference on AIDS Abstracts, 478C, Yokohama, Japan.

Rojanapithayakorn, W. & Hanenberg, R (1996). The 100% Condom Program in Thailand. *AIDS* 1996, 10, 1-7.

Santana, S., Fass, L., Wald, K. (1991). Human immunodeficiency virus in Cuba: The public health response of a Third World country. International Journal of Health Services, 21, 511-537.

Santana, S. (1997). AIDS prevention, treatment and care in Cuba. In G. Bond, J. Kreniske, I. Susser, & J. Vincent (Eds.) AIDS in Africa and the Caribbean, Boulder: Westview Press, 65-84.

Scheper-Hughes, N. (1993). AIDS, public health and human rights in Cuba. *Lancet*, 342 (8877), 965-967.

Schoepf, B.G. (1988). Women, AIDS, and economic crisis in Central Africa. *Canadian Journal of African Studies*, 22, 625-644.

Schoepf, B.G. (1992a). Gender relations and development: Political economy and culture. In A. Seidman & F. Anang (Eds.) Twenty-First Century Africa: Towards a New Vision of Sustainable Development, Trenton, N.J.: African World Press.

Schoepf, B.G. (1992b). Women at risk: Case studies from Zaire. In G. Herdt & S. Lindenbaum (Eds.) The Time of AIDS: Social Analysis, Theory and Method, Beverly Hills, California: Sage Publications, 259-286.

Schoepf, B.G. (1993). Gender, development, and AIDS: a political economy and culture framework. In R. Gallin, A. Ferguson, & J. Harper (Eds.) Women and International Development, Vol 3., Boulder, CO: Westview Press, 53-85.

Schoepf, B.G., Engundu, W., Nkera, W.A., Ntsomo, P., & Schoepf, P. (1991). Gender, power, and risk of AIDS in Central Africa. In M. Turshen (Ed.) Women and Health in Africa, Trenton, N.J.: Africa World Press, 187-203.

Schuler, S.R. & Syed, H. (1994). Credit programs, women's empowerment, and contraceptive use in rural Bangladesh. *Studies in Family Planning*, 25, 65-76

SHARAN. (1995). Annual Report, New Dehli.

Shreshtha, D.M., Shreshtha, N.M. & Gautama, K. (1995). Methadone treatment programme in Nepal: A one-year experience. *Journal of the Nepal Medical Association*, 33, 33-46.

Shuey, D. & Bagarukayo, H. (1996). AIDS: Despair, or a stimulus to reform? In J. Mann and D.J.M. Tarantola (Eds.) AIDS in the World II, Oxford: Oxford University Press, 122-124.

Singer, M. (Ed.) (1998). The Political Economy of AIDS, New York: Baywood.Publishing Company.

Stein, Z. (1990). HIV prevention: The need for methods women can use. *American Journal of Public Health*, 80, 460-462.

Stein, Z. (1995). Editorial: More on women and the prevention of HIV infection. *American Journal of Public Health*, 85, 1485-1488.

Stimson, G.V. (1992). The global diffusion of injecting drug use: implications for HIV infection. VIII International Conference on AIDS, Amsterdam, Abstract No. 1748.

Stimson, G.V. (1994). Reconstruction of subregional diffusion of HIV infection among injecting drug users in Southeast Asia: Implications for early interventions. *AIDS*, 8, 1630-1632.

Stimson, G.V. & Choopanya, K. (1998). Global perspectives on drug injecting. In G.V. Stimson, D.C. Des Jarlais & A.L. Ball (Eds.) Drug Injecting and HIV Infection: Global Dimensions and Local Responses, London: University College London Press.

Strarthdee, S.A., van Ameijden, E., Mesquita, F., Wodak, A., Rana, S., & Vlahov, D. (1998). Can HIV epidemics among injection drug users be prevented? *AIDS*, 12 (suppl A), S71-79.

Susser, I. & Kreniske, J. (1997). Community organizing around HIV prevention in rural Puerto Rico. In G. Bond, J. Kreniske, I. Susser, & J. Vincent (Eds.) AIDS in Africa and the Caribbean, Boulder: Westview Press, 51-64.

Sweat, M.D. & Denison, J.A. (1995). Reducing HIV incidence in developing countries with structural and environmental Interventions. *AIDS*, 9 (suppl A), S251-S257.

Symonds, P.V. (1998). Political economy and cultural logics of HIV/AIDS among the Hmong in Northern Thailand. In M. Singer (Ed.) The Political Economy of AIDS, New York: Baywood Publishing Company, 205-226.

Tan, M.L. (1993). Socio-economic impact of HIV/AIDS in the Philippines. *AIDS Care* 1993, 5, 283-288.

Tawil, O., Vertser, A., & O'Reilly, K. (1995). Enabling approaches for HIV prevention: Can we modify the environment and minimize the risk? *AIDS*, 9, 1299-1306.

Ten Brommelhuis, H. & Herdt, G. (Eds). (1995). Culture and Sexual Risk: Anthropological Perspectives on AIDS, Amsterdam: Gordon and Breach Publications.

Turner, C.F., Miller, H.G., & Moses, L.E. (Eds.). (1989). AIDS: Sexual Behavior and Intravenous Drug Use, Washington, D.C.: National Academy Press.

Turshen, M. (1992). US Aid to AIDS in Africa. *Review of African Political Economy*, 55, 95-101.

Turshen, M. (1995). Societal instability in international perspective: Relevance to HIV/AIDS prevention. National Academy of Sciences/Institute of Medicine Workshop on the Social and Behavioral Science Base for HIV/AIDS Prevention and Intervention, Washington, D.C., 117-128.

Turshen, M. (1998). The political ecology of AIDS in Africa. In M. Singer (Ed.) The Political Economy of AIDS, New York: Baywood Publishing Company, 169-184.

Wallace, R. (1998). A synergism of plagues: "Planned shrinkage," contagious housing destruction, and AIDS in the Bronx. *Environmental Research*, 47, 1-33.

Wallace, R., Fullilove, M., Fullivove, R., Gould, P., & Wallace, D. (1992). Will AIDS be contained within U.S. Minority Urban Populations? *Social Science and Medicine*, 8, 1051-1062.

Watney, S. (1994). Practices of Freedom: Selected Writings on HIV/AIDS, Durham: Duke University Press.

Webb, D. (1997). HIV and AIDS in Africa, London: Pluto Press.

Williams, E., Lamson, N, Efem, S. *et al.* (1992). Implementation of an AIDS prevention program among prostitutes in the Cross River State of Nigeria. *AIDS*, 6, 229-230.

Wilson, D., Sibanda, B., Mboyi, L., Msimanga, S., & Dube, G. (1990). A pilot study for an HIV prevention programme among commercial sex workers in Bulawayo, Zimbabwe. *Social Science and Medicine*, 5, 609-618.

Wilson, D., Sibanda, A., Nyathi, B., Lamson, N., & Sibanda, T. (1994). Ethnographic and quantitative research to design a community intervention among long-distance truck drivers in Zimbabwe. In Focusing Interventions among Vulnerable Groups for HIV Infection: Experiences from Eastern and Southern Africa. Nairobi: NARESA Monograph 99-118.

Wodak, M.B., Strathdee, S.A., Friedman, S.R., & Byrne, J. (1998). The global response to the threat of HIV infection among and from injecting drug users. *AIDS Targeted Information*, 12 (6), R41-R44.

Zoysa, I., Sweat, M.D. & Denison, J. (1996). Faithful but fearful: reducing HIV transmission in stable relationship. *AIDS*, 10 (suppl A), S197-S203.

Chapter 3

Female-Controlled Prevention Technologies

Janet S. Moore and Martha Rogers
Division of HIV/AIDS Prevention, National Center for HIV, STD and TB Prevention, Centers for Disease Control and Prevention, Atlanta Georgia

1. HIV INFECTION AND WOMEN

The Joint United Nations Program on HIV/AIDS estimates that AIDS has claimed 13.9 million lives worldwide and 3.4 million people are currently living with HIV/AIDS (Joint United Nations Programme on HIV/AIDS [UNAIDS], December 1998). Approximately 5.8 million new infections occurred throughout the world in 1998 alone and 16,000 new infections occur daily. In sub-Saharan Africa, the region of the world most affected by the epidemic, an estimated 34 million people have been infected with HIV and approximately 11.5 million of those have already died. In some southern African countries between 20% and 26% of the general population aged 15-49 are reported to be living with HIV. In the United States, HIV infection is now the third leading cause of death among women age 25-44 and the leading cause of death among African American women in this age category (National Center for Health Statistics, 1997).

The majority of newly acquired HIV infections throughout the world are the result of heterosexual transmission (UNAIDS, December, 1998). In sub-Saharan Africa, heterosexual sex and perinatal transmission account for almost all cases of HIV infection (UNAIDS, June, 1998). In the United States the proportion of HIV infections attributable to heterosexual transmission has increased sharply among women; approximately 40% of new AIDS cases and 57% of new HIV infections are attributed to heterosexual transmission (Centers for Disease Control and Prevention [CDC], 1999), an increase from 15% of reported AIDS cases among women in 1983 (CDC, 1997). The current public health recommendations to reduce sexual transmission of HIV include 1) treatment of sexually transmitted diseases (STDs) associated with acquisition and transmission of HIV; 2) limiting number of sex partners; and 3) correct and consistent use of condoms. Each of these prevention strategies has been shown to have limitations in stemming the epidemic, particularly among women. First, although observational studies have shown that certain STDs are associated with the transmission and acquisition of HIV (Laga, 1993; Waserheit, 1992), the efficacy of treating them as a method for limiting HIV transmission has not been clearly demonstrated. One randomized community trial providing enhanced syndromic treatment of STDs showed that treatment can decrease HIV incidence at the community level (Grosskurth et al., 1995). Another study of mass STD treatment, however, showed no effect on HIV incidence (Wawer et al., 1998). Even if mass STD treatment were an effective means of HIV prevention, most resource poor countries do not have the health care infrastructures to deliver such a large-scale, ongoing medical intervention, thereby limiting its applicability to countries where HIV prevention is most needed. Syndromic treatment of STDs is not a realistic prevention strategy for women, particularly in developing countries, because they do not receive routine gynecologic care where STDs might be detected. In addition, women often are not symptomatic and do not seek treatment until the disease is quite advanced.

Limiting number of sex partners also is a prevention strategy that is not likely to have a major impact on the HIV epidemic, particularly among women. Partner restriction is not a realistic option for women or men whose livelihood depends on commercial sex work. Additionally, many women who acquire HIV heterosexually do not have multiple sex partners; they are infected by their sole male partner (Grinstead, Faigeles, Binson, & Eversley, 1993; Kost & Forrest, 1992). For example, in a sample of HIV-positive women in the United States, Diaz et al. (1994) found that 35% reported having just one partner in the past five years. Approximately 31% of women reported with AIDS to the Centers for Disease Control and Prevention in 1999 had no identified risk for HIV (CDC, 1999). At least a portion of these cases represent women who were heterosexually infected by their sole male partner whose HIV status or risk history was unknown to the woman. The strategy for avoiding HIV infection by limiting number of partners should be a part of all prevention plans, but clearly is not sufficient to combat the HIV epidemic, particularly among women. Correct and consistent use of condoms has the potential to be a highly effective means of HIV control. Laboratory studies show that latex male condoms provide a mechanical barrier to bacterial and viral sexually transmitted diseases, including HIV (Carey et al., 1992; CDC, 1993). In vivo studies have confirmed that the male condom is an effective means of reducing risk of HIV transmission (Cates & Stone, 1992; Weller, 1993). In studies of heterosexual HIV serodiscordant couples, correct and consistent use of male condoms has been shown to be highly effective in preventing transmission to the uninfected partner (Saracco et al., 1993; de Vincenzi, 1994). Despite their efficacy, widespread consistent male condom use has been difficult to achieve particularly among heterosexuals. Interventions in both the developing and developed world have been somewhat successful at increasing self-reported condom use in heterosexual populations and several studies have shown concommitant reductions in transmission of HIV infection and other STDs (Kamb et al., 1998; Nelson et al., 1996). In particular, interventions among commercial sex workers have increased the proportion of paid and casual sexual encounters in which condoms are used (Asamoah-Adu et al., 1994; Bhave et al., 1995; Laga et al., 1994). Among heterosexual couples receiving HIV counseling and testing, increases in consistent condom use have been reported (Allen, Serufilira, et al., 1992), particularly among couples found to be HIV serodiscordant (Allen, Tice, et al., 1992: Kamenga et al., 1991; Padian, O'Brien, Chang, Glass, & Francis, 1993; The Voluntary HIV-1 Counseling and Testing Efficacy Study Group, 2000). Nonetheless, male condom use even among the highest risk persons is far from universal (consistent use rates even in the highest risk situations rarely exceed 60%) and is difficult to sustain over long periods of time. For example, HIV seroincidence rates as high as 3 to 5 per 100 person years has been found among sex workers receiving an intensive condom promotion program (Allen, Serufilira, et al., 1992; Laga et al., 1994). In studies that counsel and give free supplies of male condoms and spermicides to sex workers, HIV seroincidence rates of 7-15 per 100 person years have been documented (Roddy et al., 1998; Van Damme, 2000). Condoms may be a particularly difficult prevention strategy for women to implement because they must rely on their male partner's cooperation to achieve HIV protection. Interventions targeting women (other than sex workers) have met with partial success; those stressing condom negotiation skills in conjunction with risk assessment, education, and skills building have been most effective (Sikkema et al., 1995; DiClemente & Wingood, 1995; Kelly et al., 1994). However, even with the most successful interventions, a sizable group of women are unable to introduce and negotiate consistent and sustained condom use with their partners, particularly in the context of primary relationships (O'leary & Wingood, 1999). Barriers to introducing condoms include the woman's reluctance to raise issues of trust and fidelity in the relationship and concerns about the male partner's reaction to condoms. Additionally, power discrepancies found in many heterosexual relationships and the cultural dictates around the role of women in sexual encounters may leave women unable or unwilling to engage in condom negotiation.

The limitations of current HIV prevention methods for women have led many human rights advocates, HIV researchers, and public health professionals to call for development of methods of HIV and other STD prevention that women can use without reliance on male partners (Elias & Coggins, 1996; Elias & Heise, 1994; Stein, 1990; Stone & Hitchcock, 1994). Many advocates of female controlled methods have suggested that the HIV epidemic among women will rage unabated without the development of a woman-controlled technology. The ideal female controlled product is one that could be used without detection by or active involvement of sex partners, could be applied in advance of sexual activity, available in contraceptive and noncontraceptive forms without prescription, effective against other STDs, easily stored, and affordable and available to women throughout the world (The Population Council & International Family Health, 2000).

Research has focused on development and testing of the female condom and products showing promise as vaginal microbicides. In this chapter we review in vitro and in vivo studies on the efficacy of these two methods for prevention of HIV and STDs and on the acceptability of these methods to women and their male partners. We also describe two female controlled methods that may hold promise as HIV prevention methods (diaphragm and cervical cap), but have received little research attention. Finally, we review ethical and methodologic challenges faced in evaluating new female controlled methods of HIV prevention.

2. FEMALE CONDOM

2.1 Description

The female condom provides a physical barrier that lines the vagina. The best studied of the female condoms is marketed as Reality in the United States and Femidon in England although several other products are in various stages of research and development (Stewart, 1998). The Reality condom is a 17 cm polyurethane vaginal sheath with two rings. The inner ring holds the device in place during intercourse. The outer ring sits on the labia and partially covers the external genitalia, possibly offering additional protection against STDS such as herpes and chancroid. The sheath is coated on the inside with a silicone-based lubricant that does not contain spermicide. The Reality condom is intended for one-time use and can be inserted up to 8 hours before intercourse.

2.2 Efficacy/Effectiveness

In 1993 the US Food and Drug Administration (FDA) approved the marketing of the Reality female condom. This approval was based on contraceptive efficacy data as there were no data on the efficacy of the device in protecting against HIV and other STDs. Bounds, Guillebaud, Stewart, & Steele (1992), conducting one of the first contraceptive efficacy trials, computed the accidental pregnancy rate of women using only the female condom for contraception and found a pregnancy rate of 15% for women followed one year. In 1994, Farr, Gabelnick, Sturgen, & Dorflinger assessed the contraceptive effectiveness of the female condom for the FDA. In this study conducted at 6 US sites and three Latin America sites, 6-month accidental pregnancy rates were 12.4 in the U.S. and 22.2 in Latin America. Under conditions of consistent and correct use of the method, pregnancy rates were 2.6 in the US and 9.5 for Latin American sites. These and other data suggest that the contraceptive efficacy of the female condom during typical use is similar to that reported for other female-controlled methods of contraception including the diaphragm, sponge, and cervical cap (Trussell, Sturgen, Strickler, & Dominik, 1994). In terms of disease protection, the polyurethane female condom is impermeable to virus-sized particles (Voeller, Coulter, & Mayhan, 1991) including HIV and cytomegalovirus (Drew, Blair, Miner, & Conant, 1990). In a study of post-coital leakage designed to detect pinholes and tears after actual condom use, 3.4% of male condoms showed leakage but less than 1% of Reality condoms leaked (Leeper & Conrady, 1989). Unless the female condom slips out of place, it theoretically should provide protection against STD exposure that is as good as that provided by male condoms. Actual data on effectiveness of the female condom to reduce transmission of HIV and other STDs are limited, however. In 1993, Soper et al. showed a reduction in recurrent vaginal trichomoniasis by compliant use of the female condom. In a more recent study of commercial sex workers in Thailand, indirect support was found for the efficacy of the female condom (Fontanet et al., 1998). Sex establishments in four cities were randomized to two study groups. In one group women were instructed to use male condoms for each act of intercourse, and in the other group women were offered the option of using the female condom when a male condom was not used. The proportion of unprotected sex acts (defined as sex acts in which condoms were not used, tore, or slipped in or out) and incidence of STDs were measured over 6 months for the two groups. The proportion of protected sex acts was greater in the male/female condom group than in the male condom only group. Additionally, although not statistically significant, there was a 34% reduction in the mean incidence of STDs in the male/female condom group compared to the male condom only group. The authors concluded that the parallel decrease in proportion of unprotect sex acts and in the incidence rate of STDs in the male/female condom group when compared to the male condom group suggested that the female condom was as effective as the male condom in reducing transmission of common STDs. Data on the efficacy of the female condom to reduce transmission of HIV are not yet available, although several studies designed to investigate this issue are underway.

2.3 Acceptability

In determining the acceptability of new HIV prevention methods, a number of factors must be considered. First, the product must be safe for the intended activities and for a wide range of use patterns. Second, users must have confidence in the product and be willing to try it. Third, persons who try the product must find it easy to use correctly, an acceptable part of sexual intercourse, and be willing to use it routinely. Fourth, the product must be acceptable to others who may influence the user; in the case of HIV prevention methods for women, this is likely to be the male sex partner. The new product should address an unmet public health need (e.g., female controlled methods should appeal to and be used by women unable or unwilling to use male condoms rather than only to women who are already good male condom users). Finally, the product must be available and affordable.

Data indicate that the female condom is safe for most users. Few reports of allergic reactions or genital irritation have been reported by women using the female condom or by their male partners (Soper, Brockwell, & Dalton, 1991; Stewart, 1998). Additionally, rates of breakage are low, generally below that reported for the male condom (Fontanet et al, 1998; Leeper & Conrady, 1989; Ruminjo, Steiner, Joanis, Mwathe, & Thagana, 1996). Women and men report confidence in the durability and effectiveness of the female condoms as a contraceptive and disease prevention method (Gollub, Stein, & El-Sadr, 1995; Klein, Eber, Crosby, Welka, & Hoffman, 1999; Sly et al., 1997). Women in particular view the thickness of the female condom in a positive light and perceive it to be a more reliable method of contraception and disease prevention than the male condom. Studies also find that many women have positive reactions to the female condom when initially introduced (Ashery, Carson, Falck, Siegal, & Wang, 1995; Gollub et al., 1995; Farr et al., 1994; Shervington, 1993; Sly et al., 1997). They find the concept of a disease prevention method that women control and use autonomously particularly appealing (Gollub et al., 1995; Klein et al., 1999; Shervington, 1993). But women and their male partners also have negative initial impressions of the female condom; they view it as large, awkward, and difficult to insert (Eldridge, St. Lawrence, Little, Shelby, & Brasfield, 1995; Jivasak-Apimas, 1991). Nonetheless, most studies report that the majority of women are willing to try the device. Studies with sex workers show a high degree of interest in and willingness to try the female condom and a generally favorable response to its use, with a majority intending to use the device in the future (Madrigal, Schifter, & Feldblum, 1998; Ray et al., 1995; Sakondhavat, 1990; Witte, El-Bassel, Wada, Gray, & Wallace, 1999). Studies of injecting drug and crack using women have reported high initial interest in and uptake of female condoms (Ashery et al., 1995; Klein et al., 1999; Stein et al., 1999), as have several studies with heterosexual couples (Bounds, Guillebaud, Stewart, & Steele, 1988; Farr et al., 1994; Musabe, Morrison, Sunkutu & Wong, 1998; Ruminjo et al., 1996; Xu et al., 1998). Positive features identified by women who have tried the female condom include perceived reliability (Sly et al., 1997), less reduction of sexual sensation than the male condom (Klein et al., 1999; Sly et al., 1997), and ability to insert in advance of a sexual encounter (Sly et al., 1997).

But studies show that favorable ratings decline with use, and in some studies willingness to use the female condom has dropped over time below willingness to use the male condom (Artz et al., 2000; Gollub et al., 1995; Kalichman, Williams, & Nachimson, 1999; Sinpisut, Chandeying, Skov, & Uahgowitchai, 1998). Reported difficulties in use include 1) outer ring of the device is driven inside the vagina by the penis (Bounds et al, 1992); 2) penis is misrouted and enters between the female condom and the vaginal wall (Bounds et al, 1992); 3) difficulty inserting (Gollub et al., 1995; Klein et al., 1999); and 4) slippage during intercourse (Gollub et al., 1995; Klein et al., 1999). Men and women also complain about diminished sensation when using the female condom compared to use of no barrier (Bounds et al, 1988; Ehrhardt, Yingling, Zawadzki, & Martinez-Ramirez, 1992; Eldridge et al., 1995; Ford and Mathie, 1993; Sly et al., 1997). Finally, although the hope was that the female condoms could be used without the cooperation, and ideally, without the knowledge of the male partner, use of the device requires cooperation from the man in routing the penis inside the sheath and in keeping the outer ring in place (Ashery et al., 1995; Bounds et al., 1992; Farr et al., 1994; Jivasak-Apimas, 1991). Additionally, men and women are often aware of the inside and outside rings of the female condom, which can detract from the sexual experience (Jivasak-Apimas, 1991; Ray et al., 1995). Several studies have attempted to determine if the female condom fills a unique HIV/STD prevention need (i.e., women unable to use male condoms or who find them unacceptable are able and willing to use the female condom). Contrary to expectations, a number of studies have found that the female condom is of greater interest and more acceptable to women who are successful male condom users than to women who are not (Cabral et al., 1999; Cecil, Perry, Seal, & Pinkerton, 1998; Gil, 1995; Sly et al., 1997; Walker et al., 1993). For example, Cabral et al (1999) found that women who had a history of using the male condom were more likely to uptake the female condom than nonusers of the male condom. Moreover, women in abusive relationships (i.e., those expected to be unable to negotiate male condom use and to desire a female-controlled prevention method) were no more interested in the female condom than women in nonabusive situations. A study by Murphy, Miller, Moore, & Clark (2000) showed that the women most interested in female-controlled methods of HIV/STD prevention participated in fewer risk behaviors and were more likely to use other means of contraception and disease prevention methods, including male condoms. The women least interested in female controlled methods were those who had higher levels of risk behavior and had used male condoms less. In several respects, the female condom does not meet the ideal criteria of a female controlled HIV prevention method. Although it is technically used by the woman the male partner is aware that the female condom is being used and must cooperate to assure that the method is used correctly. Recent evidence suggests that the male partner's reaction to the female condom is highly influential in determining the woman's attitude toward the device (Cabral et al., 1999; Eldridge et al., 1995; Farr et al., 1994; Jivasak-Apimas, 1991; Sly et al., 1997). Several studies report dissatisfaction by the male partner, as the primary reason women are unwilling to try or discontinue use of the female condom (Ford & Mathie, 1993; Gil, 1995; Jivasak-Apimas, 1991; Sakondkavat & Potter, 1990). Although not meeting all criteria for a female- controlled prevention method, the female condom may be a feasible and preferred prevention method for some women and certainly should be included as an alternative in all HIV/STD prevention interventions. Studies have shown that when women present their male partners with the choice of using a male or female condom, the number of protected sex acts increase (Artz et al., 2000; Fontanent et al., 1998; Latka, Gollub, French, & Stein, 2000; Musabe et al., 1998). This increase is due in part to the use of female condoms but also to the increased use of the male condom when a choice is offered; the female condom becomes a negotiation tool for the woman, resulting in greater uptake of the male condom by the partner (Ashery et al., 1995; Latka et al., 2000). A more recent article by these authors found, however, that the recurrence of trichomonas did not differ for groups offered multiple prevention options in a hierarchy compared to women offered a single prevention method (Gollub et al., 2000).

Finally, to meet acceptability criteria, an HIV prevention method must be available and accessible to those who need it most. The female condom is currently available in pharmacies throughout the world. However, it is much more expensive than the male condom and is too expensive for most women to purchase for routine use. Because of the cost, female condoms typically are not distributed by governmental or nongovernmental community agencies. Efforts are underway to make the female condom more available and affordable (Stewart, 1998). One aspect of cost reduction involves reuse of the female condom. Research is currently underway to determine if the structural integrity of the female condom is maintained through multiple washings and if soap and water eliminate retention of microbes.

2.4 Research Needs

Despite the number of studies on the female condom, few large, well-controlled, longitudinal studies have examined its efficacy or acceptability. More information is needed on the characteristics of women who prefer and continue to use the female condom so that marketing efforts can be targeted to that group. More research also is needed to determine if and how the female condom is used by women as a negotiation tool with male partners and if this negotiation results in more male and/or female condom use. If so, then both methods should be made available to women in HIV prevention interventions and they should be offered training on their use as negotiation tools.

3. DIAPHRAGM AND CERVICAL CAP

3.1 Description

The diaphragm and the cervical cap are two female-controlled barrier contraceptive devices that may have some applicability to HIV/STD prevention. The diaphragm is a dome-shaped rubber cup with a flexible rim. The dome covers the cervix and spermicidal cream is placed inside the dome before insertion. The diaphragm provides effective contraceptive protection for up to 6 hours. The cervical cap is a soft deep rubber cup with a firm round rim, which is sealed against the surface of the cervix. Spermicide is used to fill the dome prior to insertion and is held in place against the cervix until the cap is removed. The cap provides continuous protection from pregnancy for up to 48 hours. Because both the diaphragm and the cervical cap cover the cervix, researchers have speculated that they may offer protection against acquisition of HIV and other STDs. (Stewart, 1998)

3.2 Efficacy / Effectiveness

The diaphragm and cervical cap are effective contraceptive devices although not as effective as the male and female condom. From 5-9% of nuliparious users and from 5-26% of parious users become pregnant during the first year of perfect use (Bernstein et al., 1986; Edleman, McIntyre, and Harper, 1984; Trussel, Strickler, & Vaughan, 1993). Data on the efficacy or effectiveness of the devices for STD prevention are limited and inconclusive. Several observational studies have suggested that the devices confer some protection against certain sexually transmitted diseases, but confounding factors in these studies have precluded a definitive interpretation of the data (d'Doro, Parazzini, Naldi, & LaVecchia, 1994; Rosenberg & Gollub, 1992). For example, a reduced risk for pelvic inflammatory disease has been found among diaphragm users (Cramer et al., 1987; Kelaghan, Rubin, Ory, & Layde, 1982). The explanation for the finding could be that protection against STDs is provided by the diaphragm. On the other hand, women who choose the diaphragm may be at lower risk for reproductive tract infections than women choosing other forms of contraception. Even if the causal role of the diaphragm and cervical cap in preventing STDs is disentangled, most researchers agree that the risk reduction they provide for STDs is only modest. No data are available on the efficacy of the devices to protect against acquisition of HIV although several studies are planned.

The role that the diaphragm and cervical cap could play in stemming the HIV epidemic among women depends, in part, on the extent to which the cervix is the primary entry point for the virus, an issue that has not been definitively determined. At least one study has shown that HIV infection can occur without the presence of a cervix (Howe, Minkoff, and Duerr, 1994; Miller, Alexander, Vogel, Anderson, & Marx, 1992), indicating that the cervix is not the only portal for the virus. If the majority of infections are acquired through the cervix, however, the diaphragm and cervical cap could have a sizable impact on the epidemic. The devices may also contribute to HIV prevention indirectly by reducing acquisition of sexually transmitted infections that invade the cervix such as gonorrhea and chlamydia (Rosenberg & Gollub, 1992).

Another determinant of the effectiveness of the diaphragm and cervical cap for HIV and STD prevention depends upon the importance of the spermicidal product used with both devices in providing protection. It may be that both devices show protective effects against STDs because the spermicidal product used with the devices has antimicrobial properties. There are no reports of studies examining the contraceptive or disease prevention efficacy of these devices when used without spermicide. Because currently available spermicidal products (those containing N-9) have been shown to be ineffective, and perhaps even harmful, as an HIV prevention method, it is not likely that further testing of these devices as methods of HIV prevention will proceed until an antimicrobial spermicide becomes available. Alternatively, the efficacy of the devices to provide HIV/STD protection even when used without a spermicide could be pursued.

3.3 Acceptability

Although several studies are planned to evaluate the acceptability of the diaphragm and cervical cap as methods of HIV/STD prevention, data on the topic are not currently available. Data on the acceptability of both as contraceptive devices have been available for years. Only rare cases of allergic reactions to the devices have been documented although some women have allergic reactions to the nonoxynol-9 spermicidal product used with them (Stewart, 1998). Some women report cramps, bladder pain, or rectal pain when wearing a diaphragm or cap. Male partners occasionally report penile pain during intercourse. Foul odor and vaginal discharge have been reported if either device is left in the vagina more than a few days. Higher rates of bacterial vaginosis and urinary tract infections have been detected among diaphragm users than among women using oral contraceptives; however, it is likely that the spermicidal product used with the diaphragm rather than the device itself is responsible for this finding (Hooton, Hillier, Johnson, Roberts, & Stamm, 1991). Both the diaphragm and the cervical cap must be fitted by a trained health care provider, adding an additional step in the distribution of these devices for HIV/STD prevention.

3.4 Research Needs

Research on the role of the cervix in HIV transmission to women is needed to determine the potential importance of methods that protect the cervix in reducing HIV transmission. If and when this issue is resolved and if the cervix plays a primary role in transmission, evaluation of barrier methods such as the diaphragm and cervical cap will be needed to determine if they are protective against HIV. As this basic biologic information is being collected, data on the acceptability of the devices to women and male partners and feasibility (e.g., issues of storage, cleaning, distribution) of using these methods should be assessed. Although acceptability is difficult to accurately assess when the efficacy of a product is unknown, preliminary investigations could determine if the products are likely to be rejected outright.

4. MICROBICIDAL PRODUCTS

4.1 Description

Topical microbicidal agents that can be applied to the surface of the vagina or rectum are promising methods of HIV prevention. Unlike the male and female condom that protect by providing a physical barrier to pathogens, microbicidal agents protect through chemical action. The common characteristic of topical microbicides is that they act superficially rather than systemically. The antimicrobial activity of some agents is specific to certain STDs whereas others provide protection against a wide range of pathogens. Some of the potential agents under development and evaluation are contraceptive, whereas others allow for pregnancy. The particular mechanism by which the agent offers protection against HIV or other STDs varies; current microbicidal candidates include products that kill or inactivate the virus, inhibit viral entry, or inhibit viral replication.

4.2 Agents That Kill Or Inactivate The Virus

These agents kill or inactivate HIV and other pathogens through membrane or envelope disruption. Two approaches have been used for developing agents in this class: testing of existing over-the-counter spermicidal products and development of new products that have potential to kill or inactivate HIV and other STD pathogens (Elias & Coggins, 1996). All currently available over-the-counter spermicidal products use detergents to disrupt cell membranes. In the United States these products contain either nonoxynol-9 or octoxynol-9. In other countries, benzalkonium chloride and menfegol are approved spermicides. Many of these products have been available as contraceptives for years and several have recently been evaluated for antimicrobial properties in Phase III efficacy trials (Kreiss et al., 1992; Roddy et al., 1998). Reformulation of existing products has also been attempted to reduce irritation to the vagina, increase coverage of the reproductive tract, and increase duration of action. Agents in this category include Col-1492, a bioadhesive formulation of nonoxynol-9 recently evaluated in a Phase III efficacy trial (Van Damme, 2000). Products that kill or inactivate HIV through mechanisms other than that used by the detergents are being investigated for their antimicrobial capacity. One group of agents includes products that keep the vagina acidic in the presence of semen. The normal vagina has an acidic pH and research has shown that HIV may not survive well in an acidic environment (Ongradi, J., Ceccherini-Nelli, Pistell, Spector, & Bendinelli, 1990). Semen, however, increases the vaginal pH making it more susceptible to some infections. Acid-buffering agents would inactivate HIV and other STDs by keeping the vagina acidic in the presence of semen. An example of this product currently under investigation is Buffer-gel which has been found to be safe for use in humans (van de Wijgert, et al., 2000) and is now being considered for Phase III efficacy trials (Alliance for Microbicide Development, 2000). Another group of products acts to resist infection by maintaining the normal vaginal ecology. The normal vaginal environment is characterized by a predominance of hydrogen peroxide-producing lactobacilli that may play a role in maintaining a low vaginal pH and resisting infection (Klebanoff, Hillier, Eschenbach, & Waltersdorph, 1991). A suppository containing lactobacilli that helps maintain the normal vaginal ecology is currently being tested for safety in humans (Alliance for Microbicide Development, 2000).

4.3 Agents That Inhibit Viral Entry

Another group of compounds works by inhibiting viral entry into mucosal cells. A number of agents in this class have shown antimicrobial activity in vitro and in animal studies and several products are ready for human safety trials (Alliance for Microbicide Development, 2000). Compounds in this category include PC515 (Carraguard) that has been shown to inhibit viral entry and cell fusion for HIV, herpes simplex virus (HSV), and chlamydia (Young et al., 2000). PC515 also provides some protection against vaginal Simian Immunodeficiency Virus (SIV) transmission in monkeys (Pauwels & De Clercq, 1996), and has been shown to be safe for humans in small Phase-I clinical trials (Coggins et al., 2000). Another product in this class of agents, PRO 2000 (Procept), inhibits HIV, HSV, and chlamydia in vitro, protects mice against HSV-2 infection, causes little or no vaginal irritation in animal studies, and appears to be safe for humans (Profy, Sonderfan, Chancellor, & McKinlay, 2000). This agent is currently being considered for Phase III efficacy trials (Alliance for Microbicide Development, 2000).

4.4 Agents that Inhibit Viral Replication

This class of compounds acts to prevent infection through inhibition of HIV replication and includes nucleoside and nonnucleoside reverse transcriptase inhibitors, post fusion inhibitors, and protease inhibitors. Most of these products are in the pre-clinical stage of development and research although one is in Phase I safety-trials. (Elias & Coggins, 1996). For example, a vaginal gel containing PMPA (a nucleoside reverse transcriptase inhibitor) has been evaluated in vivo and has been shown to confer some protection against SIV in the macaque (Haney, 1996). Plans are underway to begin Phase I safety trials on this product.

4.5 Efficacy / Effectiveness

Efficacy trials (Phase III clinical trials) have been conducted only on commercially marketed spermicides (nonoxynol-9) to determine if these agents reduce HIV transmission in women. N-9 products are effective contraceptives with accidental pregnancy rates during typical use ranging from 5 to 50% (Cates & Raymond, 1999). N-9 inactivates HIV and other STD pathogens in vitro (Judson, Ehret, Bodin, Levin, & Reitmeijer, 1989; Malkovsky, Newell, & Dalgleish, 1988). Additionally, N-9 has been shown to partially protect macaques against SIV transmission (Miller, Alexander, Gettie, Hendrickx, & Marx, 1992; Miller et al., 1990). As early as 1987, observational studies suggested that N-9 had antimicrobial properties for preventing certain STDs including gonococcal and chlamydial infections (Louv, Austin, Alexander, Stagno, & Cheeks, 1988; Niruthisard, Roddy, & Chutivongse, 1992; Rosenberg, Rojanapithayakorn, Feldblum & Higgins, 1987; Weir, Feldblum, Zekeng, & Roddy, 1994). Based on these early findings, N-9 appeared to be a promising microbicidal agent and interest was turned to evaluating its efficacy. The first N-9 Phase III HIV prevention trial was conducted with female sex workers in Kenya (Kreiss et al., 1992). One-half of the women were randomly assigned to use a vaginal sponge with 1,000 mg of N-9 and one-half to the placebo condition that used a vaginal suppository containing mineral oil. Use of the N-9 sponge was associated with an increased risk for genital ulcers and vulvitis and a reduced risk of gonococcal cervicitis. Additionally, there was a trend toward an increased incidence of HIV among the N-9 users; 45% of women in the N-9 group became infected compared to 36% in the placebo control group. Because of the potentially harmful effect of the N-9, the study was discontinued although problems with study design made results difficult to interpret. For example, the increased HIV incidence in the N-9 group may have been the result of increased epithelial disruption caused by the large dose of N-9 contained in the contraceptive sponge. However, more women in the N-9 than the placebo group had genital ulcers at baseline, and thus may have been more susceptible to becoming HIV infected before using the N-9 sponge. Because results of this study were inconclusive, additional studies were conducted to examine the effect of N-9 on HIV transmission.

In 1993, an observational study (Zekeng, Feldblum, Oliver, & Kaptue, 1993) suggested that N-9 offered some protection against HIV among Cameroon sex workers after controlling for condom use. A lower rate of HIV infection occurred among women consistently using N-9 suppositories compared to women using them less consistently. A reanalysis of these data was conducted and published by the authors with findings consistent with the original conclusions (Feldblum & Weir, 1994). As a result of these promising observational findings, a randomized controlled trial of N-9 was conducted among Cameroon Sex workers (Roddy et al., 1998). This study attempted to deal with design problems that plagued the efficacy trial conducted in Kenya. In a double blind, placebo-controlled study, women used either a 70mg N-9 vaginal film or a placebo film. All women were supplied with male condoms and instructed to use them for each act of intercourse. They also were instructed to use the vaginal film for every act of intercourse. The investigators reasoned that when partners would not use male condoms, women would use the vaginal film (N-9 or placebo), thereby providing a test of the efficacy of the N-9 film when used alone. The investigators found that the rate of genital lesions was slightly higher among women using the N-9 than among those in the placebo condition. However, the rate of HIV seroconversion was the same in the two groups (6.7 per 100 woman years in the N-9 group and 6.6 per 100 woman years in the placebo group), as were the rates of gonorrhea and chlamydia. A number of explanations were offered for the failure of this study to detect a difference in the N-9 and placebo groups including the high reported use of male condoms by women in both groups and the potential failure of the film to provide sufficient vaginal coverage.

Despite the disappointing results from the Cameroon trial, the decision was made to continue an ongoing Phase III clinical trial of another N-9 product marketed as COL1492 in Europe and Advantage-S in the U.S. This decision was made because COL1492, although having a lower concentration of N-9 (52mg) than the product used in Cameroon (72mg), is a gel rather than a film (as used in the Cameroon study), and thus, was expected to provide better vaginal coverage. The study was conducted among sex workers in five African countries and two sites in Thailand. Study subjects were instructed to use male condoms and the spermicidal product for each and every act of intercourse. Trial results were announced at the XIII International AIDS Conference (Van Damme, 2000). Contrary to predictions, the incidence of HIV seroconversion was significantly higher in the COL-1492 group (15.5) than in the placebo condition (10.1). Additionally, there was a dose effect for N-9 on HIV acquisition; the more women used the product the more likely they were to become HIV infected. Women receiving the N-9 product were more likely to develop genital ulcers than women in the placebo condition that may have been responsible for the higher incidence of HIV infection in the treatment group. Some women in this study applied the N-9 product or the placebo multiple times per day. It is not known if the product would have a similar disruptive effect on epithelial tissue if used less frequently. No protective effect of N-9 was seen for chlamydia and gonorrhea. The continued failure of N-9 to demonstrate a protective effect, and possibly to have harmful effect on HIV transmission has eliminated interest in this agent as a potential means of HIV prevention. The Centers for Disease Control and Prevention (CDC) issued a statement after the COL1492 results were released recommending that N-9 products not be included as an option in hierarchies of prevention methods and that N-9 products not be used as lubricants for anal sex (H.D. Gayle, personal communication, August 4, 2000). CDC plans to convene a meeting to discuss if N-9 lubricated condoms pose a risk for HIV transmission although it is anticipated that the small concentration of N-9 available in condoms (<0.05%) is not harmful.

Attention in the area of microbicide research and development has turned to agents, other than N-9, that kill or inactivate HIV and to agents that inhibit viral entry or replication. Thirty-five potential microbicidal products are currently in preclinical stages of research (i.e, animal model data and in vitro data have been or are being collected). Twenty-two products are in various stages of clinical evaluation; the safety of 17 products is being evaluated in Phase I studies, 3 products are in Phase II, and two products (Buffer gel and PRO 2000) are ready for Phase III efficacy trials (Alliance for Microbicide Development, 2000).

4.6 Acceptability

Spermicidal N-9 products, available over-the-counter for years, are safe at low doses with typical patterns of use (Martin et al., 1997; Roddy Cordero, Cordero, & Fortney, 1993; Van Damme et al., 1998). Nononxynol-9, however, appears to have a relatively narrow margin of safety with higher and more frequent doses resulting in irritation and epithelial disruption (Bird, 1991; Kreiss et al., 1992; Niruthisard, Roddy, & Chutivongse, 1991; Roddy et al., 1993; Van Damme, 2000). Roddy et al. (1993), found that the rate of epithelial disruption among women using N-9 every other day was no different than the rate among placebo users. However, the rate of epithelial disruption in one/day and two/day users was 2.5 times greater than among placebo users and five times greater among women using N-9 four times per day. The findings from the efficacy trial of COL-1492 also showed a dosing effect; women using the N-9 more frequently were more likely to become HIV infected, possibly because of an increase in genital ulcers with more frequent use of N-9 (Van Damme, 2000). Final analyses have not been completed, however, these findings have caused such concern about the safety of N-9 among researchers and public health professionals that the agent is no longer considered a viable candidate for use as a vaginal microbicide.

Few data are available on other aspects of acceptability of candidate microbicides. The sparse data that are available suggest that both women and men have favorable responses to demonstrations of the products and indicate a willingness and eagerness to try them (Hammett et al., 2000; Moon et al., 2000; Pool et al., 2000). Responses after a period of product trial also are typically positive. In safety and efficacy trials, microbicide use is reportedly high throughout the trial and generally women report no difficulties using the product (Roddy et al., 1998; Rustomjee, Karim, Karim, Laga, & Stein, 1999; Van Damme, 2000). In a study of 520 Cameroonian sex workers participating in a clinical trial of N-9 film, the majority of women liked the film with over 80% willing to use the product in the future if it were found to be efficacious (Visness, Ulin, Pfannenschmidt & Zekeng, 1998). In a safety study of twenty sex workers in South Africa almost all women reported positive experiences with N-9 film including feeling clean and fresh-tasting and smelling good, and feeling tight and dry. They reported no difficulty inserting N-9 vaginal film (Rustomjee et al., 1999). Women report liking microbicidal products because 1) they provide them with an opportunity to control their own protection, 2) the product can be used without the partner's knowledge, and 3) microbicides allow direct physical contact during sex (Visness et al., 1998). Despite women's stated interest in using microbicides without their partner's knowledge, several studies have found that the majority of women want their partners to know and often tell them when they use the product. In a study reported by Hammett et al. (2000), 80% of women said they would want their regular partners to know they were using a microbicide, and 42% said they would want their paying customers to know. Pool et al. (2000), found that although many women said they wanted a product they could use secretly, most informed their partners when they used the microbicide. Scarlett, Macaluso, and Duerr (1997) also found that most (80%) women participating in a study on preferences for HIV prevention methods told their partners they were using a microbicide.

Several studies have investigated men's attitudes toward candidate microbicides to be used by their female partners and have found mixed results. Generally, studies have found men to be either positive or unconcerned about women using microbicides (Ramjee, Meyer, Andrews, & Gouws, 2000; Srirak et al., 2000). In a study of sex workers about one-half of the women told their partners they were using a microbicide and none experienced negative reactions from the partner (Rustomjee et al., 1999). But men have voiced concerns about microbicides including the fear that they give women too much autonomy (Pool et al., 2000) and concerns about the amount of lubrication they cause during sex. (Ramjee et al, 2000). In cultural groups where dry sex is preferred, microbicidal products that lubricate may be unacceptable, particularly to men.

Data on women's willingness to continue using microbicidal products outside clinical trials and over long periods of time are not available and are not likely to be collected until a product with a satisfactory level of efficacy is available. One group of investigators (Cohen, Reardon, Alleyne, Murthy, & Linton, 1995) were able to demonstrate that a brief intervention delivered in the waiting room of public health family planning clinics in the US can significantly influence attitudes toward and use of spermicidal products for HIV/STD protection. The frequency and duration of actual product use were not reported, however.

4.7 Research Needs

More information is needed on the biologic mechanism of HIV transmission to women. First, determining whether HIV transmission involves cell-associated virus in the semen, cell-free virus, or both is important in developing effective antimicrobial agents. Second, understanding the precise cells, tissues and location within the reproductive tract that are infected during transmission would be very helpful in the development of agents that block transmission. Additionally; a better understanding of vaginal ecology is needed as any substance introduced vaginally is likely to disrupt the normal vaginal flora, pH, and immune functioning and may inadvertently increase HIV risk. In the clinical domain, randomized controlled trials of promising agents are urgently needed to definitively determine which products are efficacious in human use. Estimating the acceptability of and demand for microbicides is difficult without an efficacious product available. Studies in which women are offered a variety of prevention options presented in a hierarchy of effectiveness show some uptake of microbicides, but less so than of male and female condoms. Given that women in these studies are informed that the efficacy of microbicidal products is unknown, it is not surprising that there is less uptake than of products with demonstrated efficacy. Because efficacy is an important factor in willingness to accept and use a product, a true measure of a product's acceptability cannot be determined as long as efficacy is unknown. However, studies on the characteristics that could make microbicidal candidates completely unacceptable and result in outright rejection regardless of efficacy (e.g., the amount of lubrication they provide during sex may be completely unacceptable in cultures where dry sex is preferred) should be conducted before extensive time and resources are invested in products for which there could be little or no market.

Should an efficacious microbicidal product be found, it remains to be seen whether it will fill a unique public health need; that is whether it will be a more acceptable prevention alternative than male or female condoms to women unable or unwilling to use condoms. Alternatively, will most up-take be among women already using HIV prevention methods? Research on these issues could offer valuable information about the characteristics and size of the market for microbicidal products. An additional issue that is likely to arise if an efficacious vaginal microbicidal product is found is the use of the product for other purposes, such as rectal use among heterosexuals and men who have sex with men. Given the differences in rectal and vaginal tissue, it cannot be assumed that a product that is safe and efficacious for vaginal use will be appropriate for rectal use. Studying the safety of microbicides for rectal use has only begun to receive attention, but will certainly be an important area for future research.

5. ETHICAL AND METHODOLOGIC ISSUES IN THE EVALUATION OF NEW HIV PREVENTION METHODS

A number of ethical and methodological issues arise when evaluating the efficacy or acceptability of new HIV prevention methods. Most researchers have ascribed to the belief that in studies of new prevention methods with unknown efficacy, participants must be offered the most appropriate currently established intervention (Council for International Organizations of Medical Sciences, 1991). Because there is an effective HIV prevention method available, the male condom, women participating in microbicide studies have been offered and encouraged to have their partners use male condoms when possible. Two prevention messages have been used to offer women both the male condom and the new prevention method being evaluated: the dual- use message and the hierarchical message. The dual-use message instructs women to use both the male condom and the new method (e.g., spermicide) each and every time they have sex. The hierarchical message instructs women to have her partner use the male condom; but if he does not, to use the new product as a back up. The hierarchical message is intended to increase the number of protected sex acts by offering women an option for times when a male condom cannot be used, thereby increasing the overall HIV protection for women. Both approaches create scientific and ethical dilemmas. First, male condom use may be so prevalent in these studies that it is difficult to evaluate the efficacy or acceptability of the new product alone. In efficacy studies, high levels of condom use result in a small proportion of sex acts protected by the new product alone, and only these acts contribute to determining its efficacy. Condom use essentially blunts the ability to assess the protective effect of the prevention method under evaluation. Even in populations with a high incidence of HIV, the incremental effect of the new product must be large and there must be a sufficient number of sex-acts protected by the new product alone to assess its efficacy. In the Roddy study of sex workers in Cameroon (1998), 90% of sex acts were reportedly protected by a male condom. Under these circumstances, it was extremely difficult to determine if the new product, NB9, was efficacious at reducing HIV/STD acquisition. At least one researcher has suggested that offering male condoms to research participants precludes an ability to evaluate new prevention methods (Potts, 2000). To circumvent this issue, he suggests an equivalency model of efficacy testing for new prevention methods (i.e., testing the new product for equivalent efficacy to the old product, male condoms). Other researchers adamantly disagree with this position, and argue that not offering persons at high risk for HIV the choice of using an effective prevention method is highly unethical (de Zoysa, Elias, & Bentley, 1998). These researchers argue that studies must have a sufficient number of participants to test the effect of a new HIV prevention method above and beyond that offered by male condoms. Another potential ethical and methodological dilemma generated by the hierarchical message is that of Acondom substitution or migration. Condom substitution occurs when persons who are using the male condom substitute a less effective method or when persons who may uptake the male condom if offered a behavioral intervention do not attempt its use and go instead to the less effective, but more easily implemented, method. The issue of condom migration or substitution has been investigated in several studies. Farr et al. (1994) randomly assigned women to receive either a male condom HIV prevention message or a hierarchical message in which they were told to use a male condom when they could, but to use a sperimicidal product when they could not use the male condom. Although the number of sex acts protected by any method was greater in the hierarchical condition, the uptake of male condoms was lower than in the group receiving only the male condom intervention. Fontanet and colleagues (1998) found similar results when women in one group were offered the male condom only and women in another group were offered the male or female condom; the number of acts protected by a male condom was lower in the hierarchical condition than in the condom only condition, but the overall number of protected sex acts was greater. In a study of behavioral intentions to use various barrier methods, women read a brochure on HIV prevention that contained either a condom only prevention message or a three level hierarchical message: use a male condom; if you can't use a male condom, use a female condom; if you can't use a female condom, use spermicide (Miller, Murphy, Clark, & Moore, 2001). Women read a description of the product, information about the efficacy of each product as an HIV prevention method, and procedures for its use. The researchers then measured the perceived efficacy of each method and women's intention to use the product. Women given the hierarchical message rated the male condom as less effective and indicated less intention to use it than did women receiving the male condom only message. Taken together these results suggest that the hierarchical message increases overall number of protected sex acts but may undermine attitudes, intentions, and behaviors related to the male condom.

When considering the impact a new prevention method could have on curtailing the HIV epidemic, the loss to condom substitution must be taken into account. The loss of male condom use through substitution must be offset by the efficacy and frequency of use of the new product. Modeling studies that have taken condom migration into account suggest that an HIV prevention method that is less effective than a male condom could nonetheless have a beneficial impact on HIV transmission with sufficient uptake (Watts, Thompson, & Heise, 1998), however, close attention should be paid to the efficacy of the new product that is needed to offset condom use. Recently, an alternative model for offering women multiple HIV prevention options was tested with women in Harare, Zimbabwe. In this two-phase study, women were first enrolled in a male condom intervention. Women who became consistent condom users (>75% of sex acts protected by a male condom) were not offered other methods of HIV prevention that were potentially less effective. Instead, male condom use was reinforced, and women were followed to determine if use continued over time. Women who did not achieve consistent condom use were enrolled in the second phase of the study during which they were offered alternative HIV prevention methods (i.e., the female condom and a spermicidal product) and were followed to determine patterns of use for all three products. The new model was designed to eliminate some of the problems generated by the dual- use and hierarchical messages. Using the two-phase model, good condom users were eliminated from the second phase of the study in which women were offered new prevention methods. Their elimination may help reduce blunting of the effect of the new product caused by consistent condom use. Second, because good condom users were eliminated from the second phase of the study and therefore not offered alternative prevention methods, condom migration to less effective products may be reduced. Evaluation of this two-phase model as a method for testing new prevention methods is currently underway.

6. SUMMARY

Many researchers and women's advocates have viewed female-controlled prevention methods as essential for stemming the HIV epidemic among women. The search for an acceptable, efficacious female-controlled HIV prevention method has not met with immediate success, however. The methods evaluated thus far have either not been efficacious (N-9 spermicidal agents) or have not met with wide acceptance (female condom). To understand the issues involved in developing an efficacious, acceptable product for women, additional biologic, clinical, behavioral, and ethical research is essential. Only through additional studies can we hope to find a method that will have a pervasive and sustained effect on the HIV epidemic in women.

REFERENCES

Allen, S., Serufilira, A., Bogaerts, J., Van de Perre, P., Nsengumuremyi, F., Lindan, C., Carael, M., Wolf, W., Coates, T., & Hulley, S. (1992). Confidential HIV Testing and Condom Promotion in Africa: Impact on HIV and gonorrhea rates. *JAMA*, 268, 333843.

Allen, S., Tice, J., Van de Perre, P., Serufilira, A., Hudes, E., Nsengumuremyi, F., Bogaerts, J., Lindan, C., & Hulley, S. (1992). Effect of serotesting with counseling on condom use and seroconversion among HIV discordant couples in Africa. *British Medical Journal*, 304, 1605-09.

Alliance for Microbicide Development (2000, November). Microbicide product development: Research overview. Author.

Artz, L., Macaluso, M., Brill, I., Kelaghan, J., Harland, A., Fleenor, M., Robey, L., & Hook, E. W. (2000). Effectiveness of an intervention promoting the female condom to patients at sexually transmitted disease clinics. *American Journal of Public Health*, 90, 237-244.

Asamoah-Adu, A., Weirs, S., Pappoe, M., Kaulisi, N., Neequaye, A., & Lamptey, P. (1994). Evaluation of a targeted AIDS prevention intervention to increase condom use among prostitutes in Ghana. *AIDS*, 8, 239-246.

Ashery, R. S., Carson, R. G., Falck, R. S., Siegal, H. A., & Wang, J. (1995). Female condom use among injection drug- and crack cocaine-using women. *American Journal of Public Health*, 85, 736-737.

Bernstein, G.S., Clark, V., Coulson, A.H., Frezieres, R.G., Kilzet, L. Moyer, D., Nakamura, R.M., & Walsh, T. (1986, July). Use effectiveness of cervical caps. Final report. (Contract No. 1-HD-1-2804). Washington DC: National Institute of Child Health and Human Development.

Bhave, G., Lindan, C., P., Hudes, E., S., Desai, S., Wagle, U., Tripathi, S.P., & Mandel, J.S. (1995). Impact of an intervention on HIV, sexually transmitted diseases, and condom use among commercial sex workers in Bombay, India. *AIDS*, 9 (suppl 1), S21-S30.

Bird, J.A. (1991). The use of spermicide containing nonoxynol-9 in the prevention of HIV infection. *AIDS*, 5, 791-796.

Bounds, W. Guillebaud, J., Stewart, L., & Newman, G. B. (1992). Female condom (Femidom). A clinical study of its use-effectiveness and patient acceptability. *British Journal of Family Planning*, 18, 36-41.

Bounds, W., Guillebaud, J., Stewart, L., & Steele, S. (1988). Female condom (Femshield): A study of its user-acceptability. *British Journal of Family Planning*, 14, 83-87.

Cabral, R.J., Pulley, L., Artz, L., Johnson, C., Stephens, R., & Macaluso, M. (1999). Women at risk of HIV/STD: Who is receptive to using the female condom? *Journal of Sex Education and Therapy*, 24, 89-98.

Carey, R., F., Herman, W., A., Retta, S., M., Rinaldi, J., E., Herman B., A., & Athey, T., W. (1992). Effectiveness of latex condoms as a barrier to human immunodeficiency virus-sized particles under conditions of simulated use. *Sexually Transmitted Diseases*, 19, 230-4.

Cates, W., & Raymond, E. G. (1999). Vaginal Spermicides. In Hatcher, R., Trussell, J., Stewart, F., Cates, W., Stewart, G., Guest, F., Kowal, D.(Eds.), Contraceptive Technologies (pp. 357-369). New York: Ardent Media, Inc.

Cates, W., & Stone, K., M. (1992). Family Planning, sexually transmitted disease, and contraceptive choice: a literature update. *Family Planning Perspectives*, 24, 75-84.

Cecil, H., Perry, M.J., Seal, D.W., & Pinkerton, S.D. (1998). The female condom: What we have learned thus far. *AIDS and Behavior*, 2, 241-256.

Centers for Disease Control and Prevention (1993). Update: Barrier protection against HIV infection and other sexually transmitted diseases. *MMWR*, 42, 589-591,597.

Centers for Disease Control and Prevention (1997). Update: Trends in AIDS incidence B United States, 1996. *MMWR*, 46, 861-867.

Centers for Disease Control and Prevention. (1999). HIV/AIDS Surveillance Report, Vol 11 (No. 2). Atlanta, GA: Author.

Coggins, C., Blanchard, K., Alvarez, F., Brache, V., Weisberg, E., Kilmarx,P.H., Lacarra, M., Massai, R., Mishell, D., Salvatierra, A., Witwatwongwana, P., Elias, C., & Ellertson, C. (2000, March). Safety and acceptability of Lambda-Carrageenan-containing vaginal microbicide gel PC-503. Paper presented at the Microbicide 2000 meeting, Washington, DC.

Cohen, D., Reardon, K., Alleyne, D., Murthy, S., & Linton, K. (1995). Influencing spermicide use among low-income minority women. *Journal of the American Medical Women's Association*, 50, 11-13.

Council for International Organizations of Medical Sciences (1991). International guidelines for ethical review of epidemiological studies. Geneva, Switzerland. Author.Cramer, D. W., Goldman, M.B., Schiff, I., Belisle, S. Albrecht, B., Stadel, B., Gibson, M., Wison, E., Stillman, R., T., & Thompson, I. (1987). The relationship of tubal infertility to barrier method and oral contraceptive use. *Journal of the American Medical Association*, 257, 2446-2450.

de Vincenzi, I., for the European Study Group on Heterosexual transmission of HIV (1994). A longitudinal study of human immunodeficiency virus transmission by heterosexual partners *The New England Journal of Medicine*, 331, 341-346.

de Zoysa, I., Elias, C.J., & Bentley, M.E. (1998). Ethical challenges in efficacy trials of vaginal microbicides for HIV prevention. *American Journal of Public Health*, 88, 571-575.

Diaz, T., Chu, S.Y., Conti, L., Sorvillo, F., Checko, P.J., Hermann, P., Fann, S.A., Frederick, M., Boyd, D., Mokotoff, E., Rietmeijer, C.A., Herr, M., & Samuel, M.C. (1994). Risk behaviors of persons with heterosexually acquired HIV infection in the United States: Results of a multistate surveillance project. *Journal of Acquired Immune Deficiency Syndromes*, 7, 958-963.

DiClemente, R., J., & Wingood, G., M., (1995). A randomized controlled trial of a community based HIV sexual risk reduction intervention for young adult African-American females. *Journal of the American Medical Association*, 274, 1271-1276.

D'Oro, L.C., Parazzini, F. Naldi, L., & LaVecchia, C. (1994). Barrier methods of contraception, spermicides, and sexually transmitted diseases: A review. *Genitourinary Medicine*, 70, 410-417.

Drew, W., L., Blair, M., Miner, R., C, & Conant, M. (1990). Evaluation of the virus permeability of a new condom for women. *Sexually Transmitted Diseases*, 17, 110-112.

Edelman, D.A., McIntyre, D. L., & Harper, J.A. (1984). A comparative trial of the Today contraceptive sponge and diaphragm. *American Journal of Obstetrics and Gynecology*, 150, 869-876.

Ehrhardt, A. A., Yingling, S., Zawadzki, R., & Martinez-Ramirez, M. (1992). Prevention of heterosexual transmission of HIV: Barriers for women. *Women and Health*, 23, 73-89.

Eldridge, G.D., St. Lawrence, J.S., Little, C. E., Shelby, M.C., & Brasfield, T.L. (1995). Barriers to condom use and barrier method preference among low-income African-American women. Women and Health, 23, 73-89.Elias, C., & Coggins, C. (1996). Female controlled methods to prevent sexual transmission of HIV. *AIDS*, 10, S43-51.

Elias, C., & Heise, L. (1994). Challenges for the development of female-controlled methods to prevent sexual transmission of HIV. *AIDS*, 8, 1-9.

Farr, G., Gabelnick, H., Sturgen, K., & Dorflinger, L. (1994). Contraceptive efficacy and acceptability of the female condom. *American Journal of Public Health*, 84, 1960-64.

Feldblum, P.J. & Weir, S.S. (1994). The protective effect of nonoxynol-9 against HIV infection [Letter]. *American Journal of Public Health*, 84, 1032-1034.

Fontanet, A., Saba, J., Chandelying, V., Sakondhavat, C., Bhiraleus, P., Rugpao, S., Chongsomchai, C, Kiriwat, O, Tovanabutra, S., Dally, L., Lange, J., Rojanapithayakorn, W. (1998). Protection against sexually transmitted diseases by granting sex workers in Thailand the choice of using the male or female condom: results from a randomized controlled trial. *AIDS*, 12, 1851-1859.

Ford, N., and Mathie, E. (1993). The acceptability and experience of the female condom, Femidom, among family planning clinic attenders. *British Journal of Family Planning*, 19, 187-192.

Gil, V.E., (1995). The new female condom: Attitudes and opinions of low income Puerto Rican women at risk for HIV/AIDS. *Qualitative Health Research*, 5, 178-203.

Gollub, E.L., French, P., Loundou, A., Latka, M., Rogers, C., & Stein, Z. (2000). A randomized trial of hierarchical counseling in a short, clinic-based intervention to reduce the risk of sexually transmitted diseases in women. *AIDS*, 14, 1249-1255.

Gollub, E.L., Stein, Z., and El-Sadr, W. (1995). Short-term acceptability of the female condom among staff and patients at a New York City hospital. *Family Planning Perspectives*, 27, 155-158.

Grinstead, J.A., Faigeles, B., Binson, D., & Eversley, R. (1993). Sexual risk for human immunodeficiency virus infection among women in high-risk cities. *Family Planning Perspectives*, 25, 252-256,277.

Grosskurth, H., Mosha, F., Todd, J., Mwijarubi, E., Klokke, A., Senkoro, K., Mayaud, P., Changalucha, J., Nicoll, A., ka-Gina, G., Newell, J., Mugeye, K., Mabey, D., & Hayes, R. (1995). Impact of improved treatment of sexually transmitted diseases on HIV infection in rural Tanzania: randomized control trial. *Lancet*, 346, 530-536.

Hammett, T., Norton, G., Mason, T., Mayer, K., Robles, R., Feudo, R., & Seage, G. (2000, March). Drug-involved women's user perspective on microbicides. Paper presented at the Microbicides 2000 meeting, Washington, DC.

Haney, D. (1996, May 20). Associated Press News Release.

Hooton, T.M., Hillier, S., Johnson, C., Roberts, P.L., & Stamm, W.E., (1991). Esherchia coli bacteriuria and contraceptive method. *Journal of the American Medical Association*, 245, 64-69

Howe, J.E., Minkoff, H.L., & Duerr, A. C. (1994). Contraceptives and HIV. *AIDS*, 8, 861-871.

Jivasak-Apimas, S. (1991). Acceptability of the vaginal sheath (Femshield) in Thai couples. *Contraception*, 44, 183-190.

Joint United Nations Programme on HIV/AIDS [UNAIDS] (1998, June). Report on Global HIV/AIDS Epidemic. Geneva, Switzerland: Author.

Joint United Nations Programme on HIV/AIDS [UNAIDS] (1998, December). *AIDS* Epidemic Update. Geneva, Switzerland: Author.

Judson, F.N., Ehret, J.M., Bodin, G.F., Levin, M. J., & Reitmeijer, A.M. (1989). In vitro evaluations of condoms with and without nonoxynol-9 as physical and chemical barriers against Chlamydia trachomatis , herpes simplex virus 2 and human immunodeficiency virus. *Sexually Transmitted Diseases*, 16, 51-56.

Kalichman, S.C., Williams, E., & Nachimson, D. (1999). Brief behavioural skills building intervention for female controlled methods of STD-HIV prevention: outcomes of a randomized clinical field trial. *International Journal of STD and AIDS*, 10, 174-181.

Kamb, M.L., Fishbein, M., Douglas, J.M., Rhodes, F., Rogers, J., Bolan, G., Zenilman, J., Hoxworth, T., Malotte, K., Iatesta, M., Kent, C., Lentz, A., Graziano, S., Byers, R.H., & Peterman, T.A., for the Project RESPECT Study Group. (1998). Efficacy of risk-reduction counseling to prevent human immunodeficiency virus and sexually transmitted diseases: a randomized control trial. *Journal of the American Medical Association*, 280, 1161-7.

Kamenga, M., Ryder, R.W., Jingu, M., Mbuyi, N., Mbu, L., Behets, F., Brown, C., & Heyward WL. (1991). Evidence of marked sexual behavior change associated with low HIV-1 seroconversion in 149 married couples with discordant HIV-1 serostatus: experience at an HIV counselling center in Zaire. *AIDS*, 5, 61-67.

Kelaghan, J., Rubin, G.L., Ory, H.W., & Layde, P. M. (1982). Barrier-method contraceptives and pelvic inflammatory disease. *Journal of the American Medical Association*, 248, 185.

Kelly, J., A., Murphy, D., A., Washington, C., D., Wilson, T., S., Koob, J., J., Davis, D., R., Ledezma, G., & Davantes, B. (1994). The effects of HIV/AIDS intervention groups for high-risk women in urban clinics. *American Journal of Public Health*, 84, 1918-1922.

Klebanoff, S. J., Hillier, S.L., Eschenbach, D.S., & Waltersdorph, S.M. (1991). Control of the microbial flora of the vagina by H2O2-generating lactobacilli. *Journal of Infectious Diseases*, 164, 94-100.

Klein, H., Eber, M., Crosby, H., Welka, D.A., & Hoffman, J.A. (1999). The acceptability of the female condom among substance-using women in Washington, DC. *Women and Health*, 29, 97-114.

Kost, K., & Forrest, J. (1992). American women's sexual behavior & exposure to risk of sexually transmitted diseases. *Family Planning Perspectives*, 24, 244-254.

Kreiss, J., Ngugi, E., Holmes, K., NdinyaAchola, J., Waiyaki, P., Roberts, P.L., Ruminjo, I., Sajabi, R., Kimata, J., Fleming, T.R., Anzala, A., Holton, D., & Plummer, F. (1992). Efficacy of nonoxynol-9 contraceptive sponge use in preventing heterosexual acquisition of HIV in Nairobi prostitutes. *Journal of the American Medical Association*, 268, 477-482.

Laga, M., Alary, M., Nzila, N., Manoka, A.T., Tuliza, M., Behets, F., Goeman, J., St Louis, M., & Piot, P. (1994). Condom promotion, sexually transmitted diseases treatment, and declining incidence of HIV-1 infection in female Zairian sex workers. *Lancet*, 344, 246-248.

Laga, M., Manoka, A., Kivuvu, M., Malele, B., Tuliza, M., Nzila, N., Goeman, J., Behets, F., Batter, V., Alary, M., Heyward, W.L., Ryder, R.W., & Piot, P. (1993). Non-ulcerative STD as risk factors for HIV infection in women: Results from a cohort study. *AIDS*. 7, 95-102.

Latka., M., Gollub, E., French, P., Stein, Z. (2000). Male and female condom use among women after counseling in a risk reduction hierarchy for STD prevention. *Sexually Transmitted Diseases*, 27, 431-437.

Leeper, M. A., & Conrady, M. (1989). Preliminary evaluationof REALITY, a condom for women to wear. *Advances in Contraception*, 5, 229-235.

Louv, W.C., Austin, H., Alexander, W.J., Stagno, S., & Cheeks, J.A. (1988). A clinical trial of nonoxynol-9 for preventing gonococcal and chlamydial infections. *Journal of Infectious Diseases*, 158, 518-523.

Madrigal, J., Schifter, J., & Feldblum, P.J. (1998). Female condom acceptability among sex workers in Costa Rica. *AIDS Education and Prevention*, 10, 105-113.

Malkovsky, M., Newell, A., & Dalgleish, A.G. (1988). Inactivation of HIV by nonoxynol-9. *Lancet*, 1, 645.

Martin, H.L., Stevens, C.E., Richardson, B.A., Rugamba, D., Nyange, P.M., Mandaliya, K., Ndinya-Achola, J., & Kreis, J.K. (1997). Safety of a nonoxynol-9 vaginal gel in Kenyan prostitutes. *Sexually Transmitted Diseases*, 24, 279-283.

Miller, C.J., Alexander, N.J., Gettie, A., Hendrickx, A.G., & Marx, P.A. (1992). The effect of contraceptives containing nonoxynol-9 on the genital transmission of simian immunodeficiency virus in rhesus macaques. *Fertility and Sterility*, 57, 1126-1128.

Miller, C.J., Alexander, N.J., Sutjipto, S., Joye, S.M., Hendrickx, A.G., Jennings, M., & Marx, P.A. (1990). Effect of virus dose and Nonoxynol-9 on the genital transmission of ZIV in rhesus macaques. *Journal of Medical Primatology*, 19, 401-409.

Miller, C., Alexander, N.J., Vogel, P., Anderson, J., & Marx, P.A.. (1992). Mechanisms of genital transmission of ZIV: A hypothesis based on transmission studies and the location of ZIV in the genital tract of chronically infected females. *Journal of Medical Primatology*, 21, 64-68.

Miller, L.C., Murphy, S.T., Clark, L.F., & Moore, J. (2001). Hierarchical messages for introducing multiple HIV prevention options: Promise and pitfalls. Unpublised manuscript.

Moon, M.W., Mbizvo, M.T., Heiman, J.E., Chirenje, Z.M., Khumalo-Sakutukwa, G., Mwale, M., Nyamapfeni, P., & Padian, N. (2000). Evaluation of the feasibility and acceptability of vaginal microbicides for the prevention of HIV/STI in Zimbabwe. *National Academies of Practive Forum*, 2, 135-139.

Murphy, S. T., Miller, C. L., Moore, J., & Clark, L.F. (2000). Preaching to the choir: Preference for female-controlled methods of HIV and Sexually Transmitted Disease Prevention. *American Journal of Public Health*, 90, 1135-1137

Musabe, E., Morrison, C.S., Sunkutu, M.R., & Wong, E. L. (1998). Long-term use of the female condom among couples at high risk of human immunodeficiency virus infection in Zambia. *Sexually Transmitted Diseases*, 25, 1-5.

National Center for Health Statistics. (1997). HealthBUnited States 1996-1997 and Injury Chartbook. (DHHS Publication No. PHS 97-1232). Hyattsville, MD: Superintendent of Documents.

Nelson, K.E., Celentano, D.D., Eiumtrakol, S., Hoover, D.R., Beyrer, C., Suprasert, S., Kuntolbutra, S., & Khamboonruang, C. (1996). Changes in sexual behavior and a decline in HIV infection among young men in Thailand. *New England Journal of Medicine*, 335, 297-303.

Niruthisard, S., Roddy, R.E., & Chutivongse, S. (1991). The effects of frequent nonoxynol9 use on the vaginal and cervical mucosa. *Sexually Transmitted Diseases*, 18, 1769.

Niruthisard, S., Roddy, R.E., & Chutivongse, S. (1992). Use of nonoxynol-9 and reduction in rate of gonococcal and chlamydial infections. *Lancet*, 339, 1371-1375.

O'Leary, A., & Wingood, G. (1999). Interventions for sexually active heterosexual women. In J.L. Peterson & R.J. DiClemente (Eds), Handbook of HIV Prevention. New York: Plenum.

Ongradi, J., Ceccherini-Nelli, L., Pistell, M., Spector, S., and Bendinelli, M. (1990). Acid sensitivity of cell-free and cell-associated HIV-1: clinical implications. *AIDS Research and Human Retroviruses*, 6, 1433-1436.

Padian, N.S., O'Brien, T.R., Chang, Y., Glass, S., & Francis, D.P. (1993). Prevention of heterosexual transmission of human immunodeficiency virus through couple counseling. *Journal of Acquired Immune Deficiency Syndromes*, 6, 1043-1048.

Pauwels, R., & De Clercq, E. (1996). Development of vaginal microbicides for the prevention of heterosexual transmission of HIV. *Journal of Acquired Immune Deficiency Syndromes and Human Retrovirology*, 11, 211-221.

Pool, R., Whitworth, J., Green, G., Mbonye, A., Harrison, S., Hart, G., & Wilkinson, J. (2000, March). Ambiguity, sexual pleasure, and the acceptability of microbicidal products in southwest Uganda. Paper presented at the Microbicides 2000 meeting, Washington, DC.

Potts, M. (2000). Thinking about vaginal microbicide testing. *American Journal of Public Health*, 90, 188-190.Profy, A., Sonderfan, A., Chancellor, T., & McKinlay, M. (2000, March). PRO 2000 gel: A candidate topical microbicide based on a naphthalene sulfonate polymer with antimicrobial and contraceptive properties. Paper presented at the Microbicides 2000 meeting, Washington, DC.

Ramjee, G., Meyer, L., Andrews, A., & Gouws, E. (2000, March) Acceptability of a vaginal microbicide among South African men. Paper presented at the Microbicides 2000 meeting, Washington, DC.

Ray, S., Bassett, M., Maposhere, C., Manangazira, P., Nicolette, J.D., Machekano, R., & Moyo, J. (1995). Acceptability of the female condom in Zimbabwe: Positive but male-centered responses. *Reproductive Health Matters*, 5, 68-79.

Roddy, R.E., Cordero, M., Cordero, C., & Fortney, J.A. (1993). A dosing study of nonoxynol-9 and genital irritation. *International Journal of STD and AIDS*, 4, 165-170.

Roddy, R.E., Zekeng, L., Ryan, K.A., Ubalk, M., Weir, S. S., and Wong, E.L. (1998). A controlled trial of nonoxynol-9 film to reduce male-to-female transmission of sexual transmitted diseases. *The New England Journal of Medicine*, 339, 504-510.

Rosenberg, M.J., & Gollub, E.L. (1992). Commentary: methods women can use that may prevent sexually transmitted disease, including HIV. *American Journal of Public Health*, 82, 1473-1478.

Rosenberg, M.J., Rojanapithayakorn,W., Feldblum, P.J., and Higgins, J.E. (1987). Effect of the contraceptive sponge on chlamydial infection, gonorrhea, and candidiasis: a comparative clinical trial. *Journal of the American Medical Association*, 257, 2308-2312.

Ruminjo, J.K., Steiner, M., Joanis, C., Mwathe, E.G., & Thagana, N. (1996). Preliminary comparison of the polyurethane female condom with the latex male condom in Kenya. *East African Medical Journal*, 73, 101-106.

Rustomjee, R., Abdool Karim, Q.A., Abdool Karim, S., Laga, M., & Stein, Z. (1999). Phase 1 trial of nonoxynol-9 film among sex workers in South Africa. AIDS, 13, 1511-1515.

Sakondhavat, C. (1990). The female condom [Letter]. *American Journal of Public Health*, 80, 498.

Sakondhavat, C., & Potter, L. (1990). Further testing of female condoms [Letter]. *British Journal of Family Planning*, 15, 129-130.

Saracco A., Musicco M., Nicolosi A., Angarano, G., Arici, C., Gavazzeni, G., Costigliola, P., Gafa, S., Gervasoni, C., Luzzati, R., Piccinino, F., Puppo, F., Salassa, B., Sinicco, A., Stellini, R., Tirelli, U., Turbessi, G., Vigevani, G.M., Visco, G., Zerboni, R., & Lazzarin, A. (1993). Man-to-woman sexual transmission of HIV; longitudinal study of 343 steady partners of infected men. *Journal of Acquired Immune Deficiency Syndrome*, 6, 497-502.

Scarlett, M., Macaluso, M., & Duerr (1997, May). Acceptability of microbicides among women attending a sexually transmitted disease clinic in Alabama [Abstract]. National Conference on Women and HIV (Abstract No. P1.13).

Shervington, D.O. (1993). The acceptability of the female condom among low-income African-American women. *Journal of the National Medical Association*, 85, 341-347.

Sikkema, K.,J., Heckman, T.,G., Kelly, J., A., Anderson, E.S., Winett, R.A., Solomon, L.J., Wagstaff, D.A., Roffman, R.A., Perry, M.J., Cargill, V., Crumble, D.A., Fuqua, R.W., Norman, A.D., & Mercer, M.B. (1995). HIV risk behaviors among women living in low-income, inner city housing developments. *American Journal of Public Health*. 86, 1123-1128.

Sinpisut, P., Chandeying, V. Skov, S., and Uahgowitchai, C. (1998). Perceptions and acceptability of the female condom [Femidom] amongst commercial sex worker in the Songkla province, Thailand. *Internation Journal of STD & AIDS*, 9, 168-172.

Sly, D. F., Quadagno, D., Harrison, D. F., Eberstein, I.W., Riehman, K., & Bailey, M. (1997). Factors associated with the use of the female condom. *Family Planning Perspectives*, 29, 181-184.

Soper, D.E., Brockwell, N.J., & Dalton, H.P. (1991). Evaluation of the effects of a female condom on the female lower genital tract. *Contraception*, 44, 21-29.

Soper, D.E., Shoupe, D., Shangold, G., A., Shangold, M.M., Gutmann, J., & Mercer, L. (1993). Prevention of vaginal trichomoniasis by compliant use of the female condom. *Sexually Transmitted Diseases*, 20, 137-139.

Srirak, N., Sirirojn, B., Wichajarn, M., Rugpao, S., Nelson, K., Celentano, D.D., & Khamboonruang, C. (2000, March). Acceptability of Thai males toward Buffergel as a vaginal microbicide in Chiang Mai, Thailand. Paper presented at the Microbicides 2000 meeting, Washington, DC.

Stein, Z.A. (1990). HIV prevention: the need for methods women can use. *American Journal of Public Health*, 80, 460-462.

Stein, Z., Saez, H., El-Sadr, W., Healton, C., Mannheimer, S., Messeri, P., Scimeca, M.M., Van Devanter, N., Zimmerman, R., & Betne, P. (1999). Safer sex strategies for women: the hierarchical model in methadone treatment clinics. *Journal of Urban Health*, 78, 62-72.

Stewart, F. (1998). Vaginal Barriers. In R. Hatcher, J. Trussell, F. Stewart, W. Cates, G. Stewart, F. Guest, & D. Kowal (Eds.), *Contraceptive Technologies* (pp. 371-404). New York: Ardent Media, Inc.

Stone, A., & Hitchcock, P. (1994). Vaginal microbicides for preventing the sexual transmission of HIV. *AIDS*, 8, S285-293.

The Population Council & International Family Health (2000). The case for microbicides: A global priority. New York: Author.

The Voluntary HIV-1 Counseling and Testing Efficacy Study Group (2000). Efficacy of Voluntary HIV-1 counseling and testing individuals and couples in Kenya, Tanzania and Trinidad: a randomised trial. *The Lancet*, 356, 103-112.

Trussell, J., Strickler, J., & Vaughan, B. (1993). Contraceptive efficacy of the diaphragm, sponge and cervical cap. Family Planning Perspectives, 26, 66-72.

Trussell, J., Sturgen, K., Strickler, J., & Dominik, R. (1994). Comparative Contraceptive Efficacy of The Female Condom and Other Barrier Methods. *Family Planning Perspectives*, 26, 66-72.

Van Damme, L. (2000, July). Advances in topical microbicides. Plenary presented at the 13th International Conference on AIDS. Durban, South Africa.

Van Damme, L., Niruthisard, S., Atisook, R., Boer, K, Dally, L., Laga, M., Lange, J., Karam, M., & Perriens, J.H. (1998). Safety evaluation of nonoxynol-9 gel in women at low risk of HIV infection. *AIDS*, 12, 433-437.

van de Wijgert, J., Nelson, K., Fullem, A., Kumwenda, N., Mehendale, S., Rugpao, S., Joglekar, N., Taha, T., Bollinger, R., Padian, N., Heagerty, P., Kelly, C., & Rosenberg, Z. (2000, March). Safety results of a multi-site international Phase I trial of the topical microbicide Buffergel. Paper presented at the Microbicides 2000 meeting, Washington, DC.

Visness, C.M., Ulin, P., Pfannenschmidt, S., & Zekeng, L. (1998). Views of Cameroonian sex workers on a woman-controlled method of contraception and disease protection. *International Journal of STD & AIDS*, 9, 695-699.

Voeller, B., Coulter, S.L., & Mayhan, K.G., (1991). Gas, dye, and viral transport through polyurethane condoms [Letter to the Editor]. *Jounal of the American Medical Association*, 266, 2986-2987.

Walker, C. K., Hitti, J., Nsubuga, P. S. J., Sembajwe, V., Katende, S., & Mbidde, E. D. (1993, June). Condom use among STD patients in Uganda [Abstract]. Ninth International Conference on AIDS (Abstract No. WS-C14-2).

Wasserheit, J.N. (1992). Epidemiological synergy: interrelationships between HIV infection and other STDs. In L. Chen, J. Sepulveda, & S. Segal, (Eds.), AIDS and Women's Health: Science for Policy and Action (pp. 42-72). New York: Plenum Press.

Watts, C., Thompson, W., & Heise, L. (1998). The effectiveness of microbicides for HIV prevention. [Meeting Abstract]. International Conference on AIDS, (Abstract No. 33161).

Wawer, M.J., Gray, R.H., Sewankambo, N.K., Serwadda, D., Paxton, L., Berkley, S., McNairn, D., Wabwire-Mangen, F., Li C., Nalugoda, F., Kiwankua, N., Lutalo, T.,

Brookmeyer, R., Kelly, R., & Quinn, T.C. (1998). A randomized community trial of intensive sexually transmitted disease control for AIDS prevention, Rakai, Uganda. *AIDS*, 12, 1211-1225.

Weir, S. W., Feldblum, P.J., Zekeng, L., & Roddy, R. (1994). The use of nonoxynol-9 for protection against cervical gonorrhea. *American Journal of Public Health*, 84, 910-914.

Weller, S., C. (1993). A meta analysis of condom effectiveness in reducing sexually transmitted HIV. *Social Science & Medicine*, 36, 1635-44.

Witte, S. S., el-Bassel, N, Wada, T., Gray, O., & Wallace, J. (1999). Acceptability of female condom use among women exchanging street sex in New York City. *International Journal of STD & AIDS*, 10, 162-168.

Xu, J. X., Leeper, M.A., Wu, Y., Zhou, X.B., Xu, S.Y., Chen, T., Yang, X.L., & Zhuang, L.Q. (1998). User acceptability of a female condom (Reality) in Shanghai. *Advances in Contraception*, 14, 193-199.

Young, N.L., Chaowanachan, T., Wasinrapee, P., Borchardt, K.A., Elias, C., Mastro, T.D., & Kilmarx, P.H. (2000, March). In vitro effect of microbicide PC-515 and placebo gels on gen-probe pace 2 and COBAS amplicor chlamydia trachomatis and neisseria gonorrhoeae tests, and on inpouch TV trichomonas vaginalis growth. Paper presented at the Microbicides 2000 meeting, Washington, DC.

Zekeng, L., Feldblum, P.J., Oliver, R.M., & Kaptue, L. (1993). Barrier contraceptive use and HIV infection among high-risk women in Cameroon. *AIDS*, 7, 725-731.

Chapter 4

STD Diagnosis and Treatment as an HIV Prevention Strategy

Sevgi O. Aral
Division of STD Prevention, National Center for HIV, STD and TB Prevention, Centers for Disease Control and Prevention, Atlanta Georgia

Thomas A. Peterman
Division of HIV/AIDS Prevention, National Center for HIV, STD and TB Prevention, Centers for Disease Control and Prevention, Atlanta Georgia

1. INTRODUCTION

STD control for HIV prevention is a controversial interface between well-financed HIV prevention programs and less wealthy STD prevention programs. STD experts are frustrated at the lack of HIV and other resources committed to this HIV prevention strategy. Some HIV experts are skeptical of the motivations of the proponents of this strategy, and think the potential for HIV prevention by STD control has been exaggerated. Between these two camps lies a huge mass of data accumulated by hundreds of studies conducted over the past 15 years. Synthesizing this data is particularly important for HIV prevention world wide, because the developing countries where STD control programs have been weak are often the countries where the AIDS epidemic has been most devastating.

While epidemiological and microbiological evidence support the existence of a two-way relationship between STDs and HIV infection, the relationship between early and appropriate diagnosis and treatment of STDs and prevention of spread of HIV needs to be further elaborated. The parameters that need to be specified in such elaboration include 1) factors related to the STI: the specific STI; whether the STI is symptomatic or asymptomatic; whether the STI is incident (new) infection or prevalent (chronic or long standing) infection; and perhaps the stage of the sexually transmitted infection; 2) factors related to the population, which may also function as multipliers of the STI effect: age-gender composition; patterns of sexual mixing and concurrency; prevalence of male circumcision; 3) factors related to the phases of the STD and HIV epidemics: for example, whether the HIV and STD epidemics are nascent or generalized epidemics; 4) factors related to the goals of the HIV prevention program: objectives related topreventing the acquisition of infection among the uninfected; objectives related to preventing the transmission of infection by the infected; objectives related to provision of services to protect the personal health of individual members of the population; objectives related to protecting public health, i.e., limiting the spread of HIV infections: objectives related to targeting primary prevention of HIV through behavior change versus primary prevention of HIV through control of co-factors. The appropriate approach to the implementation of STD control for HIV prevention in a specific setting depends on the values of all of the above factors. In addition, many of the above factors are interdependent, and it is important to consider their reciprocal influences.

In this chapter we critically review some of the evidence that support the reciprocal relationship between STDs and HIV infection, the so-called epidemiological synergy (Wasserheit 1992; Fleming and Wasserheit 1999). We introduce the concept of sociological synergy — the demographic, social, behavioral, attitudinal, and belief patterns that surround the dissemination of STD and HIV in a population and which exert synergistic influences on the spread of both epidemics. We discuss the significance of coinfection with both STD and HIV from the epidemiologic and the behavioral perspectives, and discuss the HIV risk to the population that is attributable to STD. Finally, we describe situations influenced by factors mentioned above, propose what may be appropriate approaches to STD control for HIV prevention in settings defined by particular combinations of these factors, and present explanations for these proposals.

Throughout the chapter we assume that STD control is a public health priority in its own right. The value of STD control per se is neither questioned nor discussed here. We focus solely on the role of STD control for HIV prevention.

2. EPIDEMIOLOGICAL SYNERGY

2.1 Impact of STD control on HIV incidence in individuals

The synergistic relationship between STD and HIV involves a two-way interaction; STD affect the acquisition and transmission of HIV while HIV influences many aspects of STD including transmission and natural history. In this chapter we focus on the role of STD in facilitating the transmission and acquisition of HIV.

Several studies exploring the biological plausibility of the observed association between HIV and other STD (Wasserheit 1992) have suggested particular biological mechanisms. HIV transmission may be enhanced by ulcerative and non-ulcerative STD which may affect both HIV infectiousness and susceptibility to HIV (Fleming and Wasserheit 1999). Other STDs increase HIV shedding in the genital tract that may promote HIV infectiousness; in addition, they recruit HIV susceptible inflammatory cells to the genital tract and disrupt mucosal barriers to infection, which may increase susceptibility to HIV. Results of studies that adjust for level of immunosuppression in data analysis or document reduced HIV shedding after STD treatment suggest that the role of STD in HIV transmission is independent of level of immunosuppression due to HIV infection. (For a detailed review of relevant studies, see Fleming and Wasserheit 1999).

Further support for STD-HIV interaction, beyond biological plausibility, can be found in studies of new HIV infections in the presence of STDs. Many of these studies followed groups of initially HIV seronegative individuals with repeated physical examinations and HIV tests to determine the temporal sequence of STD acquisition and HIV seroconversion, they also adjusted for potential confounding effects of sexual behavior, but they could not adjust for exposure to HIV. These studies yield risk estimates that range from 2.0 to 23.5, most of which fall between 2 and 5 (Fleming and Wasserheit 1999). These studies suggest that ulcerative STD increase the risk of acquiring or transmitting HIV, regardless of which partner has the ulcer. Non-ulcerative STD appears to increase HIV risk primarily for the receptive partner. However, since non-ulcerative STD is more frequent than ulcerative STD in most populations, they may account for a greater number of HIV infections globally (a detailed review of these studies can also be found in Fleming and Wasserheit 1999).

Most studies of new HIV infections in the presence of STDs are observational studies that are subject to a number of potential biases (Mertens 1990). Considering different study designs can help identify how the designs influence bias (this thought experiment should not be construed as implying a particular study should be done). In this context, the pertinent research question is: during sex with an infected partner, who is more likely to acquire HIV, a person with an STD or a person with no STD? In the least biased (but unethical) approach to answer this one would randomize persons to receive vs not receive a STD and then, while the STD is present, have sex with a randomly selected HIV-infected partner. Alternatively, one could randomize some individuals to have sex with HIV and STD infected persons (exposed) and others to have sex with HIV infected persons who do not have other STD (unexposed). We cannot tell from non-randomized studies if persons with/without STD were equally likely to have sex with an HIV-infected partner or if the STD was present at the time that they were exposed to the person with HIV. Both of these factors introduce potential bias into observational studies, and it is difficult to determine the likely directions and magnitudes of these biases. Many studies have found associations between HIV and other STDs, so persons who acquired an STD are more likely to have been exposed to HIV than persons who did not acquire an STD, but it is difficult to know if the transmission of HIV occurred when the STD was present (Figure 1).

Figure 1.

RCT			
	Exposure		Outcome in exposed
Randomize --->		---> Follow --->	
	No exposure		Outcome in unexposed
Cohort			
	Exposure		Outcome in exposed
		---> Follow --->	
	No exposure		Outcome in unexposed
Case-Control			
	Exposure		Case
		<--- Look back <---	
	No exposure		Control

Theoretical Study Design	Reality
Randomized trials would randomize some individuals to have sex with HIV-infected persons with STD (Exposed) and others to have sex with HIV-infected persons without STD (Unexposed)	Not ethical. Should not be done.
Cohort studies would not randomize, but would look at individuals who chose to have sex with HIV-infected persons with STD (Exposed) and compare them to other individuals who chose to have sex with HIV-infected persons without STD (Unexposed)	Few "cohort studies" are studies of people with known exposure to HIV. Some HIV discordant couples have been followed, but not in sufficient detail to know if they had intercourse while one partner had an STD.
Case-control studies would compare the histories of HIV-infected cases with HIV-uninfected controls. Exposure would be difficult to determine because most individuals in the study would not know if their partners had HIV or STD at the time they had sex.	Most studies are in this category. They assume uniform exposure to HIV among cases and controls, or assume they can adjust for the likelihood of exposure. They also assume any STD in the past was present during sex with the HIV-infected person.

Thought experiment considering theoretical and realistic study designs to determine the relative risk for HIV transmission from person s with versus without an STD.

Transmission of HIV is facilitated if a person with an STD is more likely to transmit HIV. A person who acquired an STD and HIV at the same time may not have detectable HIV antibody at the time the STD was diagnosed. By the time a subsequent HIV test is positive, the infected person may have had other potentially infected sex partners, so it is difficult to be certain that HIV was acquired from a person who had the STD. Moreover, in some instances where transmission was facilitated by an STD, that STD may not be transmitted.

Acquisition of HIV is facilitated if a person with an STD is more likely than a person with no STD to acquire HIV during sex with an HIV-infected partner. In this scenario, the STD and HIV are acquired at different times. This would also be difficult to detect because the time of infections would be uncertain. If the STD is symptomatic, the symptoms will be present before HIV antibodies are detectable. If the STD remains asymptomatic, it is difficult to ascertain that the STD preceded the acquisition of HIV.

One of the critical concerns in the interpretation of results from observational studies is that it is difficult to control or adjust for the potential confounding effects of sexual behavior adequately. There are at least two reasons for this. First, measurement of sexual behavior presents a multitude of problems and the variables used in adjusting for the effects of sexual behavior tend to be subject to considerable measurement error. Second, sexual behavior is multidimensional, and most studies attempt to measure only a few of these dimensions. Number of sex partners, condom use, casual/regular partners, exchange of sex for money or drugs, number of new partners, concurrency of partnerships, behavioral characteristics of partners, networkcharacteristics of respondents and their sex partners, and mixing patterns are all important correlates of STD/HIV acquisition and transmission. However, most studies of STD and/or HIV transmission attempt to measure only the first four or five of these variables. Thus, in analyses, even under the best circumstances, only some of the many dimensions of sexual behavior are adjusted for. The unmeasured dimensions of sexual behavior such as network characteristics, mixing patterns and partner characteristics may be more important than the measured dimensions, such as number of partners. Consequently it is difficult to ensure that confounding effects of sexual behavior are adequately adjusted for in analyses of data from observational studies.

Despite all these considerations of potential bias in the design of observational studies, available data suggest that, at the individual level, there is a cofactor effect of STDs for HIV transmission. The size of this cofactor effect may vary depending on other factors and is difficult to determine exactly (Plummer 1998). Nevertheless, having an STD is associated with a 2 to 5 fold increase in HIV risk at the individual level, and adequate STD diagnosis and treatment must be provided to assure the protection of individuals (Gray et al 1999). In other words, STD clinical services may be indicated in relation to an individual's health even if they are not indicated for their impact on STD or HIV transmission in the community.

These individual level studies do not provide sufficient information to estimate the potential impact of STD diagnosis and treatment on HIV spread in a population. Such impact may be influenced by a number of factors including the phase of the HIV epidemic (Wasserheit and Aral 1996), the extent of overlap between the HIV and STD epidemics, the particular STDs that are prevalent in the population, the quality of the existing STD program including its coverage and the attributable risk for STD.

2.2 Impact of STD control on HIV incidence in populations

Most information on the impact of other STDs on HIV transmission in populations is based on mathematical modelling (May and Anderson 1987; Boily and Anderson 1996; Boily 1996). This body of work suggests that the impact of STDs on HIV spread in populations may be underestimated by analytic epidemiologic methods that do not take into account the dynamic nature of spread of infectious diseases. Mathematical models indicate that

STD diagnosis and treatment is more effective in preventing HIV transmission during earlier phases of the HIV epidemic, when HIV infection is concentrated in particular subpopulations (Garnett and Anderson 1995; Over and Piot 1996; World Bank 1997; Robinson et al 1997) and that diagnosis and treatment of STDs among individuals who are most likely to transmit HIV infection to uninfected persons is more effective (as well as cost effective) than providing STD care to other members of the population (World Bank 1997; Koopman 1998).

Several cohort studies of commercial sex workers have shown that provision of STD clinical care combined with condom promotion may lead to reductions in HIV incidence in these populations. However, these studies have not measured HIV incidence in the larger population. Only two studies have measured the impact of STD control on HIV incidence in the population — the Mwanza trial (Grosskurth et al 1995) and the Rakai trial (Wawer 1999).

A community randomized trial of STD diagnosis and treatment for HIV prevention was conducted in the Mwanza region of Tanzania (Grosskurth 1995). Six pairs of rural communities were randomized to intervention and treatment arms. The intervention was the provision of continuous access to improved treatment for symptomatic STDs through existing primary care clinics. Improved treatment was realized through training of staff from health centers and dispensaries in STD diagnosis and treatment using syndromic algorithms, assuring a regular supply of drugs, implementing regular supervisory visits to health facilities, and establishing an STD reference clinic and laboratory. Individuals in intervention areas also received visits from health educators who provided information on STDs focusing on the availability of effective treatment and emphasizing the importance of prompt treatment for symptomatic STDs. The trial continued for 24 months and during this period no efforts were made to alter the STD care that existed in comparison communities. At the end of the trial period the intervention was implemented in the comparison communities.

At the end of the 24 months, a 38% reduction was observed in HIV incidence in intervention communities compared to control communities. The greatest impact of the intervention was in women aged 15-24 years and men aged 25-34. These are the groups in which HIV incidence was highest in comparison communities.

An economic analysis of the STD treatment intervention in Mwanza showed that it was cost effective in preventing HIV infection (Gilson 1997). The cost was US $10 per disability adjusted life year (DALY) saved and US $218 per HIV infection averted. These figures compare favorably to interventions like childhood immunization that cost US $12-17 per DALY saved.

In Rakai, Uganda another approach to STD treatment for HIV prevention was tested (Wawer 1999). Intervention communities were grouped into five clusters of four to seven villages each, reflecting social and sexual networks. In intervention communities' mass treatment was provided for curable STDs at ten-month intervals, in people's homes. Single dose antibiotics were used for this purpose. In control-communities mass treatment for conditions other than STDs was provided in people's homes using low dose multivitamins, iron folate and an antihelminth. Individuals with STD symptoms in control communities were referred for STD care to mobile clinics that were in these communities during mass treatment rounds. Condoms, HIV prevention education and counseling, and free general health care were offered to all study subjects. HIV incidence was similar in intervention and control communities after three mass treatment rounds.

The apparently contradictory results of the two community randomized trials discussed above have lead many to speculate on possible reasons for the different outcomes. Some suggest that the relative importance of STD diagnosis and treatment for HIV prevention may vary depending on the characteristics of the STD and HIV epidemics; and that some approaches to STD diagnosis and treatment may be more effective in preventing HIV transmission than others (Fleming and Wasserheit, 1999). STDs may be relatively more important in HIV transmission during earlier phases of the HIV epidemic; if prevalence of curable bacterial STD such as chlamydia, gonorrhea and syphilis are relatively higher; if prevalence of HIV is relatively lower; and efforts to diagnose and treat STD target symptomatic STD cases. In addition, provision of STD clinical services on a continuous basis may be more effective than provision of mass treatment at ten-month intervals, for HIV prevention.

3. THE ATTRIBUTABLE RISK QUESTION

It would be impossible to test the effects of STD control for HIV prevention in every community with a high incidence of HIV. Theoretically, the potential impact of an STD control program on HIV incidence could be calculated using two variables. The formula for determining the percent of HIV transmission risk attributable to STD is $AR\%=P(RR-1) / [P(RR-1)+1] \times 100\%$, where P is the prevalence of the STD in the population and RR is the relative risk for acquiring HIV for persons with (versus without) an STD. The difficulties in estimating the relative risk have been discussed. Additional difficulties are encountered when estimating the prevalence of STD.

A major problem with measuring the prevalence is that the attributable risk calculation assumes an even distribution of the disease (HIV) and risk factor (STD) in the population. This is clearly not the case because HIV and STD tend to cluster, especially early in an epidemic. Consider a hypothetical example that applies the finding from a research study that STDs increase the RR for HIV by 4. (Table I.)

In a population of 1,000,000 with 45,000 HIV incident infections in a year, and an STD prevalence of 0.1, the formula states that 23% or 10,350 HIV infections are attributable to STD. In a larger, low prevalence population of 100,000,000 with 5,000 HIV incident infections in a year and an STD prevalence of 0.0001, the formula tells us that 0.03% or 1.5 of the HIV infections were attributable to STD. When the two populations are combined; the total population is 101,000,000 with 50,000 HIV incident infections and an STD prevalence of 0.001. The formula tells us that 0.3% or 150 HIV infections were attributable to STD whereas a total of 10,351.5 HIV infections were attributable to STD in the preceding stratified analysis.

Table 1. HIV incident

Population	Infections	STD Prevalence	HIV Attributable to STD
1,000,000	45,000	0.1	10,350
100,000,000	5,000	0.0001	1.5
101,000,000	50,000	0.001	150

HIV transmission attributable to STD in three populations. Note that if the third population was made up of the two very different sub-populations above it, a stratified analysis would have identified 10,351.5 HIV infections attributable to STD.

This problem suggests that the traditional approach to attributable risk will not be of much use in assessing the contribution of STD to HIV transmission. How can we ever know all the strata in a population, much less the prevalence of STD and HIV in those groups? There may be a way to estimate. All HIV transmission is from HIV-infected persons, so we need to know the prevalence of STD among the HIV-infected individuals. Actually, the HIV-infected individuals who are not having sex with an uninfected partner should also be excluded from our calculations. A few studies have looked for STDs in persons receiving treatment for HIV, in one study the prevalence of gonorrhea based on urine testing was 1.6 percent among HIV infected people in HIV primary care (Erbelding et al, 2000). Persons who are not receiving treatment for HIV, and especially those who do not even know that they are HIV-infected, may have a much higher prevalence of gonorrhea, in some studies this has been as high as 14% (Farley et al, 2000). If the prevalence of gonorrhea is 12% and an HIV-infected person with gonorrhea is 4 times more likely to transmit than an

HIV-infected person who does not have gonorrhea, the atributable risk would be 26%.

STD might also facilitate HIV acquisition. In this instance, the population of interest is the population having sex with HIV-infected persons. They are much harder to identify. One way to estimate is to assume that they have the same prevalence of STD as their HIV-infected partners and use the prevalence estimates from the HIV-infected persons.

Thus, an important determinant of the role of STD control for HIV prevention will be the prevalence of STD in HIV-infected persons. The extent of overlap between these infections will determine their potential for epidemiologic synergy.

4. SOCIOLOGIC SYNERGY

STD and sexually transmitted HIV are similarly influenced by a number of demographic, economic, social, behavioral and attitudinal factors which interact with each other synergistically and impact the rates of other STD and HIV. A youthful age composition in a population - with large percentages being in sexually active age groups - is conducive to high rates of STD and HIV. A sex ratio that deviates from unity with an excess of men or women is conducive to both STD and HIV transmission. An economy with high proportions of the population in poverty is conducive to both STD and HIV transmission. Similarly, economies marked by high levels of inequality are conducive to high rates of both STD and HIV. Youthful age composition, high or low sex ratios, poverty, high levels of inequality tend to occur together in societies and mutually reinforce each other.

Individuals that engage in high-risk sexual behaviors with other high-risk individuals tend to be at risk for both other STD and HIV. Individuals who practice high-risk behaviors tend to seek out others like themselves and these persons are often found in the same social and sexual networks - mutually reinforcing each other's risk for STD and HIV. None of the studies that have focused on STD/HIV interactions to date have adjusted for the potentially confounding effects of sexual network membership. Social structural properties such as sexual mixing (Laumann and Youm, 1999; Aral, 1999a; Aral, 1999b), presence of concurrent partnerships and bridge populations (Morris, 1997; Gorbach, 2000; Aral, 2000), and network properties such as the presence of radial versus linear networks (Wylie and Jolly, 2000) influence the rate of spread of STD and HIV similarly. Studies of STD/HIV interactions have not adjusted for these social structural parameters, which synergistically influence STD and HIV rates.

Societal attitudes toward sexuality and sexually transmitted diseases constitute another set of factors that affect both STD and HIV similarly and synergistically. Lack of open conversation about sexuality and STD hinders primary prevention efforts, and effective health care seeking and acceptable health service provision for STD, which in turn mutually reinforce their negative impact on higher STD rates (Eng and Butler, 1997).

Finally, recent research highlights the importance of circumcision as a preventive factor in both HIV transmission and HIV acquisition (Quinn, 2000). Circumcision is also preventive against STD acquisition (Aral and Holmes, 1999). Thus, culturally prescribed practices such as circumcision contribute to the sociological synergy that similarly influences rates of spread of STD and HIV.

5. STD/HIV CO-INFECTIONS AS SENTINEL EVENTS

From a public health perspective, co-infected persons represent much more than an opportunity for biologic facilitation of transmission. They represent persons who are likely to be transmitting HIV. They represent persons who are probably not getting all of the treatment, social, and psychological support that they need to deal with their infection.

Persons who are co-infected with HIV and STD are sentinel events--they tell us where HIV and STD prevention is failing. HIV infected persons should know that they are infected, and should be taking precautions to avoid transmitting to others. Persons discovered to have HIV in an STD clinic may provide insight regarding HIV-infected persons who are unaware of their HIV infection. Persons who are known to be HIV-infected, but acquire an STD represent infected individuals who need support to avoid transmitting HIV.

HIV-STD co-infected persons are tremendously important for reflecting the convergence of the epidemics and the potential contribution of STD to HIV transmission. Interestingly, we have a pretty good idea of the HIV prevalence and the STD incidence in different areas, but rarely do we know how often co-infection occurs--perhaps because people responsible for controlling HIV and those responsible for controlling STD are in different organizational units (Belongia 1997).

6. CONCLUSIONS

Uncertainty about some aspects of HIV-STD interactions should not lead to inaction in areas where there is sufficient information or where the answers to the questions are unlikely to change the decisions.

Here are some observations and recommendations that we believe are well supported by evidence:

- Some HIV-infected persons will acquire STD. These STD will facilitate HIV transmission. Since most bacterial STD are asymptomatic, HIV infected persons should be periodically screened for STD.
- Careful evaluation of HIV infected persons who acquired an STD will provide valuable information about where HIV is being transmitted in a community.
- HIV-uninfected persons who get an STD are at higher risk of getting HIV than others in the community. This risk is related to the types of partners they are having sex with and the facilitation of HIV transmission by the presence of an STD. Quality counseling has been shown to reduce the risk of acquiring a new STD. Persons diagnosed with an STD should be screened in six months, because many will have new asymptomatic infections.
- Communities with high rates of STD often have high rates of HIV. This suggests a biologic interaction, but high rates in these areas of many other diseases not transmitted sexually, suggest that other factors contribute broadly to human illness. Basic public health research into the root cause of disease clustering may identify interventions.

ACKNOWLEDGMENT:

The authors would like to acknowledge Patricia Jackson for her outstanding support in the preparation of this manuscript.

REFERENCES

Aral SO, Holmes KK. Social and behavioral determinants of the epidemiology of STDs: industrialized and developing countries. *Sex Transm Dis*, KK Holmes, PF Sparling, P-A Mardh, SM Lemon, WE Stamm, P Piot, JN Wasserheit (Eds), third edition, McGraw Hill, 1999;39-76.

Aral SO. Behavioral aspects of STD: Core groups and bridge populations. *Sex Transm Dis* 2000 (In Press).

Aral SO. Sexual network patterns as determinants of STD rates: Paradigm shift in the behavioral epidemiology of STDs made visible. *Sex Transm Dis*, 1999a;26(5):262-264.

Aral SO, Hughes JP, Stoner B, Whittington W, Handsfield HH, Anderson RM, Holmes KK. Sexual mixing patterns in the spread of gonococcal and chlamydial infections. *American Journal of Public Health* 1999b;89(6):825-833.

Belongia EA, Danila RN, Angamuthu V, Hickman CD, DeBoer JM, MacDonald KL, Osterholm MT. A population-based study of sexually transmitted disease incidence and risk factors in human immunodeficiency virus-infected people. *Sex Transm Dis* 1997;24(5):251-256.

Boily MC. Transmission dynamics of co-existing chlamydial and HIV infections in the United States. In: *The hidden epidemic: confronting sexually transmitted diseases*. Washington, DC: National Academy Press, 1996;C1-13.

Boily MC, Anderson RM. Human immunodeficiency virus transmission and the role of other sexually transmitted diseases. Measures of association and study design. *Sex Transm Dis* 1996;23:312-32.

Brody S. Potterat JJ. Is there really a heterosexual AIDS epidemic in the United States? Findings from a multisite validation study, 1992-1995. *American Journal of Epidemiology* 1999;150(4):429-30.

Eng TR and Butler WT, *Editors*. The hidden epidemic: confronting sexually transmitted diseases. Institute of Medicine, National Academy Press, Washington, DC 1997.

Erbelding EE, Stanton D, Quinn TC, Rompalo A. Behavioral and biologic evidence of persistent high-risk behavior in an HIV primary care population. *AIDS* 2000;14:297-301.

Farley T, Sanders L, Elkin W, Cohen D. Lack of sysmptoms is the primary reason non-ulcerative STDs are untreated in the US: Implications for prevention of HIV infection. 13th International AIDS Conference, Durban, South Africa, July 9-14, 2000.

Fleming DT, Wasserheit JN. From epidemiological synergy to public health policy and practice: the contribution of other sexually transmitted diseases to sexual transmission of HIV infection. *Sex Transm Inf* 1999;75:3-17.

Garnett GP, Anderson RM. Strategies for limiting the spread of HIV in developing countries: conclusions based on studies of the transmission dynamics of the virus. J *Acquir Immun Defic Syndr Hum Retrovirol* 1995;9:500-13.

Gilson I, Mkanje R, Grosskurth H, et al. Cost-effectiveness of improved treatment services for sexually transmitted diseases in preventing HIV-1 infection in Mwanza region, Tanzania. Lancet 1997;350:1805-9.

Gorbach PM, Sopheab H, Phalla T, Leng HB, Mills S, Bennett A, Holmes KK. Sexual bridging by Cambodian Men: Potential importance for general population spread of STDS/HIV epidemics. *Sex Transm Dis* 2000 (In Press).

Gray RH, Wawer MJ, Sewankambo NK, et al. Relative risks and population attributable fraction of incident HIV associated with symptoms of sexually transmitted diseases and treatable symptomatic sexually transmitted diseases in Rakai District, Uganda. *AIDS* 1999;13:2113-2123.

Grosskurth H, Mosha F, Todd J, *et al.* Impact of improved treatment of sexually transmitted diseases on HIV infection in rural Tanzania: randomised controlled trial. *Lancet* 1995;346:530-6.

Koopman J, Kwon JW. The effect of HIV treatment on population infection levels is robustly dependent upon the rate of epidemic rise. Abstract presented at the 12th World AIDS Conference, Geneva June 28-July 3, 1998, Poster Sessions, Track C #33257.

Laumann EO, Youm Y. Racial/ethnic group differences in the prevalence of sexually transmitted diseases in the United States: A network explanation. Sexually Transmitted Diseases 1999;26:250-261.

May R, Anderson R. Transmission dynamics of HIV infection. *Nature* 1987;326:137-42.

Mertens TE, Hayes RJ, Smith PG. Epidemiological methods to study the interaction between HIV infection and other sexually transmitted diseases. AIDS 1990;4:57-65.

Morris M. and Kretzchmar M. Concurrent partnerships and the spread of HIV. *AIDS* 1997;11:641-648.

Over M, Piot P. Human immunodeficiency virus infection and other sexually transmitted diseases in developing countries: public health importance and priorities for resource allocation. *J Infect Dis* 1996;174(Suppl 2):162-75.

Plummer FA. Heterosexual transmission of human immunodeficiency virus type 1 (HIV): interactions of conventional sexually transmitted diseases, hormonal contraception and HIV-1. *AIDS Research and Human Retroviruses* 1998;15(suppl 1):S5-S10.

Quinn TC, Wawer MJ, Sewankambo N, Serwadda D, Li C, Wabwire-Mangen F, Meehan MO, Lutalo T, Gray RH, for the Rakai Project Study Group. Viral load and heterosexual transmission of human immunodeficiency virus type 1. *The New England Journal of Medicine* 2000;342(13):921-929.

Robinson NJ, Mulder DW, Auvert B, *et al.* Proportion of HIV infections attributable to other sexually transmitted diseases in a rural Ugandan population: simulation model estimates. *Int J Epidemiol* 1997;26:180-9.

Wasserheit JN. Epidemiological synergy. Interrelationships between human immunodeficiency virus infection and other sexually transmitted diseases. *Sex Transm Dis* 1992;19:61-77.

Wasserheit JN, Aral SO. The Dynamic Topology of Sexually Transmitted Disease Epidemics: Implications for STD Prevention Strategies. *Journal of Infectious Diseases* 1996;174(Suppl 2):S201-13.

Wawer MJ, Gray RH, Sewankambo NK, *et al.* Results of a randomized, community trial of STD control for AIDS prevention, Rakai District, Uganda: reductions in STDs are not associated with reduced HIV incidence. *Lancet* 1999;353:52-53.

World Bank. *Confronting AIDS: public priorities in a global epidemic*. Washington, DC: International Bank for Reconstruction and Development/World Bank 1997;1-14.

Wylie JL, Jolly A. Sexual network analysis of chlamydia and gonorrhea transmission in Manitoba, Canada. *Sex Transm Dis* 2000 (In Press).

Chapter 5

HIV Treatment Advances as Prevention

Lynn Paxton and Robert Janssen
Division of HIV/AIDS Prevention, National Center for HIV, STD and TB Prevention, Centers for Disease Control and Prevention, Atlanta Georgia.

1. INTRODUCTION

In the industrialized world, 1996 is widely considered to have marked a turning point in the AIDS epidemic. In that year protease inhibitors were introduced and quickly became, in combination with reverse transcriptase inhibitors, the foundation of the most potent anti-HIV drug combination available to date, Highly Active Antiretroviral Therapy (HAART). Large population studies demonstrated that combination therapy with three drugs reduced the risk of death by 85% and directly linked declining trends in the incidence of specific opportunistic infections to the intensity of antiretroviral treatment (McNaghten et al, 1999; Palella et al, 1998). Early studies demonstrating the powerful ability of HAART to reduce study participants' serum viral burden to undetectable or near undetectable levels were so encouraging that for the first time since the beginning of the epidemic there was talk of the possibility of transforming AIDS from a fatal into merely a chronic disease. There were even hopes that HAART might reduce an individual's viral burden and facilitate reconstitution of the immune system to the point where it could eradicate the virus. This optimism was bolstered by very steep declines in AIDS incidence and mortality among populations with access to HAART: In 1997, the first full year following the introduction of HAART, deaths in the US from AIDS decreased 42% and AIDS incidence decreased by 18%. In the ensuing years AIDS mortality and incidence have continued to decline in the US albeit at a slower rate. While expanded use of prophylaxis against opportunistic infections has contributed to this trend, (Kaplan et al, 2000) there is no doubt that the bulk of the decreases shown are related to the expanded use of antiretroviral therapy. To say that HAART has changed the face of AIDS in the industrialized world is not an exaggeration, however, the early optimism about its potential to eliminate HIV in an individual was fairly quickly dispelled. Clinical experience has revealed that, with rare exceptions, even patients who achieve optimum viral suppression on long term HAART experience return of their viral burden to pre-treatment levels when the drug regimen is stopped (Havlir et al, 1998; Pialoux et al, 1998). It has also been shown that HIV can and does remain dormant in various cells of the body for many years and possibly for the person's lifetime. Thus viral reactivation may occur years after initial infection even when antiretroviral therapy has been optimal. Another problem is that HIV mutates frequently within an infected individual and drug resistant strains can rapidly develop, particularly in the setting of imperfect adherence to therapy. Worrisome trends have already been observed. Concurrent with larger numbers of people receiving antiretroviral therapy there has been documented transmission of drug-resistant virus, which means that resistance will not remain a problem limited only to those who have been on HAART. One study documented genetic mutations conferring resistance to one or more antiretroviral drug in 16% of newly infected persons studied (Boden et al, 1999). Another, which looked at persons within 12 months of seroconversion, found that 26% had strains of HIV with reduced antiretroviral susceptibility (Little et al, 1999). Even though hopes of eradicating HIV from individuals that are already infected have dimmed many believe that HAART has enormous untapped potential to decrease HIV transmission. HAART's primary biologic effect is to reduce the amount of virus (commonly referred to as the HIV viral load or burden) present in an individual. Higher viral load has consistently been shown to be associated with higher risk for all forms of transmission. In a study of pregnant HIV-infected women in Thailand mothers who transmitted HIV to their infants had a median viral load that was 4.3 times higher than that among women who did not transmit and the risk increased in a linear fashion from the lowest to the highest quintiles of viral load. Significantly, no transmissions occurred at less than 2000 copies/ml (Shaffer et al, 1999). Similarly, among heterosexual discordant couples in a Ugandan cohort viral load was the chief predictor of transmission and each log increment in viral load was associated with a risk ratio increase of 2.4. Again there were no transmissions at the lowest viral loads of less than 1500 copies/ml (Quinn et al, 2000). A Zambian cohort showed almost identical findings (Fideli et al, 2000). Antiretroviral therapy, particularly

HAART, tends to dramatically reduce viremia, or the amount of virus in the blood stream. This decline in blood viral load is usually paralleled by similar declines in genital viral load (Barroso, et al, 2000; Gupta et al 1997). Given that lower viral load has been associated with lower risk for transmission it is therefore highly plausible that the widespread use of HAART could through this mechanism result in lowered transmission risk. Several years before protease inhibitors were introduced and even before the link between viral load and transmission was known, antiretroviral therapy was looked to as a means of preventing transmission. HIV-infected pregnant women and their offspring have always been priority populations in which to study the use of ART since the risk of HIV transmission from an infected mother to her baby in the absence of therapy is known to be extremely high, in the range of 25-33%. Published in 1994, the landmark AIDS Clinical Trials Group 076 study was the first to demonstrate the efficacy of zidovudine monotherapy in decreasing HIV transmission from 25% to 8% (Connor et al, 1994). Newer studies comparing combination therapy with zidovudine and lamivudine found a further reduction in transmission from 6.5% to 2.6% (Blanche et al, 1999) and there are indications that combination therapy with protease inhibitors (HAART) might be even more effective (Morris et al, 1999). In the United States expanded efforts to identify and treat pregnant HIV-infected women have resulted in a marked decrease in the birth of HIV-infected babies to fewer than 200 annually.

2. HAART AND SEXUAL TRANSMISSION

Unfortunately, despite the success of antiretrovirals in reducing perinatal transmission, to date this remarkable achievement has not been matched by a measurable decrease in sexual or injection drug use (IDU) related HIV transmission in the US population. Even before HAART came into widespread use examination of US surveillance data by back calculation from reported AIDS cases showed that HIV incidence began to decline in the late 1980's in many population groups, particularly older men who have sex with men (MSM). Incidence in IDUs and in heterosexuals (with the exception of African-American women) declined also, albeit not to the same degree as for MSM. Available case surveillance and survey studies (Schwarcz-Kaplan, 1999) indicate that HIV incidence has remained stable at approximately 40,000 cases per year throughout the 1990's and that there has not been a significant decline in HIV incidence commensurate with those seen in AIDS incidence and mortality (Centers for Disease Control and Prevention, 1999). While there is no one clear explanation for the lack of any notable decrease in sexual and injection-drug related transmission attributable to HAART there are several potential factors that deserve consideration. Perhaps the most important is the fact that many infected persons are unaware of their infection status and may unknowingly account for the bulk of HIV transmission. According to CDC estimates, more than 225,000 infected people in the United States have not been diagnosed. In addition, a significant proportion of these undiagnosed people may be in an early and perhaps more infectious stage of their illness. In the usual course of HIV infection the viral burden is very high within the first weeks after infection, not uncommonly in the range of several hundred thousand viral copies per milliliter of plasma. Some theorize that individuals who are in the very earliest stages of infection, around the time of seroconversion, may contribute a disproportionate amount to overall population transmission because they are both highly contagious and unlikely to modify their sexual behavior since they are unaware of their infection. Other researchers dispute the importance of the contribution of the newly infected to population transmission dynamics. It is not, however, only the undiagnosed who are at risk of transmitting HIV. Studies show that more than 70% of seropositive men and women engage in oral, vaginal, or anal sex after they become aware of their infection. Most feel a responsibility to protect sexual partners and adopt safer sexual behaviors, particularly with known seronegative partners. Nevertheless, a sizable percentage engage in unprotected sexual intercourse with partners of unknown or negative serostatus (Marks et al, 1999). For infected persons who are on HAART additional factors must be considered. In sexual transmission it is the virus present in the genital tract that is transmitted. HAART clearly lowers plasma viral loads yet studies have shown that despite a general correlation, plasma viral load does not always accurately reflect the viral load in the genital compartment (Zhang et al, 1998; Hart et al, 1999). Thus, even persons with an undetectable plasma viral load may remain capable of transmitting infection although presumably at lower levels than in the untreated state. The absolute number of HIV infected persons has risen, in part because more are living longer and feeling better because of HAART. Even if the per-sexual act transmission rate is lowered by HAART that may be counterbalanced by the increase in HIV prevalence and consequent absolute increase in unprotected sexual acts resulting in higher HIV incidence. There are also disturbing indications that certain complacency has set in among those infected with or at risk of HIV.

Rates of sexually transmitted diseases have risen significantly among MSM in certain areas of the United States, particularly among men in their twenties (Centers for Disease Control and Prevention, MMWR, 1999). Other studies have shown that the proportion of MSM engaging in unprotected anal intercourse with partners of unknown serostatus has risen as well and that a number of men who engage in risky sex report that the availability of HAART has rendered AIDS less of a perceived threat. (Murphy et al, 1998; DiClemente et al, 1998; Lehman et al, 2000) In any given population, if the sole change is an increase in risky behaviors then this will invariably lead to more HIV infections. Similarly, if the sole population change is a decrease in the contagiousness of the infected individual (as presumably occurs with HAART) this should lead to fewer infections. In populations that have access to HAART these two factors are usually acting simultaneously and their relative interactions can be extremely difficult to distinguish. US population based surveillance data has not shown any declines in HIV incidence attributable to HAART but this therapy has only been available for the past four years and many people who meet clinical criteria for its use are not currently receiving it. Recently, Blower and colleagues attempted to predict the potential epidemic-level effects if antiretroviral usage were to be expanded in San Francisco, a city where 30% of the gay population is HIV infected and of whom only about 50% are currently on HAART (Blower et al, 2000). They looked at various projections using a mathematical transmission model coupled with a statistical approach that incorporated increases in risky sexual behavior and emergence of drug resistance. Their 'best case' scenario assumed that the rate of resistance emergence would remain constant and low at approximately 10% per year and that risk behavior would not increase. Their 'worst-case' scenario assumed that the rate of drug resistance would increase from 10 to 60% per year and that risk behavior would double. Under the optimistic scenario their model predicted that after 10 years of ART 40% of new infections would be prevented. Their pessimistic scenario predicted that the incidence rate would initially increase but that over time ART would decrease the incidence rate. At ten years, even under this 'worst-case' scenario ART's effect on decreasing incidence would finally compensate for the initial rise in incidence and ultimately, infections would be lower than if treatment had not been expanded. The authors concluded that their model shows that expanding use of viral suppressing agents to more infected men in San Francisco will always reduce HIV incidence compared to not expanding treatment, no matter what the rate of drug resistance or risk behavior. HAART has been available in the US for four years and even though there are indications that there may have been an increase in risky behavior in some risk groups, most notably young MSM, it does not appear that the overall rate has doubled. Assuming that the conclusions of Blower and her colleagues are correct, why then has there not been any change in HIV incidence? There are several explanations that could fit their theory. One is that we are simply too early on the curve and that we will soon see significant decreases at the population level. Another is the fact that many infected persons are either not aware of their seropositivity or are not being treated for some other reason. In that case the recent public health emphasis on early diagnosis and treatment of HIV infected persons such as the CDC sponsored Sero-status Approach to Fighting the Epidemic (SAFE) initiative should eventually lead not only to decreased morbidity and mortality for those treated but also will decrease the net rate of HIV transmission in the population.

Discussion continues on how best to actively prove the hypothesis that the use of HAART can decrease sexual transmission. Some debate whether in the developed world this question deserves active investigation since the goal of getting every HIV infected person into treatment has already been established and thus any potential effects of HAART on sexual transmission good be considered as a welcome but merely adjunctive benefit. Some research proposals include 'look-back' studies in which recent seroconverters would be identified along with their source partners. These 'transmitting pairs' would then be compared to matched 'control' pairs in which no transmission occurred to evaluate any differences in antiretroviral use. Other research designs rely on a more prospective approach and would involve studies of persons on HAART and their sexual partners and would look at HAART- associated suppression of plasma and genital viral load and any subsequent transmission. As previously stated there is continued uncertainty about the relative contribution to HIV transmission of the newly infected and there is much thought being given to the optimal time of initiation of HAART therapy. Valuable information may be gained about the effectiveness of early HAART as a prevention strategy as research continues among such populations. The primary goal of current research is to determine whether early HAART is beneficial to the primary patient and whether this benefit will be maintained over many years, perhaps decades of use. Proposed adjunctive studies would look at transmission to sexual partners. Should it be shown that early HAART produces both a long-lasting benefit to the primary patient and also decreases transmission to partners then this could be considered a 'win-win' situation. Conversely, if it is shown that early HAART is ultimately detrimental to the primary patient then clearly it would not be advocated.

If, however, it turns out that early HAART results in no added benefit to the primary patient but does decrease the risk of transmission to others then this brings up the ethical dilemma of whether it is proper to advise a patient to take potentially toxic medications primarily for the benefit of others. Aside from potential adverse drug reactions this strategy would also have a substantial downside in that it would be expensive and would run the risk of undermining condom promotion interventions as seropositive patients might feel that the HAART use alone could supplant condoms.

3. POST EXPOSURE PROPHYLAXIS

While investigators struggle to define how HAART use among seropositives might affect sexual HIV transmission there is much attention also being given to HAART use by the other side of the transmission equation: the exposed HIV negative partner. The strategy of giving ART after exposure to HIV, usually referred to as post-exposure prophylaxis (PEP), was first studied among healthcare workers (HCW) with percutaneous exposures. The average risk associated with a percutaneous needlestick has been estimated at 0.3% (Gerberding, 1994; Henderson et al, 1990; Tokars et al, 1993), which is 100-fold less than that for vertical transmission. An attempt was made to conduct a prospective, placebo-controlled trial of post-exposure prophylaxis (PEP) with zidovudine prevention but it had to be abandoned due to poor enrollment. It was replaced by a pooled case-control study among patients reported to several surveillance systems in the US and Europe (Cardo et al, 1997). To date, this has been the largest study of occupational exposures with 33 cases and 679 controls. Unfortunately, there were many confounding factors and in univariate analysis there was no difference in zidovudine use between cases and controls. With logistic regression and multivariate analysis zidovudine use was shown to be associated with an 81% reduction in risk. The study had several limitations, most notably the fact that it was retrospective in nature, cases were relatively few, and cases and controls were drawn from different populations. Nevertheless, it is essentially the only occupational efficacy data available and it has become the basis of US Public Health Service (USPHS) recommendations to routinely offer HIV post-exposure prophylaxis to healthcare workers with occupational exposures (CDC MMWR, 1998).

Since publication of the healthcare worker data and the subsequent USPHS recommendations, the issue of PEP for sexual exposures has taken on increased prominence. A comparison by McCullough and Boag of published estimates of single exposure transmission risk by type of exposure places the risk for percutaneous exposures below that for receptive anal intercourse and above that for receptive vaginal intercourse. (Table taken from McCullough and Boag, Journal of HIV Therapy, Vol 5, No.1, Feb 2000).

Table 1. Probability of transmission of HIV from a single exposure

Per Episode	Infection rate
One transfusion of a single unit of infected whole blood	0.95
Intravenous needle/syringe exposure	0.0067
Percutaneous exposure	0.0032
Receptive penile-anal intercourse	0.008-0.032
Receptive vaginal intercourse	0.0005-0.0015
Insertive vaginal intercourse	0.0003-0.0009

Unfortunately, these estimates for sexual exposure risk mask considerable uncertainty and variability. Most studies of per-contact risk have been done among serodiscordant couples in stable partnerships and assumed a constant rate of infectivity. However, constant infectivity is probably the exception, not the rule and these estimates probably seriously underestimate the risk of serotransmission after a few contacts while seriously overestimating that associated with a large number of contacts (Downs and De Vincenzi, 1996). In addition, these estimates do not take into account other factors that might affect infectivity including characteristics of the virus and the host such as, viral load and presence of other sexually transmitted infections, or characteristics of the exposure such as mucosal injury associated with sexual assault.

Given the HCW data and the success of the perinatal efficacy studies it is very plausible that PEP can be effective in preventing sexual transmission of HIV. There has been a successful efficacy study of intravenous ART after vaginal exposure to HIV-2 in a pig-tailed macaque model (Otten et al, 2000). Unfortunately, human efficacy data is completely lacking. Since the mechanism and determinants of sexual transmission have not been completely elucidated a certain degree of caution is necessary when extrapolating from studies of vertical and occupational exposures, as they are quite distinct in significant respects. The absolute level of risk for sexual exposures is more similar to that seen in HCW exposures than to that for perinatal transmission. A notable difference when comparing these two groups is that sexual transmission occurs primarily through the mucous membranes whereas all patients in the HCW study had a documented percutaneous exposure to HIV-infected blood by a needle stick or a cut with a sharp object. It is quite likely, however, that the absolute amount of virus transferred may be comparable and that similar immunological responses might occur in both mucosal and transcutaneous exposures (Blauvelt, 1997). HCW exposures are usually solitary incidents, their annual number is relatively small, the HIV infection status of the source is often already known or easily ascertained and treatment can usually be started very soon after the exposure. This is in marked contrast to the annual number of sexual exposures which probably number in the hundred thousands if not millions. They often take place in the context of ongoing risk behavior and the infection status of the potential source is often not known or cannot be easily ascertained. Some researchers argue that providing PEP for sexual exposures under these conditions is not cost-effective and may have a considerable downside in that it exposes many recipients who are at no or low risk to adverse drug effects and, perhaps most importantly, may encourage risky behaviors that will result in more infections than were prevented by PEP (Evans, Darbyshire and Cartledge, 1998). Others consider this reticence to be unwarranted. There have been no human efficacy trials and a randomized, placebo-controlled trial is likely to have enrollment problems similar to those in the HCW study and thus is unlikely to ever take place. Some claim that it is discriminatory to routinely offer PEP to healthcare workers and not to those who are sexually exposed. They point out that the risk of seroconversion after a high-risk sexual act such as receptive anal intercourse with either a known HIV positive partner or a partner of unknown serostatus in an area of high prevalence may in fact be higher than that for many occupational exposures. Others also discount the issue of cost-effectiveness of PEP for sexual exposures and cite the obligation of the practitioner to act 'in the best interests' of the individual patient (Lurie et al, 1998).

Sexual exposure occurring as a result of sexual assault appears to fall into a gray area in this ongoing debate. For one thing, we know even less about HIV transmission due to non-consensual intercourse than to consensual intercourse among discordant couples. Although there are certainly documented cases of HIV transmission as a result of rape in the medical literature there have been no studies, observational or otherwise, that have been able to even attempt to estimate the incidence of HIV seroconversion after rape. Sexual assault can and often does encompass single or multiple assailants and many potential routes of exposure (oral, vaginal, anal) all of which can substantially affect risk. Moreover, a substantial number of assaults involve violence and injury to mucosal tissues which probably increases transmission risk but to an unknown degree. Analogous to HCW exposures, sexual assault is usually not an ongoing occurrence and thus worries about PEP encouraging continued risky behavior do not apply but unlike for HCW, it is exceedingly rare that the infection status of the potential source can be determined in a timely manner. Survivors of sexual assault have already been traumatized and there are many who argue that it is 'victimizing the victim' to not offer PEP under these circumstances even if the efficacy of PEP is unproven. Of great significance is that in those places that have tried to institute routine recommendation of PEP to rape survivors (San Francisco, New York, and Vancouver) acceptance rates have been surprisingly low and the rates of completion have been even lower. For example, during a 16 month study in Vancouver only 71 of 258 victims accepted PEP and only 8 completed a full course (Wiebe et al,, 2000). One speculation as to the reason for such low rates is that survivors may be psychologically unable to deal simultaneously with the aftermath of the rape and the exigencies of PEP. In 1997 the Centers for Disease Control and Prevention convened a meeting of external consultants to address the subject of PEP for non-occupational exposures. The subsequent report was published in 1998 (CDC, 1998). This report summarized the available data about PEP and the potential risks including drug toxicity, the potential for undermining behavioral prevention efforts, the theoretic possibility of acquisition of antiretroviral resistant HIV strains and the possible diversion of already scarce public resources. Due to the lack of efficacy data no recommendation was made either for or against the use of PEP for sexual exposures. When deciding whether or not to recommend PEP for an individual patient CDC advises physicians and other health care providers to carefully evaluate the likelihood that the source patient was HIV infected and the specifics of the risk event, the time elapsed since the event and presentation for care, and the frequency of the individual's ongoing HIV exposures. Monitoring of drug toxicity is essential for those patients for whom the provider recommends antiretroviral therapy and who elect to take it. All patients, whether PEP is recommended or not, should receive supportive counseling and prevention services. The report concluded by recognizing that much research is needed about the use and efficacy of PEP in non-occupational exposures. In order to gather more information in July 1999 the CDC established the National Nonoccupational PEP Registry. This registry, similar to the one previously established for occupational PEP, is a prospective surveillance system to collect data on the utilization, safety and outcome of PEP use. Healthcare providers throughout the US who prescribe or consider PEP for a patient are asked to report to this anonymous registry. Other countries have established similar registries

(Switzerland, France, Belgium, Italy, Catalonia-*Spain*, Australia) and others will soon begin (England, Greece, Portugal, Denmark, Holland, Austria, Germany). Eventually, as was done for the HCW study, data from these multinational registries might be combined to draw conclusions about PEP efficacy. Since the publication of the CDC recommendations for non-occupational exposures there have been attempts to explore the feasibility of PEP provision. The largest study of this type to date was the San Francisco PEP Study (Martin et al, 2000). Information about the study was disseminated at locations frequented by persons with high risk for HIV exposure. Participants who reported receptive or insertive anal or vaginal intercourse, receptive oral intercourse with ejaculation, sharing of injection drugs or other muco-cutaneous exposures with partners known or at risk for HIV exposure were evaluated at various clinical sites and given four weeks of antiretroviral medications along with risk reduction and medication adherence counseling. They were also urged to refer the source of their exposure to the study for HIV testing and interview. The trial was non-randomized and participants were followed for six months. Of the 401 persons enrolled (90% males) the majority (94%) had sexual exposures and the most commonly reported acts were receptive and insertive anal intercourse. Seventy-eight percent completed the four-week medication regimen and there were no seroconversions among the 300 participants who returned for repeat HIV testing during the follow-up period. Many patients reported adverse physical effects from the medications including nausea, fatigue, headache and diarrhea but relatively few developed any laboratory abnormalities. While 43% stated that they knew their partner was seropositive most participants were uncertain of their partner's HIV status. Only 67 source partners were recruited and of those 50 (76%) were found to be HIV infected. Most participants reported that the event that prompted them to seek PEP was a lapse in their usual safer sex practices and not habitual behavior. Of particular note is that six months following the initial exposure 12% of participants sought repeat PEP for another exposure. Although no conclusion can be drawn from this study about PEP efficacy it indicates that in a city with a reasonable healthcare infrastructure PEP can feasibly be delivered. However, this study also confirmed many of the potential drawbacks of PEP as an intervention, notably the difficulty in determining the source patient's HIV status, the considerable subjective toxicity associated with the medications and the fact that some patients will probably continue to engage in risky behavior as evidenced by the 12% who returned for a repeat course of PEP within six months despite intensive behavioral risk counseling. The study also confirmed suspicions that a randomized placebo-controlled efficacy trial may not be possible: despite being told that there is no evidence that PEP is efficacious for sexual exposures only 4 of the 401 participants elected not to take medications.

4. HAART AND THE DEVELOPING WORLD

When we consider the impact that HAART has already had on AIDS epidemiology and its potential impact on transmission essentially two pictures present themselves: the one in the industrialized world where HAART is available to many although not all, and the other in the developing world which cannot afford the costly therapy and where ninety-five percent of HIV infected persons live. According to estimates from the Joint United Nations Programme on HIV/AIDS (UNAIDS) and the World Health Organization (WHO) (UNAIDS, 1999), 33.6 million people will be living with HIV by the end of 1999. Sub-Saharan Africa continues to bear the brunt of the epidemic and is home to almost 70% of HIV infected persons. Much of Africa is in an extremely precarious situation, struggling with poor economic management and corruption, crippling external debt, armed conflicts, ecological disasters, and weak infrastructure. Inequitable distribution of resources is the rule rather than the exception and expenditures on health tend to be only a small fraction of governmental budgets usually in the range of one to three percent of their gross domestic product (GDP). In many countries this amounts to a per capita health care expenditure ranging from 6 to 40 dollars per year. Nations in the industrialized world are able to spend considerably more with the majority allocating between seven and ten percent of their GDP to health care. The United States spends the most at 13.5%, which amounted to $3,925 per capita in 1997. (National Center for Health Statistics, 1999). Bozzette et al. estimated the annual direct expenditures for the care of HIV infected persons in 1996 to be $6.7 billion or about $20,000 per patient per year. (Bozzette et al, 1998) As evidence mounts for HAART's beneficial effects there have been ever increasing demands to make it more widely available in the developing world. Recent studies of short-course zidovudine and nevirapine lend credence to the belief that cost-effective therapy to prevent mother-to-child transmission may soon be within the reach of many of the poorer nations. However, the availability of HAART for treatment of persons who are already seropositive remains problematic. The currently very high costs of the drugs represent a formidable, but not the only challenge. Safe storage and delivery of the drugs requires a functioning healthcare delivery system. Moreover, antiretroviral use demands regular monitoring of the person's immune system, his or her response to the drugs and the development of resistant strains of HIV. The ancillary tests necessary for this can amount to several hundred dollars per year and require trained personnel and relatively sophisticated equipment that is usually available only in a very few sites in a developing country, if at all. Recently, several pharmaceutical companies have announced that they plan to reduce the costs of their medications in the developing world and there have been discussions about manufacturing some antiretrovirals off patent and at greatly reduced cost. These innovations are very welcome but are only a preliminary step. For widespread HAART use to become feasible in the developing world, in addition to drastic reductions in drug costs, the healthcare infrastructures need to be substantially improved and the drugs themselves need to be improved so as to reduce toxicity and to shorten the dosing schedule thereby facilitating their use by patients without easy access to medical care. The HIV/AIDS epidemic is raging in the developing world and efforts will continue to make HAART more widely available yet the above-mentioned practical realities make large-scale HAART provision in the near future a distant dream. If HAART is not generally available for treatment then its potential impact on sexual transmission of HIV will be limited. Because of the magnitude of the AIDS epidemic in the developing world and the importance of sexual transmission in its spread there is currently debate over whether emphasis should be put initially on strategies that might minimize the potential of sexual transmission. Under this scenario persons who are either at particularly high risk of transmitting infection due to high viral loads (such as recent seroconverters), or persons who come in contact with many partners (such as commercial sex workers) would be identified and prioritized for treatment. Other potential recipients could be persons with an identifiable at-risk sexual partner, such as occurs in stable serodiscordant relationships. From the population standpoint targeted intervention could ultimately offer great benefit: If transmission from certain high-frequency transmitters could be stopped or significantly reduced then eventually the rate of new infections would fall below the threshold necessary to sustain the epidemic. That said such a strategy would require extremely careful implementation and consideration of the numerous potential problems that could arise. Prominent among these is the issue of fairness. When so many people are affected how do you pick some to receive potentially life-saving therapy while denying it to so many others? Also, unless HAART recipients are very closely monitored for adherence (which as noted above, can be very difficult in the absence of a highly functioning health care system) then there is the very real risk of the eventual development of widespread antiretroviral resistance, which could counteract any beneficial gains from this strategy. There is also the fear that promoting the use of HAART as a means to decrease transmission has the potential of undermining gains made in condom promotion.

5. CONCLUSION

Without question HAART has been the most significant therapeutic advance in HIV/AIDS care to date. As a direct result of its use AIDS is no longer among the top ten causes of mortality in the United States and many people who would have otherwise sickened and died of the disease are living longer lives in better health. Unfortunately, this combination therapy is not a panacea. Other than in the case of perinatal transmission, we have not seen declines in HIV transmission that can be directly attributed to its use and we are starting to see a slowing down in the rates of decline in AIDS incidence and mortality. Nevertheless, HAART is still the most powerful weapon in our biomedical arsenal and we must continue to expand its use and improve its effectiveness. The public health challenge is substantial. Access to quality care varies enormously in the United States with ethnic minority groups such as African-Americans and Hispanics, women, the poor, and behavioral sub-groups such as injection drug users tending to have less access (Shapiro et al, 1999). Currently, many people who might benefit from HAART are not receiving it, either because they are not aware that they are seropositive or because they lack access to adequate therapy. First and foremost, we must improve efforts to get more people to be HIV tested and, for those who are seropositive, improve their access to quality care. For those who are already in care and receiving HAART we need to improve their likelihood of adherence by developing drugs with less toxic side effects and simpler dosing schedules. Concurrently, the emergence of drug resistance must be closely monitored and emphasis placed on the development of newer drugs that act at different stages of the viral replication cycle. At the behavioral level we need to find more effective ways of encouraging safer sexual practices among both the infected and the uninfected and modify our prevention messages to counteract the complacency about the threat of AIDS that has arisen in relation to HAART.

However, as HAART will continue to remain out-of-reach to the vast majority of HIV-infected persons, we must keep in mind that AIDS care is much more than HAART and in the absence of an effective vaccine prevention efforts must focus on behavioral change. The disease needs to be destigmatized so more people will seek testing and adopt prevention behaviors. For those who are already infected, access to care including opportunistic infection prophylaxis and hospice care should be improved. As has been shown in countries such as Senegal, Uganda, and Thailand, concerted public health prevention efforts with active and energetic governmental support can have a significant effect on HIV incidence. We should learn from such successes and apply them to other settings so that future generations will no longer live in the shadow of AIDS.

REFERENCES

Barroso PF, Schecter M, Gupta P, Melo M, Vieira M, Murta F, Souza Y and L Harrison. Effect of antiretroviral therapy on HIV shedding in semen. *Ann Intern Med.* 2000; 133: 280-284.

Blanche S, Rouzioux C, Mandelbrot L, Delfraissy JF and Mayaux MJ. Zidovudine-lamivudine for prevention of mother to child HIV-1 transmission. 6th Annual Conference on Retroviruses and Opportunistic Infections, Chicago, 1999. Abstract no. 267.

Blauvelt A. A role of skin dendritic cells in the initiation of human immunodeficiency virus infection. *Am J Med* 1997; 102:16-20.

Blower SM, Gershengorn HB and Grant RM. A tale of two futures: HIV and antiretroviral therapy in San Francisco. *Science*, January 28, 2000, 287, 650-654.

Boden D, Hurley A, Zhang L, Cao Y, Guo Y, Jones E, Tsay J, Ip J, Farthing C, Limoli K, Parkin N, Markowitz M. HIV-1 drug resistance in newly infected individuals. *JAMA*, 1999, 282(12), 1135-1141.

Bozzette S, Berry S, Duan N, Frankel MR, Leibowitz AA, Lefkowitz D, Emmons CA, Senterfitt JW, Berk ML, Morton SC, Shapiro MF. The care of HIV-infected adults in the United States. *N Engl J Med*, 1998, 339, 1897-904

Cardo DM, Culver DH, Ciesielski CA, Srivastava PU, Marcus R, Abiteboul D, Heptonstall J, Ippolito G, Lot F, McKibben PS, Bell DM. A case-control study of HIV seroconversion in health care workers after percutaneous exposure. *N Engl J Me*d 1997; 337:1485-90.

Centers for Disease Control and Prevention. Guidelines for national human immunodeficiency virus case surveillance, including monitoring for human immunodeficiency virus infection and acquired immunodeficiency syndrome. *MMWR*, 1999, 48 (No, RR-13)

Centers for Disease Control and Prevention. Resurgent bacterial sexually transmitted disease among men who have sex with men–King County, Washington, 1997-1999. *MMWR*, September 10, 1999, 48 (35), 773-777.

Centers for Disease Control and Prevention. Increases in unsafe sex and rectal gonorrhea among men who have sex with men--San Francisco, 1994-1997. MMWR 1999;48:45-8.

Centers for Disease Control and Prevention. Public Health Service guidelines for the management of health-care worker exposures to HIV and recommendations for postexposure prophylaxis. *MMWR*, 1998, 47 (RR 7); 1-33

Centers for Disease Control and Prevention. Management of possible sexual, injecting-drug-use, or other nonoccupational exposure to HIV, including considerations related to antiretroviral therapy public health service statement. *MMWR*, 1998, 47 (RR17); 1-14

Connor EM, Sperling RS, Gelber R, Kiselev P, Scott G, O'Sullivan MJ, VanDyke R, Bey M, Shearer W, Jacobson RL, *et al.* Reduction of maternal-infant transmission of human immunodeficiency virus type 1 with zidovudine treatment. *N Engl J* Med, 1994, 331, 1173.

DiClemente, Funkhouser E, Wingood G, Fawal H, Vermund S. Russian roulette: are persons being treated with protease inhibitors gambling with high risk sex? *Int Conf AIDS*, 1998, 12:211 (abstract no. 14143)}.

Downs AM and De Vincenzi I for the European Study Group in Heterosexual Transmission of HIV. Probability of heterosexual transmission of HIV: relationship to the number of unprotected sexual contacts. *J Acquir Immun Def Synd and Hum Retro* 1996; 11:388-395.

Evans B, Darbyshire J, and Cartledge J. Should preventive antiretroviral treatment be offered following sexual exposure to HIV? Not Yet! *Sex Transm Infect,* 1998, 74, 146.

Fideli U, Allen S, Musonda R, Meinzen-Derr J, Decker D, Li L, and Aldrovandi GM. Virologic Determinants of Heterosexual Transmission in Africa. 7th Annual Conference on Retroviruses and Opportunistic Infections, San Francisco, 2000. Abstract no. 194.

Gerberding JL. Incidence and prevalence of human immunodeficiency virus, hepatitis B virus, hepatitis C virus, and cytomegalovirus among health care personnel at risk for blood exposure: final report from a longitudinal study. *J Infect Dis* 1994. 170:1410-7.

Gupta P, Mellors J, Kingsley L, Riddler, Mandaleshwar K, Schreiber S, Cronin M and C Rinaldo. High viral load in semen of human immunodeficiency virus type1 infected men at all stages of disease and its reduction by therapy with protease and nonnucleoside reverse transcriptase inhibitors. *J Virol.* 1997 Aug;71(8):62715.

Hart C, Lennox J, Pratt-Palmore M, Wright TC, Schinazi RF, EvansStrickfaden T, Bush TJ, Schnell C, Conley LJ, Clancy KA, Ellerbrock TV. Correlation of human immunodeficiency virus type 1 RNA levels in blood and the female genital tract. *J Infect Dis*, 1999, 179 (4), 871-882.

Havlir DV, Marschner IC, Hirsch MS, Collier AC, Tebas P, Bassett RL, Ioannidis JP, Holohan MK, Leavitt R, Boone G, Richman DD. Maintenance antiretroviral therapies in HIV-infected subjects with undetectable plasma HIV RNA after triple-drug therapy. *N Engl J Med*, 1998, 339, 1261-1268

Henderson DK, Fahey BJ, Willy M, Schmitt JM, Carey K, Koziol DE, Lane HC, Fedio J, Saah AJ. Risk for occupational transmission of human immunodeficiency virus type 1 (HIV-1) associated with clinical exposures: a prospective evaluation. *Ann Intern Med* 1990; 113:740-6.

Kaplan J, Hanson D, Dworkin M, Frederick T, Bertolli J, Lindegren ML, Holmberg S, Jones JL. Epidemiology of human immunodeficiency virus-associated opportunistic infections in the United States in the era of highly active antiretroviral therapy. *Clin Infect Dis*, 2000; 30,S5-14.

Lehman JS, Hecht FM, Wortley P, Lansky A, Stevens M, Fleming P. Are at-risk populations less concerned about HIV infection in the HAART era? In: Program and Abstracts of the 7th Conference on Retroviruses and Opportunistic Infections, San Francisco, CA; January 30-February 2, 2000. Abstract 198:112.

Little SJ, Daar ES, D'Aquila RT, Keiser PH, Connick E, Whitcomb JM, Hellmann NS, Petropoulos CJ, Sutton L, Pitt JA, Rosenberg ES, Koup RA, Walker BD, Richman DD. Reduced antiretroviral drug susceptibility among patients with primary HIV infection. *JAMA* 1999, 282 (12), 1142-1149.

Lurie P, Miller S, Hecht F, Chesney M, and Lo B. Postexposure prophylaxis after nonoccupational HIV exposure: Clinical, ethical, and policy considerations. *JAMA,* 1998; 280:1769-1773

Marks G, Burris S, and Peterman T. Reducing sexual transmission of HIV from those who know they are infected: the need for personal and collective responsibility. *AIDS*, 1999, 13, 297-306.

Martin N, Roland ME, Bamberger JD, Chesney MA, Waldo C, Unick J, Lay C, Katz MH, Coates TJ, and JO Kahn. Post-exposure prophylaxis after sexual or drug-use exposure to HIV: final results from the San Francisco post-exposure prevention (PEP) project. Presented at the 7th Conference on Retroviruses and Opportunistic Infections, San Francisco, CA; January 30-February 2, 2000. Abstract 196.

McNaghten AD, Hanson D, Jones J, Dworkin MS, Ward JW. Effects of antiretroviral therapy and opportunistic illness primary chemoprophylaxis on survival after AIDS diagnosis. *AIDS*, 1999, 13, 1687-1695.Morris A, Zorrilla C, Vajaranant M, Dobles A, Cu-Uvin S, Jones T, Harwell J, Carlan S, Allen D. A review of protease inhibitors (PI) Use in 89 pregnancies. 6th Annual Conference on Retroviruses and Opportunistic Infections, Chicago, 1999. Abstract no. 686.

Murphy S, Miller L, Appleby R, Marks G and Mansergh G. Antiretroviral drugs and sexual behavior in gay and bisexual men: when optimism enhances risk *Int Conf AIDS*, 1998, 12:211 (abstract no. 14137).

National Center for Health Statistics. Health, United States, 1999 with Health and Aging Chartbook. Hyattsville, Maryland: 1999.

Otten RA, Smith DK, Adams DR, Pullium JK, Jackson E, Kim CN, Jaffe H, Janssen R, Butera S, Folks TM. Efficacy of postexposure prophylaxis after intravaginal exposure of pigtailed macaques to a humanderived retrovirus (human immunodeficiency virus type 2). *J Virol.* 2000 Oct;74(20):97715.

Palella F, Delaney M, Moorman A, Loveless MO, Fuhrer J, Satten GA, Aschman DJ, Holmberg SD. Declining morbidity and mortality among patients with advanced human immunodeficiency virus infection. *N Engl J Med*, 1998, 338, 853-860.

Pialoux G, Raffi F, BrunVezinet F, Meiffredy V, Flandre P, Gastaut JA, Dellamonica P, Yeni P, Delfraissy JF, Aboulker JP. A randomized trial of three maintenance regimens given after three months of induction therapy with zidovudine, lamivudine, and indinavir in previously untreated HIV1infected patients. *N Engl J Med*, 1998, 339, 1269-1276

Quinn TC, Wawer MJ, Sewankambo N, Serwadda D, Li C, WabwireMangen F, Meehan MO, Lutalo T, Gray RH. Viral load and heterosexual transmission of human immunodeficiency virus type 1. *N Engl J Med* 2000;342:921-9.

Schwarcz-Kaplan S. Trends in HIV incidence among STD clients in the San Francisco Health Department-1989-98. Presented at National HIV Prevention Conference, 1999, August 29-September 1, Atlanta, Georgia.

Shaffer N, Roongpisuthipong A, Siriwasin W, Chotpitayasunondh T, Chearskul S, Young NL, Parekh B, Mock PA, Bhadrakom C, Chinayon P, Kalish ML, Phillips SK, Granade TC, Subbarao S, Weniger BG, Mastro TD. Maternal viral load and perinatal HIV-1 subtype E transmission, Bangkok, Thailand. *J Infect Dis, 1999,* 179, 590-599.

Shapiro M, Morton S, McCafrey D, Senterfitt J, Fleishman J, Perlman J, Athey L, Keesey J, Goldman D, Berry S, Bozzette S *et al.* Variations in the care of HIV-infected adults in the United States. Results from the HIV cost and services utilization study. *JAMA*, June 23/30, 1999, 281:24, 2305-2315.

Tokars JI, Marcus R, Culver DH, Schable CA, McKibben PS, Bandea CI, Bell DM. Surveillance of HIV infection and zidovudine use among health care workers after occupational exposure to HIV-infected blood. *Ann Intern Med* 1993; 118:913-9.

UNAIDS/99.53E-WHO/CDS/CSR/EDC/99.9-WHO/FCH/HSI/99.6 AIDS epidemic update: December 1999.

Wiebe ER; Comay SE; McGregor M; Ducceschi S. Offering HIV prophylaxis to people who have been sexually assaulted: 16 months' experience in a sexual assault service. *CMAJ* 2000 Mar 7;162(5):6415

Zhang H, Geethanjali D, Beumont M, Livornese L, Uitert B, Henning K and Pomerantz R. Human Immunodeficiency virus type 1 in the semen of men receiving highly active antiretroviral therapy. *N Engl J Med.* 1998, 339, 1803-1809.

Chapter 6

The Abstinence Strategy for Reducing Sexual Risk Behavior

John B. Jemmott III and Dana Fry
University of Pennsylvania
Annenberg School for Communication

1. THE ABSTINENCE STRATEGY FOR REDUCING SEXUAL RISK BEHAVIOR

One of the most contentious issues in HIV prevention efforts is the effectiveness and appropriateness of abstinence, the sexual-risk reduction strategy that encourages adolescents to delay sexual intercourse, if they are not sexually experienced, and to cease having sexual intercourse, if they are sexually active. The use of this strategy has been vigorously debated among educators, public health experts, parents, and other advocates for youth. Abstinence intervention proponents suggest that unless the sole message is abstinence, sex education encourages adolescents to have sexual intercourse. Opponents of the abstinence-only approach suggest that abstinence interventions are ineffective and unrealistic given the pervasiveness of sexual involvement among adolescents.

The appeal of the abstinence approach is that abstaining from sexual involvement eliminates the possibility of unintended pregnancy and sexual transmitted disease (STD), including HIV infection. Moreover, adolescents, particularly young adolescents, may not have the knowledge and judgment to make informed choices about methods to protect themselves from these ominous possibilities or to grapple with their adverse consequences. Young adolescents may lack the cognitive and emotional ability to accept their sexuality and to think about their sexuality in the objective and rational manner that is necessary to plan for sexual intercourse (Cvetkovich & Grote,

1983). Using condoms requires the skill to use them correctly and the motivation to use them consistently to maximize their effectiveness. Practicing abstinence eliminates these considerations. Consistent with this sentiment, the U.S. Congress as part of the Welfare Reform Act of 1996 has allocated $50 million per year for 1998-2002 for educational programs that teach the social, psychological, and health benefits of abstaining from sexual activity. All 50 states have applied for funding. Because this entitlement program includes a 75% cost-sharing provision with the states, over $400 million may be spent on abstinence programs during the 5-year period.

Recommending abstinence raises the question of whether the strategy is realistic. It may be reasonable to admonish young people to abstain from alcohol and drug use or cigarette smoking. To be sure, interventions to discourage such behaviors have been effective. But asking adolescents to abstain from sexual intercourse may be qualitatively different. They could never engage in these other risk behaviors during a lifetime, but at some point in their life, they will have sexual intercourse as they make the transition to adulthood. In this respect, sexual intercourse differs from many other kinds of risk behaviors. Sexual involvement is a part of adulthood. In this connection, the fact that the appropriateness of the federal abstinence-only spending initiative has been questioned is not surprising. The American Medical Association (AMA), for instance, recently released a report recommending against abstinence-only programs and in favor of comprehensive, developmentally appropriate sex education programs (Shelton, 2000). In a similar vein, DiClemente (1998) suggests that the allocation of extensive financial and personnel resources to delivering abstinence programs without empirical support appears to be an outcome of "a clash of ideology and science."

Although the abstinence strategy is very much a part of public policy, a systematic consideration of the effectiveness of abstinence interventions has been absent. Pushing polemics and politics aside, what does the scientific evidence say about the efficacy of the abstinence strategy in reducing sexual risk behavior? What are the long-term effects of abstinence interventions? Are abstinence interventions more effective in some populations than in other populations? Answers to these questions would inform the current public policy debate. This chapter is an effort to address these issues. It reviews the literature on the efficacy of abstinence interventions in reducing sexual risk behavior.

2. SEXUAL ACTIVITY AMONG ADOLESCENTS

Sexual involvement of adolescents and the consequences of such involvement are the pressing problems that abstinence interventions are designed to address. About 56% of adolescent women and 73% of adolescent men have had sexual intercourse by the time they are 18 years of age (Alan Guttmacher Institute, 1994). Age, gender, race, and ethnicity are all related to sexual activity. Older adolescents are much more likely to have initiated sexual intercourse and to report recent sexual activity. Adolescent men begin having sexual intercourse at a younger age than do adolescent women. In addition, African Americans initiate sexual intercourse at a younger age than do Latinos who initiate sexual intercourse at a younger age than do whites (Kann et al., 1998).

Although the use of latex condoms can substantially reduce the risk of STD, including HIV (Cates & Stone, 1992; CDC, 1988, 1993), most sexually active adolescents do not use condoms consistently (Hingson et al., 1990; Keller et al., 1991; Sonenstein et al., 1989). African American adolescents are more likely to use condoms than are Latinos and whites. Condom use is also related to age. Failure to use condoms is especially likely among adolescents who have been sexually active during early adolescence (Zelnik, Kantner, & Ford, 1981; Pratt, Mosher, Bachrach, & Horn, 1984; Taylor, Kagay, & Leichenko, 1986). The younger adolescents are the first time they have sexual intercourse, the less likely they are to use condoms on that occasion (Sonenstein et al., 1989). Only 27% of Black males, who were younger than 12 at first intercourse, used condoms on that occasion. Among Black males who were between the ages of 12 and 14 years, the percentage increased to 39%, and among those 15 to 17 years of age, the figure was 57%. This pattern of findings suggests that delaying the onset of intercourse may increase the likelihood that adolescents will use condoms when they initiate intercourse. If we expand the analysis to the use of <u>any</u> kind of contraceptive method, the age of onset is highly related to the likelihood of using contraception, from 27% for those under 12 years, to 43% for those 12-14 years old, to 66% for those 15-17.

The 1970s and 1980s witnessed an upward trend in the rates of sexual intercourse among adolescents. However, this trend has abated and actually reversed in recent years. Data from the Youth Risk Behavior Survey indicate that the percentage of high school students who had ever had sexual intercourse decreased by 11% between 1991 and 1997. More children are practicing abstinence by delaying the initiation of sexual intercourse. In addition, the prevalence of condom use among currently sexually active students increased 23% during that same period (CDC, 1998). Although these reductions in risk behavior are exciting, it remains the case that far too many adolescents still fail to use condoms consistently and have sexual intercourse with multiple partners.

Statistics on STD and unintended pregnancy provide clear evidence of the consequences of unprotected sexual intercourse among adolescents. Each year one in four sexually active adolescents (totaling three million per year) contracts a STD (Alan Guttmacher Institute, 1994; Eng & Butler, 1997). Although the adolescent birth rate dropped 5% between 1991 and 1994, the rate was still higher in 1994 than in any year during the period from 1974 to 1989. Moreover, despite the decline, the adolescent birth rate in the United States is still among the highest in developed countries (Singh & Darroch, 2000). Interestingly, a recent analysis suggests that increased abstinence among adolescent women made a substantial contribution to the decline in the U. S. adolescent birth rates (Darroch & Singh, 1999).

Adolescents are also at risk for sexually transmitted HIV infection. Although adolescents represent less than 1% of the total reported AIDS cases in the United States, about 17% of reported AIDS cases involve young adults 20 to 29 years of age (CDC, 1999a). Many of them were infected during adolescence because about 10 to 12 years typically elapse between the time a person is infected with HIV and the appearance of the clinical signs sufficient to warrant a diagnosis of AIDS. Newly diagnosed cases of HIV infection, while limited to the 29 states with confidential reporting, also help to clarify the risk of AIDS among adolescents. Individuals 13 to 24 years of age comprised 15% of the HIV infections reported through June 1999 (CDC, 1999a).

The proportion of female AIDS and HIV cases is much greater among young people than among adults. Among adults, the overwhelming majority of cases have been among men, whereas among adolescents, the gender split has been more even. In addition, the proportion of cases among females has increased steadily over time. In fact, in 1998, for the first time, slightly more AIDS cases were reported among women 13 to 19 years of age than among their male counterparts. The most common mode of transmission among adolescent women was heterosexual exposure (CDC, 1999b). These data on sexual behavior, unplanned pregnancy, and STD make a strong case that interventions are needed to reduce sexual risks among adolescents.

3. CHALLENGES IN ABSTINENCE INTERVENTION RESEARCH

Interventions to encourage adolescents to practice abstinence face several challenges. Adolescents often feel invulnerable and do not perceive themselves to be at risk (Sanderson & Jemmott, 1996; Walter & Vaughan,

1993; Stanton et al., 1996). Accordingly, it may be difficult to convince them that their sexual involvement at a young age may have adverse consequences for them personally. It may be difficult to persuade adolescents to practice abstinence if they have decided to be sexually active. Adolescents also may not practice abstinence if they hold negative beliefs about its consequences, including the belief that they might lose their romantic partner, or if it conflicts with their community or social norms. For example, it may be difficult to persuade adolescents to practice sexual abstinence if they perceive that all their friends are having sexual intercourse. Sexual abstinence may be an especially difficult behavior to induce when compared with increased condom use. Adolescents are likely to face far more pressure from peers and will be exposed to far more messages in the media that encourage them to have sexual intercourse compared with pressure and messages encouraging them not to use condoms. Thus, an abstinence intervention's message must compete with an onslaught of explicit and implicit countervailing influences to which adolescents are exposed. Even if an intervention successfully surmounts these obstacles, it may not have detectable effects on sexual behavior if that behavior is sporadic, which is often true of the young adolescents who are the prime targets of abstinence interventions.

4. CRITERIA FOR ESTABLISHING THAT INTERVENTIONS HAVE INFLUENCED BEHAVIOR

A number of methodological requirements must be satisfied before we can conclude that an intervention has influenced sexual risk behavior. Correlational studies, by their very design, cannot establish causal relations between interventions and outcome measures of sexual behavior. Random assignment to intervention and control groups is required to draw causal inferences. To establish that apparent effects are due to the content of the interventions rather than nonspecific factors such as special attention or group interaction per se, studies should include an attentional control group. In this way, alternative explanations in terms of Hawthorne effects can be ruled out (Cook & Campbell, 1979). The intervention should be implemented with fidelity so that significant effects or the lack of significant effects can be attributed to the intervention content rather than extraneous factors, including characteristics of the facilitators or health educators. The postintervention follow-up period should be long enough to detect intervention effects. In other words, there has to be sufficient time to observe the behavior of interest. Adolescents' sexual behavior is sporadic. A sufficient number of participants must be studied to provide statistical power. A sufficient proportion of participants must be retained at follow-up to draw unbiased conclusions about intervention effects. As we shall see, the majority of the abstinence intervention studies do not meet these criteria.

5. CHARACTERISTICS OF ABSTINENCE INTERVENTION STUDIES

We identified 9 published reports of 11 abstinence intervention studies with adolescents that included a control group and a measure of sexual behavior as an outcome variable. We excluded abstinence intervention studies that did not have a control group or sexual behavior outcome measure (e.g., Olsen, Weed, Daly, & Jensen 1992). We treated as multiple studies a single article reporting results on separate samples that participated in distinct experimental designs. For example, one article reported intervention trials with three different designs testing the same interventions (Kirby, Korpi, Barth, & Cagampang, 1997). Table 1 presents characteristics of the studies.

Table 1. [Characteristics of Abstinence Intervention Studies Conducted with Adolescents]

Author (year)	Setting	N (% women)	Race-ethnicity (%)	Conditions
Randomized Controlled Trials—Individuals as the Unit				
Jemmott et al. (1998)	Community	659 (53%), mean age = 11.8	100% African American	1. 2-session, 8-hour safe sex AIDS intervention 2. 2-session, 8-hou abstinence-based AIDS intervention 3. 2-session, 8-hou general healt promotion control
Kirby, Korpi, Barth et al. (1997, Design 3)	Community	516 (56%), mean age = 12.8	3% African American, 50% Asian, 20% Latino, 1% Native American , 8% white	1. 5-session, 4.5-hou adult-led abstinence only intervention 2. No-treatment control
Miller et al. (1993)	Home	548 families, mean age = 13.9	97% white, Mormons	1. Video 2. Video and printe material 3. No-treatment control
Kirby, Korpi,	School	4653 (56%),	9% African	1. 5-session 4 hour adul

Author (year)	Setting	N (% women)	Race-ethnicity (%)	Conditions
Barth et al. (1997, Design 1)		mean age = 12.8	American, 10% Asian, 34% Latino, 5% Native American, 34% white	led abstinence-only intervention 2. 5-session 4 hour peer-led abstinence-only intervention 3. No-treatment control
Kirby, Korpi, Barth et al. (1997, Design 2)	School	5431 (56%), mean age = 12.8	9% African American, 13% Asian, 30% Latino, 5% Native American, 39% white	1. 5-session 4 hour adult-led abstinence-only intervention 2. No-treatment control
St. Pierre et al. (1995)	Community	359 (25%), mean age = 13.6	42% African American, 14% Latino, 45% white	1. .3-session, 4.5 hour abstinence-only intervention 2. No-treatment control
Christopher & Roosa (1990)	School	320 (61%), mean age = 12.8	21% African American, 69% Latino, 2% Native American, 8% white	1. 6-session, 4.5 hour abstinence-only intervention 2. No-treatment control
Howard & McCabe (1990)	School	536, mean age = 13.5	99% African American	1. 5-session, 4 hour abstinence-only intervention 2. No-treatment control
Jorgensen et al. (1993)	School	91 (53%), mean age = 14.4	43% African American, 7% Latino, 45% white	1. 9-session, 7-hour abstinence-based intervention 2. No-treatment control
Roosa & Christopher (1990)	School	528 (57%), mean age = 13.0	15% African American, 64% Latino, 12% white, 5% Indian	1. 6-session, 4.5 hour abstinence-only intervention 2. No-treatment control
Young et al. (1992)	School	209 7th and 8th graders		1. 24-session, 18 hour abstinence-oriented intervention 2. Health education control 3. No-treatment control

The abstinence intervention studies varied along several dimensions, including design, setting, study population, and abstinence message. Randomized controlled trials provide the most internally valid test of the efficacy of interventions. Randomization was at the level of the individual in some studies (3 studies). In other studies, it was at the level of the group, including classrooms or entire schools (2 studies). There were also nonrandomized correlational studies that included a control group and preintervention and postintervention assessments (6 studies), which is one of the most internally valid of the quasi-experimental designs (Cook & Campbell, 1979).

The studies were conducted in a variety of settings, including schools (7 studies), community (3 studies), and home (1 study). The predominant ethnic group was white in four studies, African American in two studies, Latino in two studies, and Asian in one study. The mean age of the adolescents in the studies ranged from 11.8 years to 14.4 years, with a median of 12.9. Adolescence is often divided into three developmental stages: early adolescence which is 11 to 13 years of age, middle adolescence which is 14 to 16 years of age, and late adolescence, which 17 to 21 years of age. Thus, these studies primarily focused on youth in early to middle adolescence. Abstinence messages are often thought to be appropriate for adolescents in this age group because they are less apt to have initiated sexual intercourse. It may be easier to delay initiation of sexual intercourse among the sexually inexperienced than to decrease sexual intercourse among the sexually active.

6. ABSTINENCE MESSAGES

Simply put, abstinence is refraining from sexual intercourse: those who have never had sexual intercourse should not initiate sexual intercourse; those who have had sexual intercourse should refrain from having further sexual intercourse. Nevertheless, there is room for variation in abstinence messages. Interventions differ in the length of time that adolescents are advised to refrain from sexual intercourse. Some interventions state that adolescents should refrain from sexual intercourse until marriage. Others promote abstinence until adulthood, or until a later time when they are mature and independent enough to handle the consequences of having sexual intercourse. One criticism of the abstinence until marriage message is that it reflects a heterosexual bias that makes it inappropriate for some adolescents (Kantor, 1992). For example, it does not apply to gay adolescents. Such interventions fail to provide gay adolescents with appropriate messages about sexual prevention.

The definition of abstinence in the federally funded program is that "abstinence from sexual activity outside of marriage is the expected standard for all school-age children." This is commonly interpreted to mean that adolescents should refrain from sexual intercourse until marriage. It would seem that another interpretation is that adolescents should refrain from sexual intercourse until marriage or until they are no longer of school age.

It should also be noted that most abstinence interventions have been primarily designed to prevent unplanned pregnancy. They do not focus on risk of STDs or HIV, and do not address non-coital risk behaviors. The focus on pregnancy prevention may, at least in part, explain some of the emphasis on abstinence until marriage. If one believes that pregnancy should occur only in the context of marriage, then it makes sense to encourage youth to abstain from sexual intercourse until marriage.

Another way in which abstinence interventions differ is in how they handle the issue of condom use. Some programs focus exclusively on abstinence and make no mention of condom use or other forms of contraception. This is the abstinence-only focus required in programs funded under the federal abstinence initiative. In this view, any mention of contraception or prophylaxis would send adolescents a mixed message, undermining the recommendation of abstinence and encouraging sexual activity.

Other programs focus on abstinence, but make brief mention of the value of condoms or contraception if or when adolescents choose to become sexually active. This approach has been called "abstinence-based." In this view, abstinence should be promoted, but birth control and disease prevention are essential to protect youth who choose to have sexual intercourse. Still, other programs, while focusing on abstinence, downplay the effectiveness of contraception, including condoms, and may even provide inaccurate information about their effectiveness (Kantor, 1992; Whatley & Trudell, 1993). Implicit in this approach is the view that by decreasing the perceived effectiveness of contraception and prophylaxis, it will be possible to increase the appeal of abstinence.

7. EFFECTS OF ABSTINENCE INTERVENTIONS

One of the earliest studies testing an abstinence intervention was reported by Christopher and Roosa (1990) who evaluated Success Express, a 5-session abstinence-only program, designed to prevent pregnancy among middle-school students. The participants were 320 low-income 6th and 7th grade adolescents (mean age = 12.8 years). In a quasi-experimental design, 191 received Success Express and 129 received no intervention before the 6-week follow-up. Intervention participants and control group participants were drawn from different classrooms in eight schools, and five schools also received a standard health curriculum that the authors did not describe. The participants were predominantly Latino (69%) and African American (21%). The 5-session curriculum focused on (a) self-esteem and family values, (b) adolescent growth and development, including reproductive knowledge, (c) pressures adolescents encounter to become sexually active, (d) communication strategies and skills to effectively say no to sexual intercourse, and (e) future life goals and goal-setting skills. Christopher and Roosa (1990) found no significant difference in self-reported sexual intercourse at 6-week follow-up between students who received Success Express and those in the control group.

Roosa and Christopher (1990) also tested the effectiveness of the Success Express curriculum. In a quasi-experimental design, they implemented the study with 20 different sites, including public and parochial schools, community-based organizations, and Indian Reservations that all expressed interest in adopting Success Express. Control group classrooms and Success Express classrooms were selected in the schools at the discretion of teachers or principals. The participants were 528 6th, 7th, and 8th grade adolescents (mean age = 13.0 years). Once again, there were no significant effects of the intervention on either attitudes or sexual behavior at 6-week follow-up. In addition, there were no significant intervention effects among students who were virgins or among students who were sexually experienced at baseline.

One problem with both of these studies is the relatively brief follow-up period. The sporadic nature of sexual activity among young adolescents may have made it difficult to detect differences in the short amount of time the adolescents were followed. On the other hand, the fact that the intervention apparently did not cause favorable changes on attitudes would seem to suggest that changes in behavior were unlikely even with longer-term follow-up.

Parents are thought to have an important impact on adolescents' sexual behavior. Parents provide models of what is appropriate by virtue of the relationships they display to their children. Parents directly teach values. Parents can provide information to their children about sexual behavior and risk reduction. There is some evidence that good parent-child communication about sexual matters is related to reduced risky sexual behavior among adolescents. Thus, one potentially useful approach to sexual risk reduction would be to involve parents. Several studies have attempted to involve parents to varying degrees in abstinence interventions.

One way to involve parents is to give the adolescent participants homework assignments to discuss abstinence with their parents. This approach was used in the Living Smart curriculum. Young, Core-Gebhart, and Marx (1992) tested the effects of the curriculum in five junior high schools in Arkansas. Using a quasi-experimental design, they assigned 209 7th and 8th grade students in intact classrooms to one of three conditions:

(a) Living Smart curriculum, (b) the standard school health curriculum, or (c) no-intervention control group. Designed to fit into 24 days of health class, the Living Smart curriculum was comprised of three units: (a) Knowing Myself, which focused on self-esteem, puberty, values, and decision making, (b) Relating to Others, which focused on communication with family, friends, dating, and sexual decision making, and (c) My Future, which focused on goal setting and life planning. Homework assignments were designed to increase discussions about sexuality between parents and adolescents.

Young et al. found that students who received the Living Smart curriculum reported more positive attitudes toward abstinence and were more likely to discuss sexuality with their parents compared with students in the standard health and control conditions. In addition, the authors performed cross-tabular chi-square analyses examining differences across the three groups in whether they reported having sex in the past month. Although they found significant differences, and they conclude that students who received the curriculum were less likely to have had sexual intercourse in the last month at 1-week follow-up, the cells that differ are small, and the authors conclude that, "Chi-Square may not be a valid test in this situation." These results are also difficult to interpret because the participants were asked at 1-week follow-up to report their sexual behavior in the previous month; hence, the reporting period for participants' sexual-behavior overlapped substantially with the intervention period. Accordingly, the study does not demonstrate that the apparent intervention effects persisted postintervention. Moreover, even if the follow-up period did not overlap with the intervention period, a 1-week period is too brief to judge accurately behavior change given the low frequency of sexual behavior and the small sample size. In addition, Young et al. did not report the race/ethnicity or gender of the participants, making it difficult to assess the generalizability of the results.

Jorgensen, Potts, & Camp (1993) tested the effects of the Project Taking Charge, which also had a parental component. Home economics classes in schools in areas of Delaware and Mississippi with low income, high adolescent pregnancy rates, and high unemployment rates were randomly assigned to Project Taking Charge or a no-intervention control condition. The participants were 91 7th graders (mean age = 14.4). About 51% were African American, 41% were white, and 3% were Hispanic. Project Taking Charge is a 6-week, 6-unit abstinence-only curriculum that covers basic development and anatomy, pregnancy, and STDs. It covered family values and communication and vocational goal setting and planning. It also included career development as a way to reinforce the abstinence message.

An innovative feature of the curriculum is the inclusion of three sessions for parents.

Jorgensen et al. (1993), reported that some parents did not attend the parental sessions, but they did not track parent participation rates. The results revealed that among the 50 adolescents who were sexually inexperienced at baseline, 77% of the Project Taking Charge group remained abstinent at six months, as compared with only 50% of the control group ($p = .051$). However, Jorgensen, et al. (1993) did not report any behavioral data for sexually experienced participants or for the sample as a whole, which makes it difficult to judge the effectiveness of the intervention. A key question for abstinence interventions is whether they are effective irrespective of sexual experience. Abstinence interventions seek to not only delay the initiation of sexual intercourse, but also curb sexual intercourse among those who are sexually experienced. Much of the criticism of such interventions revolves around the issue of whether an abstinence intervention would work with those who are already sexually experienced. The Jorgensen et al. report leaves unanswered several important questions: Was the intervention effective ignoring sexual experience? Was it effective with those who were sexually experienced? Was it significantly more effective with sexually inexperienced adolescents as compared with sexually experienced adolescents?

Another way to involve parents is to fully integrate them into the intervention. Miller et al. (1993), tested the effects of Facts & feelings, a home-based abstinence-only video sex education curriculum. They randomly assigned 548 families with 7th or 8th grade adolescents to receive (a) the videotape sex education curriculum with mailed newsletters, (b) the videotapes without newsletters, or (c) neither. The FACTS & feelings material was divided into six units—"Changes," "Values," "Facts," "Meanings," "Choices," and "Skills"—designed to be viewed in six sessions. Each unit consisted of a 15- to 20-minute video. During the three months after the materials were distributed, telephone calls were made biweekly to the participants in the two intervention conditions to encourage their use of the program material and to collect usage data. Both the video material and printed materials were designed to be used at home by parents and adolescents jointly. This feature of the curriculum would seem to serve to encourage the parents to actively participate in the intervention.

The study was conducted in Utah, and over 90% of the parents were white and over 85% were Mormon. Parents and adolescents completed questionnaires before materials were distributed, immediately after the 3-month period of biweekly telephone calls (posttest), and one year after the materials were distributed (9-month follow-up). About 92% of the families that completed the pretest also completed the delayed posttest one year later. Attrition did not differ by condition.

The intervention groups showed significantly larger increases in parent-adolescent communication regarding sexual topics at posttest than did the control group. However, the differences were no longer significant at 9-month follow-up. In addition, there were no significant effects on self-reported sexual behavior or intentions for such behavior. Although this was a well-designed and well-executed study, one difficulty was that the percentage of participants who reported sexual intercourse was small, ranging from only 3% to 5%. Thus, the relatively low level of sexual involvement may have constrained the ability to detect intervention effects. As Miller et al. noted, a longer-term follow-up and increased sample size would have provided a more powerful test. Nevertheless, this randomized controlled trial does show that a home-based video program can be used by families and can increase parent-adolescent communication about sexual issues, which has been related to adolescents' sexual behavior.

Although there is a growing consensus that it is possible to change sexual risk behavior in a variety of populations, a key question that has emerged is how to maintain behavior change in the long term. It would seem that the need for strategies to maintain long-term behavior change would be particularly acute for abstinence interventions targeting young adolescents. As mentioned earlier, adolescents are likely to be exposed to peer pressure and media messages that contradict the abstinence message. Four studies we identified had follow-ups of at least 12 months.

The first study, conducted by St. Pierre et al. (1995), tested a strategy for increasing the duration of behavior change. Booster sessions attempt to reinforce and reinstate the information and skills critical for behavior change. St. Pierre et al (1995), incorporated booster sessions in an investigation of the effectiveness of Stay Smart, a 9-session abstinence-only curriculum. The curriculum was part of a more general health-risk program that included alcohol, drug, and smoking prevention. Stay Smart is implemented by adults and takes a personal and social competence approach to prevention, a broader version of the social influence model (St. Pierre, et al., 1995). Specifically, it emphasized not only peer and other social influences to engage in negative health behaviors, but also an array of general personal and social skills for coping with life.

To evaluate the curriculum, 14 Boys and Girls clubs across the U.S participated in a pretest-posttest, nonequivalent groups design. Five were in the Stay Smart Only condition and received the 9-session Stay Smart curriculum, five were in the Stay Smart Plus a 2-year Booster Program condition and received the Stay Smart plus seven booster sessions, and four were in the no-intervention control condition. The two treatment conditions were assigned based on specialized training that their staffs had previously received in order to participate in another program called "Smart Moves." The adolescent participants (mean age = 13.6) were 161 whites (45%), African Americans (42%), and Latinos (14%). About 25% were women. Unlike studies in schools, participants attend these clubs voluntarily, and the program context is one of promoting resiliency among youths at risk (i.e., their motto, "the club that beats the streets"). Data were collected preintervention and at 3-, 15-, and 27-month follow up. The results were reported only for those adolescents who completed measures at all four data collection periods.

St. Pierre et al. found that, at the 15-month follow-up, sexually experienced adolescents who received the Stay Smart intervention had marginally lower rates of sexual activity than did those in the control group ($p < .10$). At 27-month follow-up, they had significantly lower rates of sexual activity than did controls and, surprisingly, those in the booster condition after 27 months. In contrast, St. Pierre et al. found no treatment effects among sexually inexperienced adolescents. This pattern of findings, conflicts with the common belief that abstinence interventions are most effective with sexually inexperienced adolescents. Although the effort to assess long-term behavior change and the use of booster sessions are strengths of this study, the results are difficult to interpret. Most important, the attrition rate was extremely high. About 58% of participants were loss to 27-month follow-up and excluded from analyses. It is unclear whether results would have been the same with those participants. There were also differential attrition rates across condition among non-virgins. Younger non-virgins in the Stay Smart Booster condition were more likely to drop out than were those in the control group. African-American non-virgins in the Stay Smart Booster condition were more likely to drop out than their counterparts in the other two conditions. White non-virgins more likely to drop out of the Stay Smart Only condition than the other two conditions. In addition, booster sessions may have been inconsistent across sites. The facilitators could chose the seven modules they used from a total of 10 booster modules. This inconsistency may have led to an underestimation of the effectiveness of the boosters.

Howard and McCabe (1990) conducted a quasi-experimental study with long-term follow-up to evaluate Postponing Sexual Involvement (PSI), an abstinence intervention that included a booster session. The program had two parts. The first part was taught by adults and consisted of five classes on reproduction, family planning, and STD, including contraception and condom use. The second part was taught by student leaders, 11th and 12th grade high school students and consisted of five classes on abstinence attitudes and skills. One to three months after the first four student-led classes, the fifth class was held as a booster to reinforce the program content after the students had time to think about the material. The intervention was based on social influence or "social inoculation" theory and the concept that young people engage in early sexual activity partly because of social influences, both general and more specifically from their peers. The model uses the public health concept of immunization as a strategy for combating social and peer pressures that encourage unhealthy behaviors.

The participants were 536 low-income African American 8th grade students in the Atlanta public schools who had participated in all five of the study's interviews. A total of 395 were from 25 program schools in Atlanta, GA and 141 were from 29 other local schools outside of the Atlanta school district that did not receive the program. There were no significant differences between program and no-program school students at baseline on background variables that would bias any outcomes in favor of the program group. Data were collected via telephone interviews conducted at the beginning, middle, and end of the 8th grade—when the program was given—and at the beginning and end of the 9th grade. Medical records of young women in both the program and no-program groups were reviewed for information regarding sexual involvement, pregnancy tests, treatment of STDs, and family planning counseling and services.

Howard and McCabe reported that among sexually inexperienced students, those who participated in the program were significantly less likely to initiate sexual intercourse than were those in no-program schools. This difference was significant at the end of 8th grade, the beginning of 9th grade, and end of 9th grade. Program women also experienced fewer pregnancies than did no-program women. In contrast, there were no significant differences in the incidence of sexual intercourse or use of contraceptives between program and no-program students who were sexually experienced before the program. Although Howard and McCabe reported that among students who were sexually inexperienced at baseline but had sexual intercourse subsequently, nearly half in the program group and close to one-third in the no-program group used contraceptives, no statistical test or significance probability was reported for this difference.

One problem with this study is that the extent to which the intervention effects were due to the five abstinence modules rather than the five sexuality classes that preceded them is unclear (Howard & McCabe, 1992; St. Pierre, 1995). In addition, although results were presented separately for sexually experienced and sexually inexperienced participants, results for the whole sample were not reported. No significance tests were reported comparing the effects of the intervention among sexually experienced and sexually inexperienced adolescents. The sexually experienced group was much smaller than was the sexually inexperienced group. Lack of significance in the smaller group might be due to having less statistical power in the sexually experienced group than in the larger sexually inexperienced group. Thus, although the study found significant intervention effects among sexually inexperienced adolescents at long-term follow-up, it had several methodological problems.

More recently, Kirby, Korpi, Barth et al. (1997) evaluated the effectiveness of Project ENABL or "Education Now and Babies Later," a modified version of the PSI curriculum, among 7th and 8th graders in California. The project used three different research designs that we will treat as three different studies. In Design 1, students within selected schools were randomly assigned by classroom to a youth-led intervention, an adult-led intervention, or a no-intervention control group. Data were collected at baseline, 3-month follow-up, and 17-month follow-up. In Design 2, schools were randomly assigned to the adult-led intervention or control group. The intervention schools also received various school-wide activities in support of the ENABL initiative, whereas the control schools received the standard human sexuality education curricula. Data were collected at baseline and 17-month follow-up. In Design 3, adolescents were recruited from community-based agencies and randomly assigned to the adult-led intervention or a no-intervention control group. Data were collected at baseline and 17-month follow-up.

The study included 10,600 adolescents from schools and community-based agencies statewide. Analyses were performed on data from the 7,340 adolescents (mean age = 12.8 years) who completed baseline and follow-up questionnaires. About 75% of the students completed both the baseline and the 17-month follow-up. Among those in the Design 1, 91% also completed the 3-month follow-up. There were no significant differences in attrition between intervention and control conditions. About 39% of the participants were Latino, 35% were white, 12% were African American, 11% were Asian, and 1% were Native American. In separate analyses on data from each of the designs, Kirby et al. found no significant effects of the interventions on initiation of sexual intercourse, frequency of sexual intercourse, number of sexual partners, condom use, or contraception use at 3-month follow-up or 17-month follow-up. In addition, analyses performed on potential mediators of intervention effects revealed relatively few significant differences.

Thus, unlike Howard and McCabe who found that the PSI was effective in reducing risk behavior, at least with sexually inexperienced adolescents, Kirby et al. found that it was ineffective. What might account for these differing results? There were several differences between the samples included in the two studies. The participants in Kirby et al. were 7th and 8th graders, whereas those in Howard and McCabe were 8th graders. However, it has been argued that abstinence interventions should be more effective with younger adolescents. Another difference is that 24% of Howard and McCabe's sample were not virgins at baseline, whereas only 11% of Kirby et al.'s sample were not virgins. This difference, along with a larger overall sample size in Kirby et al.'s replication, suggests that the latter study would have had even more power to find treatment effects among virgins than did Howard and McCabe. Only 12% of the participants in Kirby et al. were African Americans, whereas 99% of the participants in Howard and McCabe were African Americans. Thus, it might be concluded that PSI may be effective only with African Americans. However, this conclusion is not supported by Kirby et al.'s finding of no significant differences in intervention effects as a function of gender, race or ethnicity, or history of serious romantic involvement. Adults led the majority Kirby et al.'s groups, whereas youth led Howard and McCabe's groups. However, Kirby et al. found that neither adult-led nor teen-led groups were effective.

In the Howard and McCabe study, the 5-session abstinence curriculum was preceded by a 5-session course in human sexuality and decision-making. In the Kirby et al. (1997) study, the participants were required to receive instruction in human sexuality before participating in the abstinence curriculum. However, they did not receive the 5-module course that the participants in the Howard and McCabe received. Because the contribution of the first five human sexuality modules to the intervention effects in Howard and McCabe's study is unknown, the contribution of the absence of these five modules to the lack of intervention effects found by Kirby et al. is also unknown.

Howard and McCabe did not report data on potential mediators of intervention effects. Therefore, the variables that might have mediated effects in their study are unknown. However, it would seem that in order to achieve behavior change there must have been significant effects on mediators. In contrast, Kirby et al. did measure potential mediators. They found scant evidence that the interventions caused positive changes on the mediators. Given the lack of effects of mediators, perhaps it is not surprising that there was a lack of effect on sexual behavior.

Kirby et al. study was much larger than was Howard and McCabe. Quality control is more difficult in a large study than in a small study, and reduced quality control could contribute to reduced intervention effectiveness. Failure to find strong intervention effects on mediators could reflect poor quality control. Another major difference was the presence in Kirby et al. of community-wide campaigns (flyer distribution, assemblies, and rallies) and statewide media campaigns delivering abstinence messages to participants in both the intervention and control conditions. To the extent that these campaigns were effective, differences between intervention and control group participants might have been reduced. In sum, the conflicting results of these two studies are difficult to explain. There were numerous differences between them, some were consistent with smaller effects in Kirby et al., but some would predict larger effects in Kirby et al.

It is often asserted that interventions for adolescents may be especially efficacious if peers implement them. Howard and McCabe's findings illustrate the successful use of peer facilitators. On the other hand, adults may generate more respect and may be perceived as more credible sources of information because of their experience and maturity. Many successful interventions have used adult facilitators. Jemmott, Jemmott, and Fong (1998) conducted a study designed to address two questions regarding sexual risk reduction interventions for adolescents: Which risk reduction messages are most effective with adolescents? Which types of individuals are likely to be the most effective in delivering those messages? The participants were 659 6th and 7th grade African American adolescents (mean age = 11.8 years). Preintervention questionnaire responses revealed that approximately 25% of the participants were sexually experienced. The participants were randomly assigned to one of three interventions: an abstinence-based intervention, a safer sex intervention, or a general health promotion intervention, which served as the control group. In addition, they were randomly assigned to a small group led by an adult facilitator or two peer co-facilitators, high school students (mean age = 16 years).

Each intervention incorporated the Be Proud! Be Responsible! theme (Jemmott, Jemmott, & McCaffree, 1995) that encouraged the participants to be proud of themselves and their community, to behave responsibly for the sake of themselves and their community, and to consider their goals for the future and how unhealthful behavior might thwart the attainment of their goals. Each intervention involved eight hours of small group discussions, videos, interactive exercises, skill-building activities, and role-playing implemented over two sessions. The two HIV interventions were based on social cognitive theory, the theory of reasoned action, and its extension the theory of planned behavior, as well as information gathered from focus groups from the study population. The abstinence intervention mentioned condom use, but stressed abstinence as the only way to eliminate risk of sexually transmitted infection, and taught skills necessary to practice abstinence. The safer sex intervention acknowledged that abstinence is the best choice, but stressed that adolescents should use condoms if they decide to have sexual intercourse, and it taught the skills to use condoms. To control for "Hawthorne effects," that is, to reduce the likelihood that effects of the HIV interventions could be attributed to nonspecific features (Cook & Campbell, 1979), the control group received a health promotion intervention regarding behaviors associated with risk of cardiovascular disease, stroke, and cancer.

A total of 25 adults and 45 high school students served as facilitators in the study. These facilitators were selected because they were capable of implementing any of the interventions. The intervention that a particular facilitator was trained to implement was determined randomly. In this way, Jemmott et al. (1998) randomized facilitator characteristics across intervention conditions. Thus, the results cannot be attributed to characteristics of the facilitators as opposed to the intervention content.

Data were collected before, immediately after, and 3, 6, and 12 months after the intervention, with 93% of participants retained at the 12-month follow-up. The results revealed construct validity for the interventions. The abstinence and safer sex interventions caused positive changes on the specific theoretical variables they were designed to influence. For instance, the abstinence intervention, compared with the control group, increased the belief that abstinence can reduce risk of pregnancy and STD and HIV, the belief that abstinence can help achieve career goals, and intentions to practice abstinence. In contrast, the safer sex intervention increased condom-use knowledge, the belief that condoms do not interfere with sexual enjoyment, and self-efficacy to use condoms, as compared with the control group.

Analyses on follow-up data revealed that adolescents who received the abstinence intervention were less likely to report engaging in sexual intercourse in the three months postintervention than were those in the control condition. However, this difference was no longer significant at 6- or 12-month follow-up. The adolescents who received the safer sex intervention reported more frequent condom use than did those in the control condition at all three follow-ups. The adolescents who received the safer sex intervention reported less unprotected sexual intercourse at 3-month follow-up, but not at 6- or 12-month follow-up. However, the effects of the safer sex intervention on unprotected sexual intercourse were moderated by the adolescents' preintervention sexual experience. The safer sex intervention was especially effective among those adolescents who were sexually experienced at baseline. Among sexually experienced adolescents, the safer sex group reported less sexual intercourse as well as less unprotected sexual intercourse than did the control group at all three follow-ups. This study did not find evidence supporting the assertion that peer facilitators are especially efficacious. The effects of the interventions on self-reported sexual behavior were not significantly different with adult facilitators as compared with peer co-facilitators.

One methodological problem in research on sexual behavior is the reliance on self-report measures. There is the possibility that participants' self-reports of their behavior might be biased due to demand characteristics. Jemmott et al. addressed this issue empirically by evaluating the influence of social desirability response bias. Contrary to the view that social desirability bias accounts for the results, analyses revealed that self-reported sexual behavior and changes in self-reported behavior were unrelated to scores on a standard measure of social desirability response bias.

8. CRITIQUE OF ABSTINENCE INTERVENTIONS

Collectively, the studies reviewed in this chapter do not provide strong evidence for the effectiveness of abstinence interventions. Of the 11 studies we reviewed, five reported significant differences favoring an abstinence intervention in at least a subgroup of the participants. However, one of the studies had a follow-up period of only one week (Young et al., 1992)—too brief to be meaningful. Two others suffered from important methodological problems, including high attrition (St. Pierre et al., 1995) and nonrandom assignment to conditions (Howard & McCabe, 1990; St. Pierre et al., 1995), rendering the results difficult to interpret. Only two of the studies had sound designs and methodology. Both were randomized controlled trials and had low attrition. However, even in these studies the effects were significant only in the short term: at 6-month follow-up in one study (Jorgensen et al., 1993) and at 3-month follow-up in the other study (Jemmott et al., 1998).

On the other hand, aside from the fact that one can never prove the null hypothesis, the research we reviewed does not provide convincing evidence that abstinence-only programs are ineffective at changing behaviors. Research has not been methodologically rigorous enough to draw such a strong conclusion. For example, many of the studies that failed to find significant effects had features that may have contributed to that failure. For example, two of the studies were nonrandomized correlational studies with follow-ups of only 6-weeks (Christopher & Roosa, 1990; Roosa & Christopher, 1990). Another study (Miller et al., 1993) suffered from extreme restriction of range on the outcome measure. Although the study was a well designed and executed randomized controlled trial, only 3% to 5% of the participants reported having sexual intercourse, which would make it extremely difficult to demonstrate behavior change.

The three studies reported by Kirby et al. can be viewed in different ways. On the one hand, they may not constitute a fair replication of the Howard and McCabe (1990) study. On the other hand, they can stand on their own merits as three large randomized controlled trials that failed to find significant effects of abstinence interventions. The fact that these studies also were ineffective in influencing mediators throws some ambiguity into the mix. Was the failure to affect mediators a weakness of the abstinence curriculum? Alternatively, was it a quality control issue—a failure to deliver the intended intervention with fidelity owing to the large size of the study?

The lack of convincing evidence on the effectiveness of abstinence interventions should not be interpreted to mean that it is impossible to delay the onset of sexual intercourse or reduce the frequency of sexual intercourse. In fact, several interventions using a safer sex message have delayed sexual onset, reduced sexual activity, or reduced unprotected sexual intercourse among adolescents (e.g. Jemmott, Jemmott, & Fong, 1992, 1998; Jemmott, Jemmott, Fong, & McCaffree, 1999; Kirby et al., 1991; Main et al., 1994; Rotheram-Borus, Gwadz, Fernandez, & Srinivasan, 1998; Rotheram-Borus, Koopman, Haignere, & Davies, 1991; Stanton et al., 1996; St. Lawrence et al., 1995). These interventions teach about abstinence as the best self-protection, but place far greater emphasize on teaching that adolescents should use condoms if they have sexual intercourse and on teaching adolescents the skills they need to practice abstinence and to use condoms. Accordingly, the failure of the abstinence programs cannot be attributed to the intractability of the behavior. Moreover, although an important rationale for abstinence-only programming is based on a fear that programs that endorse condom use may unwittingly increase adolescent sexual activity, the interventions used in these studies did not increase sexual activity. Instead, they decreased it, and when adolescents had sexual intercourse, they were more likely to protect themselves by using condoms.

9. FUTURE RESEARCH DIRECTIONS

9.1 Methodological Issues

Based on our review of the literature, we would suggest a number of directions for research on abstinence interventions. Future studies should measure as outcome variables not only abstinence or frequency of sexual intercourse, but also condom use and frequency of unprotected intercourse. Although abstinence interventions seek to affect sexual involvement, it is important that the effects on condom use, contraceptive use, and unprotected sexual intercourse also be examined. This is because one of the chief concerns and criticisms of abstinence interventions is that they do not give adolescents the information they need to be safe if they initiate sexual intercourse and some even emphasize condom or contraceptive failure.

In this view, despite intervention, many young people will have sexual intercourse during adolescence, and it is important to prepare them to have sexual intercourse responsibly and safely, in order to minimize the negative consequences adolescents experience from their sexual behavior. Because abstinence interventions may lead adolescents to have negative beliefs about contraception, it is important to determine that such interventions do not have adverse effects on contraceptive use when adolescents do become sexually active.

In addition, future research should include attentional control groups. Attentional control groups are needed to confirm the specificity of the intervention effects as opposed to Hawthorne effects. Only one published abstinence intervention study to date has included such a control group (Jemmott et al., 1998). Future studies should also be designed to have sufficient statistical power to detect intervention effects. The investigators should pay particular attention to the expected amount of sexual activity among the participants. If sexual activity will be rare, it will be difficult to overcome floor effects unless the sample is extraordinarily large.

9.2 Comprehensive Interventions versus Mixed Messages

Additional research is also needed on the effects of combining and integrating the abstinence strategy with the safer sex strategy in the same intervention. Combining abstinence and safer sex approaches within a single curriculum is strongly advocated by many researchers and public interest groups (e.g., AMA; SIECUS), who believe that such comprehensive sexuality education programs are the most efficacious in reducing HIV/AIDS sexual risk behavior among adolescents. Despite the plausibility of this position, there is currently an inadequate empirical basis to conclusively demonstrate the veracity of this position. Although some, if not most, successful sexual-risk interventions incorporate content from both approaches, such efforts are typically not systematic.

Even if a combined abstinence and safer sex intervention is successful when compared with an attentional control group (e.g., Jemmott, Jemmott, & Fong, 1992, 1998; Jemmott, Jemmott, Fong, & McCaffree, 1999), the significant intervention effect cannot logically be attributed to the use of the combination approach, unless it is compared with single-approach interventions—abstinence-only and safer sex-only. As far as we know, no randomized controlled trials that have specifically tested the critical assumption that an intervention that combines abstinence and safer sex approaches is more efficacious than either an abstinence-only or a safer sex-only intervention. It may be the case, as is pointed out by many abstinence proponents, that teaching young adolescents about both abstinence and safer sex may constitute a "mixed message"—one that might be less effective than teaching them about a single set of behavioral principles as conveyed in a single-component intervention.

9.3 Gender

There are several moderator variables, including gender, age, race, ethnicity, and sexual experience, that might be considered in future abstinence intervention research. The sex of participants is of great relevance. We know that adolescent women as compared with adolescent men are consistently older at initiation of sexual intercourse, often hold stronger normative beliefs supporting abstinence, and are more vulnerable to direct negative sexual consequences, including pregnancy and sexually transmitted infection (CDC, 1998, Kann et al., 1998; DeGaston, Weed, & Jensen, 1996). Accordingly, it would be important to know whether abstinence interventions are more effective with adolescent women than with adolescent men, as well as the mediators of any differential intervention effects across gender. If abstinence programs were known to be effective with both males and females, this lack of information would not be problematic. However, since efforts to delay and decrease sexual intercourse among adolescents have been mostly unsuccessful, it may be that we need to better understand how these gender differences relate to abstinence messages.

9.4 Age and Developmental Concerns

Research is needed on how age and developmental issues moderate the effectiveness of abstinence interventions. Howard (1992) concluded from findings in the PSI intervention that since sexually inexperienced adolescents showed treatment effects, that abstinence messages might be more appropriate for younger adolescents in order to reach them before they have sexual intercourse. What is interesting about Howard's finding is that it leads to an important question: that is, whether sexual abstinence at younger ages is the same behavior as sexual abstinence at older ages. For example, 11-year old virgins are more likely to be physically pre-pubertal, affiliating almost entirely with same-sex peers, and unexposed to pressures to have sexual intercourse. They are not necessarily wedded to abstinence behavior at all, but just in a life stage more typical of childhood than adolescence, as compared with 15- or 16-year old virgins. With this conceptualization, it is possible that PSI worked best not as a behavior change program, but as a behavior maintenance program for older adolescents who already practiced abstinence. It reinforced the sexual health strategy they already used. Systematic investigation of treatment effects among sexually inexperienced adolescents at different ages is needed in order to investigate this further. This would include well-designed measures to assess how much adolescents who are sexually inexperienced actively intend to practice abstinence at different ages, further analysis of extant data, and randomized controlled studies assigning adolescents at different ages to different curricula.

9.5 Sexually Experienced versus Sexually Inexperienced Adolescents

The abstinence literature is rife with the belief that abstinence programs will work better with virgins (Olsen, 1987) because it is easier to prevent adolescents from initiating sexual intercourse than it is to convince those who have started having sexual intercourse to stop (Thomas, 1999). For example, Postponing Sexual Involvement (PSI) was found to be effective with sexually inexperienced 8th graders (13-14 year olds), but ineffective with participants who had sexual intercourse prior to the intervention (Howard, 1992). Jorgensen et al. reported significant effects of an abstinence intervention with virgins, but did not report results with nonvirgins. The findings are not so clear, though, particularly if the target is decreased sexual intercourse rather than ceased sexual intercourse among the non-virgins. In contrast to prevailing beliefs, St. Pierre et al. (1995) reported the opposite effect: an abstinence program decreased sexual intercourse among sexually experienced adolescents, but had no effect among those who were virgins at baseline.

Future research should continue to investigate this issue using analyses that appropriately test for interactions between baseline sexual experience and effects of abstinence interventions. Simply performing separate analyses on virgins and nonvirgins and finding that results are significant in one group but not the other, does not address the question of the differential effectiveness of an intervention. Determining the differential effectiveness of an intervention requires a statistical test of whether the effects of the intervention are significantly stronger in one group than in the other (Baron & Kenny, 1986) of intervention effectiveness. Another consideration in designing future studies is to ensure that there are enough participants who are sexually inexperienced and sexually experienced at baseline to generate adequate power to detect moderator effects. Because it stands to reason that the sexually inexperienced participants will have less behavior to measure initially, longer-term outcomes and higher numbers of inexperienced participants at baseline are essential to measuring these effects. The only study to report such a test was Jemmott, Jemmott, and Fong (1998).

Although they did not find a significant interaction at 3-month follow-up, they did find significant interactions at 6-month and 12-month follow-up. These interactions suggested that the safer sex intervention was more effective with sexually experienced adolescents than with sexually inexperienced adolescents. Besides the differential effects of abstinence interventions on both sexual behavior and mediators of sexual behavior as a function of sexual experience, future studies should also explore the psychological receptiveness of differently experienced adolescents to abstinence-only and safer sex messages.

9.6 Culture and Ethnicity

Future studies should also consider whether abstinence interventions may be especially effective in certain cultural or ethnic groups. Abstinence messages must anticipate the fact that adolescents are members of subcultures with specific meanings for and sensibilities about sexual behaviors. For example, urban gay runaways have markedly different meanings and sensibilities about sexual behaviors than do rural youth in Utah. One example of differing cultural meanings is captured in the comment by Olsen et al. (1992) indicating that sexual behavior in their Utah population may reflect a nexus of more general deviant behavior, as conceptualized by Jessor and Jessor (1977). In fact, for this population, where only 5% to 8% had premarital sexual intercourse, the assertion that sexual intercourse is deviant is true, at least statistically. However, labeling sexual intercourse as deviant in other adolescent populations, where the majority of adolescents do have sexual intercourse, would be in error.

Abstinence messages may be more consonant or dissonant with different cultural contexts. Among groups that tend to initiate sexual activity at a later age, for instance, white and Latino adolescents (particularly Latino female adolescents) in comparison with African American adolescents, abstinence messages may be culturally consonant and effective. Among groups that tend to initiate sexual activity at an early age, abstinence messages may be viewed as culturally dissonant. Particularly for these adolescents, abstinence messages need to be framed in a culturally relevant way because, although it may be a dissonant message, it still may be a valuable message.

9.7 Maintaining Long-Term Behavior Change

According to the NIH Consensus Development Panel (Interventions to Prevent HIV Risk Behaviors, 1997), intervention programs need to be improved to achieve "long-term maintenance of the reduction in risky behavior" among high-risk young people. Those who would promote abstinence until marriage also have a vested interest in long-term maintenance. Although short-term gains may be useful in decreasing the societal costs associated with early sexual debut among American adolescents, if abstinence messages are going to have an important impact on the lives of adolescents, then we must increase the longevity of the effects of abstinence-based interventions. Intervention maintenance efforts such as booster sessions and telephone counseling may be particularly important and valuable in extending the effects of abstinence interventions over time. Additional research on these and other approaches to long-term maintenance is needed.

10. A FINAL WORD

In conclusion, evidence from several sources can be marshaled to make a strong case that adolescents are having sexual intercourse at an early age and are suffering the adverse consequences of this behavior. Unplanned pregnancy and STDs, including HIV, have afflicted far too many young people. The abstinence approach is logically defensible. By practicing abstinence, adolescents can eliminate the risk of unintended pregnancy and sexually transmitted infection. Empirically, the abstinence approach has not found cogent support. Relatively few studies have demonstrated significant effects of abstinence interventions. Those that have demonstrated such effects were plagued by methodological difficulties, had brief follow-up periods, or revealed that intervention effects were short lived, disappearing at long-term follow-up.

Although the data are not conclusive, at present there is scant evidence to support the effectiveness of abstinence programs. This does not mean, though, that we can completely rule out the potential effectiveness of abstinence programs at this stage of the research. More data are needed to understand if abstinence interventions can, in fact, postpone and decrease sexual activity over the long-term and whether the effects of those interventions vary among subpopulations of adolescents defined by age, development, gender, race, ethnic, and sexual experience. Part of that research should be geared toward further exploration of which types of educational messages promote those outcomes, as our review suggests that other approaches besides abstinence messages may also have this effect. Research along these lines should reduce the adverse consequences that many adolescents are confronting.

ACKNOWLEDGMENTS

Preparation of this chapter was supported in part by National Institute of Mental Health grants R01-MH55442 and R01-MH61226 and National Institute of Child Health and Human Development grant R01-HD38443.

Correspondence regarding this manuscript should be sent to Professor John B. Jemmott, III, University of Pennsylvania, Annenberg School for Communication, 3535 Market Street, Philadelphia, PA 19104-3309. Telephone: 215-573-9366. Fax: 215-573-9303. E-mail: jjemmott@asc.upenn.edu.

REFERENCES

Alan Guttmacher Institute. (1994). Sex and America's Teenagers. Washington DC: The Alan Guttmacher Institute.

Baron, R. M., & Kenny, D. A. (1986). The moderator-mediator variable distinction in social psychological research. *Journal of Personality and Social Psychology*, 51, 1173-1182.

Brown, S. V. (1985). Premarital sexual permissiveness among black adolescent females. *Social Psychology Quarterly*, 48, 381-387.

Cates, W., & Stone, K. M. (1992). Family planning, sexually transmitted diseases and contraceptive choice: a literature update - Part I. *Family Planning Perspectives*, 24, 75-84.

Centers for Disease Control and Prevention (CDC). (1988). Condoms for the prevention of sexually transmitted diseases. *Morbidity and Mortality Weekly Report*, 37, 133-137.

Centers for Disease Control and Prevention. (1993). Update: barrier protection against HIV infection and other sexually transmitted diseases. *Journal of the American Medical Association*, 270, 933-934.

Centers for Disease Control and Prevention. (1998). Trends in sexual risk behaviors among high school students—United States, 1991-1997. *Morbidity and Mortality Weekly Report*, 47(36), 749-752.

Centers for Disease Control and Prevention. (1999a). *HIV/AIDS Surveillance Report*, 11(1), 1-44.

Centers for Disease Control and Prevention (1999b). *HIV/AIDS Surveillance Supplemental Report*, 5(no. 3), 1-12.

Christopher, F. S., & Roosa, M. W. (1990). An evaluation of an adolescent pregnancy prevention program: Is "just say no" enough? *Family Relations*, 39, 68-72.

Cook T. D., & Campbell D. T. (1979). Quasi-experimentation: Design and analysis issues for field settings. Chicago: Rand McNally.

Cvetkovich, G., & Grote, B. (1983). Adolescent development and teenage fertility. In D. Byrne, & W. A. Fisher (Eds.), Adolescents, sex, and contraception (pp. 112-124). Hillsdale, NJ: Erlbaum.

Darroch, J. E., & Singh, S. (1999). Why is teenager pregnancy declining? The roles of abstinence, sexual activity and contraceptive use. Occasional Report No. 1. New York: The Alan Guttmacher Institute.

DiClemente, R. J. (1998). Preventing sexually transmitted infections among adolescents: A clash of ideology and science. *Journal of the American Medical Association*, 279, 1574-1575.

Eng, T. R., & Butler, W. T. (1997). The hidden epidemic: Confronting sexually transmitted diseases. Washington, DC: National Academy Press.

Fisher, J. D., & Fisher, W. A. (1992). Changing AIDS risk behavior. *Psychological Bulletin*, 111, 455-474.

Howard, M. (1992). Delaying the start of intercourse among adolescents. *Adolescent Medicine*, 3, 181-193.

Howard, M., & McCabe, J. B. (1990). Helping teenagers postpone sexual involvement. *Family Planning Perspectives*, 22, 21-26.

Howard, M., & McCabe, J. B. (1992). An information and skills approach for younger teens: Postponing Sexual Involvement Program. In B. C. Miller, J. J. Card, R. L. Paikoff, & J. L. Peterson (Eds.), Preventing adolescent pregnancy: Model programs and evaluations (pp. 83-109). Newberry Park, CA: Sage.

Jemmott, J. B. III, Jemmott, L. S., & Fong, G. T. (1992). Reductions in HIV risk-associated sexual behaviors among Black male adolescents: Effects of an AIDS prevention intervention. *American Journal of Public Health*, 82, 372-377.

Jemmott, J. B. III, Jemmott, L. S., & Fong, G. T. (1998). Abstinence and safer sex HIV risk-reduction interventions for African American adolescents: A randomized controlled trial. *Journal of the American Medical Association*, 279, 1529-1536.

Jemmott, J. B. III, Jemmott, L. S., Fong, G. T., & McCaffree, K. (1999). Reducing HIV risk-associated sexual behavior among African American adolescents: Testing the generality of intervention effects. *American Journal of Community Psychology*, 27(2), 161-187.

Jemmott, L. S., Jemmott, J. B. III. & McCaffree, K. (1995). Be proud! Be responsible! Strategies to empower youth to reduce their risk for AIDS. New York, NY: Select Media Publications.

Jessor, R. & Jessor, S. L. (1977). Problem behavior and psychosocial development: A longitudinal study of youth. New York: Academic Press.

Jorgensen, S. R., Potts, V., & Camp, B. (1993). Project Taking Charge: Six-month follow-up of a pregnancy prevention program for early adolescents. *Family Relations*, 40, 401-406.

Kann, L., Kinchen, S. A., Williams, B., Ross, J. G., Lowry, R., Hill, C. V., Grunbaum, J. A., Blumson, P. S., Collins, J. L., Kolbe, L., & State and Local YRBSS Coordinators. (1998). Youth risk behavior surveillance--United States, 1997. CDC Surveillance Summaries, *Mortality and Mortality Weekly Report*, 47 (No. SS-3), 1-89.

Kantor, L. M. (1992-93). Scared chaste? Fear-based educational curricula. *SIECUS Report*, 21, (2), 1-3.

Keller, S. E., Barlett, J. A., Schleifer, S. J., Johnson, R. L., Pinner, E., & Delaney, B. (1991). HIV-relevant sexual behavior among a healthy inner-city heterosexual adolescent population in an endemic area of HIV. *Journal of Adolescent Health*, 12, 44-48.

Kirby, D., Barth, R. P., Leland, N., & Fetro, J. V. (1991). Reducing the risk: Impact of a new curriculum on sexual risk-taking. *Family Planning Perspectives*, 23, 253-262.

Kirby, D., Korpi, M., Adivi, C., & Weissman, J. (1997). An impact evaluation of Project Snapp, an AIDS-and pregnancy-prevention middle school program. *AIDS Education and Prevention*, 9(1 Suppl), 44-61.

Kirby, D., Korpi, M., Barth, R. P., & Cagampang, H. H. (1997). The impact of the Postponing Sexual Involvement curriculum among youths in California. *Family Planning Perspectives*, 29, 100-108.

Main, D. S., Iverson, D. C., McGloin, J., Banspach, S. W., Collins, J. L., Rugg, D. L., & Kolbe, L. J. (1994). Preventing HIV infection among adolescents: Evaluation of a school-based education program. *Preventive Medicine*, 23, 409-417.

Miller, B. C., Norton, M. C., Jenson, G. O., Lee, T. R., Christopherson, C., & King, P. K. (1993). Impact evaluation of FACTS & feelings: A home-based video sex education curriculum. *Family Relations*, 42, 392-400.

Pratt W, Mosher W, Bachrach C, Horn M. (1984). Understanding U. S. fertility: findings from the National Survey of Family Growth Cycle III. *Population Bulletin*, 39, 1-42.

Roosa, M. W., & Christopher, F. S. (1990). Evaluation of an abstinence-only adolescent pregnancy prevention program: A replication. *Family Relations*, 39, 363-367.

Rotheram-Borus, M. J., Gwadz, M., Fernandez, M. I., & Srinivasan, S. (1998). Timing of HIV interventions on reductions in sexual risk among adolescents. *American Journal of Community Psychology*, 26, 73-96.

Rotheram-Borus, M. J., Koopman, C., Haignere, C., & Davies, M. (1991). Reducing HIV sexual risk behaviors among runaway adolescents. *Journal of the American Medical Association*, 266, 1237-1241.

Sanderson CA, Jemmott III JB. Moderation and mediation of HIV prevention interventions: Relationship status, intentions, and condom use among college students. *Journal of Applied Social Psychology*. 1996;26:2076-2099.

Shelton, D. L. (2000). Does sex ed focused on abstinence work? *American Medical News*, January 17, 2000 (www.ama-assn.org/sci-pubs/amnews).

Singh, S., & Darroch, J. E. (2000). Adolescent pregnancy and childbearing: levels and trends in developed countries. *Family Planning Perspectives*, 32(1), 14-23.

Sonenstein, F. L., Pleck, J. H., & Ku, L. C. (1989). Sexual activity, condom use and AIDS awareness among adolescent males. *Family Planning Perspectives*, 21, 152-158.

St. Lawrence, J., Brasfield, T., Jefferson, K., Alleyne, E., & O'Brannon, R. A. III (1995). Cognitive-behavioral intervention to reduce African-American adolescents' risk for HIV infection. *Journal of Consulting and Clinical Psychology*, 63, 221-237.

St. Pierre, T. L., Mark, M. M., Kaltreider, D. L., & Aikin, K. J. (1995). A 27-month evaluation of a sexual activity prevention program in Boys & Girls Clubs across the nation. *Family Relations*, 44, 69-77.

Stanton, B. F., Li, Z., Ricardo, I., Galbraith, J., Feigelman, S., & Kaljee, L. (1996). A randomized, controlled effectiveness trial of an AIDS prevention program for low-income African-American youths. *Archives of Pediatric and Adolescent Medicine*, 150, 363-372.

Taylor, H., Kagay, M., & Leichenko, S. (1986). American teens speak: Sex myths, TV, and birth control. Planned Parenthood Federation of America, Inc.

Walter, H. J., & Vaughan, R. D. (1993). AIDS risk reduction among a multiethnic sample of urban high school students. *Journal of the American Medical Association*, 270, 725-730.

Whatley, M. H. & Trudell, B. K. (1993). Teen-Aid: Another problematic sexuality curriculum. *Journal of Sex Education and Therapy*, 19, 251-271.

Young, M., Core-Gebhart, P., & Marx, D. (1992). Abstinence-oriented sexuality education: Initial field test results of the Living Smart curriculum. *Family Life Educator*, Summer, 4-8.

Zelnik, M., Kantner, J. F, & Ford, K. (1981). Sex and pregnancy in adolescence. Beverly Hills, CA: Sage.

Chapter 7

Assessing the Cost-effectiveness of Alternative Approaches to HIV Prevention

Steven D. Pinkerton
Center for AIDS Intervention Research
Department of Psychiatry and Behavioral Medicine
Medical College of Wisconsin

And

David R. Holtgrave
Division of HIV/AIDS Prevention, National Center for HIV, STD and TB Prevention, Centers for Disease Control and Prevention, Atlanta Georgia

1. INTRODUCTION

Regardless of the setting—whether in the developed or developing world—the economic resources available for HIV prevention are necessary limited. Consequently, not all worthwhile interventions can be funded. HIV prevention interventions must compete with other health care and health promotion programs and procedures, as well as with other HIV prevention interventions for the limited resources available. If the goal of health-care and health promotion spending is to optimize the health of the population, then only the most economically efficient, or cost-effective, interventions should be funded (informally, an intervention is "cost-effective" if it provides good health-related "bang for the buck").

Of course, real-world funding decisions must take into account myriad political and social factors, hence economic concerns sometimes may be secondary (Paltiel & Stinnett, 1998). Nevertheless, cost-effectiveness analyses, which attempt to quantify the cost per unit of health-related benefit of health care and health promotion programs, can help inform the decision making process by making explicit the trade-off between costs and health benefits (Holtgrave, 1994a; Kahn & Haynes-Sanstad, 1997). In the U.S., for example, most federal HIV prevention resources are allocated with input from local community planning groups composed of representatives of affected populations, behavioral/social scientists, epidemiologists, HIV/AIDS prevention service providers, health department staff, and others (Valdiserri, Aultman, & Curran, 1995). One of the main tasks these groups are charged with is to identify science-based HIV prevention interventions to address unmet HIV prevention needs in their communities and to develop comprehensive HIV prevention plans that prioritize needs and interventions (Centers for Disease Control, 1993). The comprehensive plan is then forwarded to the state or local health department, which develops a funding application to be submitted to the federal Centers for Disease Control and Prevention. In preparing their prioritization recommendations, community-planning groups are required to take into consideration a number of factors, including the "cost effectiveness of proposed strategies and interventions (either demonstrated or probable)" (Centers for Disease Control, 1993). Thus, although cost-effectiveness is not the sole criterion upon which HIV prevention resource allocation decision are based, the economic efficiency of different interventions is an important factor in the decision making process (Holtgrave, 1994b; Pinkerton, Holtgrave, Willingham, & Goldstein, 1998).

A substantial HIV prevention economic evaluation literature now exists and continues to grow. Several reviews and other guides to this literature are available (Holtgrave, 1998; Holtgrave & Pinkerton, in press; Holtgrave, Qualls, & Graham, 1996; Schrappe & Lauterbach, 1998). Many if not most of the cost-effectiveness studies that have been published to-date have examined interventions that help participants to alter the behaviors that place them at risk for HIV infection, or that help make available the resources—such as condoms, bleach, and sterile syringes—needed to enact safer behaviors. With regard specifically to the sexual risk reduction interventions that are the focus of the present chapter, numerous economic efficiency analyses have been conducted of small-group counseling interventions that promote safer sexual practices, community-level interventions that attempt to change social norms as well as individual behaviors, and condom social marketing programs. Often, these interventions have multiple goals other than increasing (male) condom use, but condom promotion remains a cornerstone of these and similar interventions.

Few economic efficiency analyses have specifically examined non-traditional approaches to reducing HIV transmission risks, such as the use of the female condom or vaginal microbicides, "alternative" behavioral strategies (such as "negotiated safety," reducing the number of sexual partners or being more careful in selecting partners, substituting safer behaviors for riskier ones, etc.), post-exposure prophylaxis with antiretroviral medications, prevention/treatment of sexually transmitted diseases (STDs), and so forth. In this chapter we present a framework for thinking about the cost-effectiveness of these alternative HIV prevention strategies. First, we provide a brief overview of cost-effectiveness analysis, specifically as it pertains to HIV prevention interventions. Next, we advance a simple mathematical model for evaluating the effectiveness of sexual risk reduction interventions. In the third section of the paper we apply this framework to several alternative sexual risk reduction strategies, highlighting what is known about the cost-effectiveness of each strategy (often, very little) and discussing how its economic efficiency is likely to be shaped by various influences.

2. BASICS OF HIV PREVENTION COST-EFFECTIVENESS ANALYSIS

The primary goal of HIV prevention interventions is obvious: to prevent the transmission of HIV. Consequently, economic evaluations of HIV prevention interventions invariably take as their starting point the number of infections averted by the intervention. This fundamental outcome measure can then be translated into estimates of ancillary economic benefits, such as medical care savings and averted economic productivity losses, and health-related benefits, such as increased longevity and improved quality of life.

Specifically, if A denotes the number of infections averted by a particular intervention and B denotes the economic or other benefits that arise from preventing a single infection, then the total benefits due to the intervention equal A*B. Hence, if the cost of implementing the intervention is C, the net cost is C – A*B. In cost-benefit analysis (CBA), one of the oldest economic evaluation techniques, the net cost of an intervention is usually called its <u>net present value</u> (Clemmer & Haddix, 1996). The net present value indicates the overall cost of, or possibly the savings due to, implementing the intervention. Cost-benefit analysis assumes that B incorporates <u>all</u> the benefits of preventing an infection, including health-related benefits as well as purely economic ones. Thus, in CBA it is necessary to assign a dollar amount to the inclusive value of preventing an

HIV infection. This is a difficult and ethically/politically contentious task because it requires, in essence, an estimate of the value of a human life. Consequently, CBA is seldom used to evaluate the economic efficiency of HIV prevention interventions.

In contrast, the other main economic efficiency evaluation technique; cost-effectiveness analysis (CEA), does not assume that the net cost necessarily includes all benefits of preventing HIV transmission. In particular, no attempt is made to monetarily quantify the health-related benefits of preventing an infection; instead, only the economic benefits of HIV prevention are included in the net cost. In CEA the main measure of economic efficiency is the ratio of net costs to an appropriate health-related outcome, such as HIV infections averted or years of life saved (Drummond, Stoddart, & Torrance, 1987; Haddix & Shaffer, 1996; Gold, Siegel, Russell, & Weinstein, 1996). Implicit in this formulation is an acknowledgment that not all health gains can be translated into a dollar equivalent and incorporated into the net cost, as is done in CBA. Of course, a negative net cost remains highly desirable. A negative net cost indicates that the economic benefits associated with the intervention exceed its cost (such as intervention is called cost-saving). Because cost-saving interventions save society money in the long run (notably, many of the economic benefits of HIV prevention accrue in the future), society should make every effort to fund them. Of course, not all interventions are cost saving. Cost-effectiveness analysis provides a basis for comparing the costs and consequences of different interventions, and thereby helping to inform the selection process (Paltiel & Stinnett, 1998).

Schematically, if A, B, and C, as above, denote the number of infections averted by the intervention, the economic benefit of preventing an infection, and the cost of implementing the intervention (respectively), and if H is the health-related benefit of preventing an infection (e.g., H might be the number of life years saved), then the cost-effectiveness ratio can be expressed as:

$$\frac{C - AB}{AH} \quad \text{(Eq. 1)}$$

(Pinkerton & Holtgrave, 1998a,b). In the special case that HIV infections are themselves the outcome of interest, the cost-effectiveness ratio ("net cost per infection averted") simplifies to $(C - AB)/A$, which can also be written, $C/A - B$. Here, the economic benefits of preventing an infection are likely to include savings in medical care costs and averted productivity losses.

The lifetime cost of treating someone with HIV disease has recently been estimated at \$195,188, after discounting at a 3% annual rate (Holtgrave & Pinkerton, 1997). (Discounting is a standard economic technique for devaluing future cost and benefits into their present value, thereby taking into account societal preferences for immediate benefits and deferred costs.) Updated estimates of the impact of HIV disease on economic productivity are lacking, but human capital estimates from the late 1980s suggest a figure between $750,000 and $1 million (Bloom & Carliner, 1988; Hardy, Rausch, Echenberg, Morgan, & Curran, 1986; Scitovsky & Rice, 1987; see also Pinkerton, Abramson, & Holtgrave, 1999). (In the human capital approach, productivity losses are estimated by calculating the lifetime wages that are foregone due to morbidity or premature mortality (Haddix & Shaffer, 1996; Hodgson, 1994; Rice, 1967; Rice & Max, 1996).) Importantly, there is considerable uncertainty regarding the impact of highly active antiretroviral therapies on HIV patients' longevity, long-term health, and economic productivity. Future advances in therapy also are likely to alter the economic course of HIV disease (Pinkerton & Holtgrave, 1999a). Therefore, these estimates of lifetime treatment costs and HIV-related productivity losses should be viewed as provisional.

In cost-utility analysis (CUA), which can be viewed as a special form of CEA, longevity and quality of life are combined into a single measure of health benefits, the number of quality-adjusted life years (QALYs) saved by preventing an infection (Fabian, 1994; Gold, Siegel, Russell, & Weinstein, 1996). (In the QALY framework, each year of life that is spent in a particular health state is multiplied by a weight between 0 and 1 that reflects the health-related quality of life experienced by someone in that health state.) Holtgrave and Pinkerton (1997) estimate that a 26-year-old who becomes infected with HIV loses 11.23 (discounted) QALYs as a result of his or her infection. Again, future advances in medical care could have a substantial impact on this estimate.

An intervention is said to be <u>cost-effective</u> if it represents a good health care "buy" in comparison with other possible uses for health-related resources. Thus, an implicit comparison is present in all statements about the cost-effectiveness of a particular intervention. In the U.S., interventions that cost less than about $50,000 per life-year or QALY saved are generally considered cost-effective (Paltiel & Stinnett, 1998). Clearly, whether or not a particular intervention is considered cost-effective depends on the resources available to fund health-related programs. The same intervention that appears highly cost-effective in the U.S. might not appear so in a resource poor country where only essential health care and health promotion services are provided. Finally, we should note that most of the analyses done to-date have compared the target intervention to a so-called "no program" option. Alternatively (and preferably), if two interventions provide comparable services to the same population, but one is more expensive and effective than the other, then they can be compared directly by evaluating the incremental cost-effectiveness ratio, which provides a measure of how much more it would cost for each additional unit of health that would be obtained by funding the more costly and effective intervention (Drummond, Stoddart, & Torrance, 1987; Gold, Siegel, Russell, & Weinstein, 1996).

The intervention cost parameter (C) should be as comprehensive as possible, subject to the particular perspective adopted by the analysis. The perspective determines which costs and consequences are to be included in the analysis and therefore should reflect the interests of the intended consumers of the analysis. Valid perspectives include the provider (hospital, physician, etc.) perspective, the insurer/managed care perspective, and the patient perspective, among others. However, the most appropriate perspective for decisions regarding the allocation of societal resources for HIV prevention is the societal perspective which includes all intervention costs and consequences, regardless of who pays for or experiences them. Thus, an analysis conducted from the societal perspective should not only include obvious program costs (such as the cost of condoms and other materials, personnel costs, and overhead), but also expenses borne by the intervention participants themselves (such as time away from work, day care, etc.) or by other social entities. Also, economic analyses should focus on the "opportunity costs" of goods and services, which reflect the true cost to society of using the goods or services for one purpose rather than another. For example, the societal cost of a condom is roughly equivalent to the cost of its production and distribution, which is typically much smaller than its retail price.

Finally, cost-effectiveness analysis requires an estimate of the number of infections prevented by the intervention. The number of infections averted, A, is simply the difference between the number of infections that occur in spite of the intervention and the number that would have been expected if the intervention had not been implemented (or, in the case of an incremental analysis, the number that would have been expected if a different intervention had been implemented instead). The "simply" in the previous sentence masks a fundamental difficulty. In developed countries the HIV incidence in most communities is (thankfully) so low that it precludes using direct measures, such as changes in seroincidence, to assess the impact of a preventive intervention. In such situations, mathematical models of HIV transmission can be used to translate behavioral data, such as reported increases in condom use or decreases in anonymous sex, into an estimate of the number of infections averted (Pinkerton, Holtgrave, Leviton, Wagstaff, & Abramson, 1998). A simple model is described in the following section to provide a framework for discussing how various interventions impact the HIV transmission rate in their target populations.

3. A FRAMEWORK FOR ASSESSING THE IMPACT OF SEXUAL BEHAVIOR CHANGES

Variants of the simple HIV transmission model described below have been used in a number of cost-effectiveness analyses (Bedimo, Pinkerton, Cohen, Gray, & Farley, under review; Holtgrave & Kelly, 1996, 1997; Johnson-Masotti, Pinkerton, Kelly, & Stevenson, in press; Moses, Plummer, Ngugi, Nagelkerke, Anzala, & Ndinya-Achola, 1991; Pinkerton, Holtgrave, DiFranceisco, Stevenson, & Kelly, 1998a,b; Pinkerton, Holtgrave, DiFranceisco, Semaan, & Coyle, under review; Pinkerton, Holtgrave, & Jemmott, under review; Pinkerton, Holtgrave, & Valdiserri, 1997). This "Bernoullian" model was recently validated in an empirical study in Africa, where the estimates of the model closely matched observed changes in seroincidence (Rehle, Saidel, Hassig, Bouey, Gaillard, & Sokal, 1998).

One of the main benefits of the model, which can be used to translate sexual behavior changes into estimates of the numbers of infections averted (or possibly caused) by these changes, is that the data it requires are routinely collected during HIV prevention interventions efficacy/effectiveness trials (Pinkerton, Holtgrave, Leviton, Wagstaff, Cecil, & Abramson, 1998). The main disadvantage of this type of model, in comparison with more elaborate epidemiological models that attempt to extrapolate the effects of the intervention beyond both the immediate intervention community (i.e., intervention participants and their partners) and the period during which intervention effectiveness was assessed, is that the individual-level model described here neglects these extended effects. Nevertheless, the model is intuitively appealing and biologically plausible (Holtgrave, Leviton, Wagstaff, & Pinkerton, 1997), and provides an excellent framework for discussing the different routes through which interventions can help individuals reduce their risk of becoming infected with HIV.

For simplicity, we will consider a hypothetical woman who engages in two sexual risk activities: vaginal and anal intercourse (alternatively, we could consider a man who engages in both insertive and receptive anal intercourse with other men, or a man who has sex with both men and women, or any one of a number of other possibilities). Suppose this hypothetical woman has $\underline{m}$ male partners, which each of whom she engages in $\underline{n}$ acts of anal intercourse and $\underline{k}$ acts of vaginal intercourse. Her risk of becoming infected as a result of this sexual activity can be estimated using the following equation:

$$P = 1 - [(1 - \pi) + \pi(1 - \alpha_n)^n (1 - \alpha_k)^{jk}]^m, \quad \text{(Eq. 2)}$$

Where α_n and α_k denote the per-act probability of HIV transmission for receptive anal and vaginal intercourse, respectively, and π represents the probability that one or more of her m partners is infected (Pinkerton & Abramson, 1998). By comparing her probability of becoming infection both before and after the intervention (or by comparing her behavior to that of a matched control), we can compute the fraction of an infection that was averted by her behavior change; aggregated over the entire intervention population, we can thereby derive an estimate of the total number of infections averted by the intervention (Pinkerton, Holtgrave, Leviton, Wagstaff, & Abramson, 1998). Specifically, let P_{pre} and P_{post} denote the average pre- and post- intervention risks, obtained using Equation 2. Then, the total number of infections averted among N intervention participants, all of whom are assumed to be susceptible to infection, is approximately $A = N(P_{pre} - P_{post})$.

4. SEXUAL RISK REDUCTION STRATEGIES

Most of the sexual risk reduction interventions that have been described in the literature and/or implemented by AIDS service providers focus on increasing condom use, which corresponds to reducing the "infectivity" (per-act transmission probability), α (see Equation 2). There are, of course, many other methods besides condom promotion by which to reduce the infectivity of the HIV virus, several of which are discussed below. Indeed, any of the several parameters in Equation 2 could be made the target of an HIV prevention intervention. Many of the less-traditional mechanisms of HIV prevention that are the focus of other chapters of this volume attempt to alter these parameters in ways that reduce the overall probability of HIV transmission. Below we discuss each of them briefly, together with some additional approaches to HIV prevention. Table 1 summarizes this discussion.

Table 1: Targets of Sexual Risk Reduction HIV Prevention Strategies

Strategies	Target*
Male condoms	α (infectivity)
Female condoms	α
Microbicides	α
Reducing the number of sex partners	m (number of partners)
Having sex only with uninfected partners ("know your	π (probability partner is infected)

Strategies	Target*
partner")	
Negotiated safety	π, with a possible increase in α
Abstinence/less sex/delaying sexual initiation	n, k, and possibly m
Substituting safer sexual activities for riskier ones	α
Sexually transmitted disease detection and treatment	α
Antiretroviral therapy for HIV disease	α
Antiretroviral post-exposure prophylaxis	α (interpreted as susceptibility)
Libido-reducing pharmacotherapy	n, k, and m
Structural and policy interventions	Macro-level factors (see text)

*See Equation 2

4.1 Male Condoms

Empirical evidence obtained from HIV transmission patterns in HIV-discordant, heterosexual couples suggests that condoms reduce the infectivity of HIV by about 90 to 95% on a per-act basis (Pinkerton & Abramson, 1997). Figure 1 illustrates how the probability of infection varies as a function of condom use for a sexually active woman who engages in 250 acts of receptive vaginal intercourse and 250 acts of receptive anal intercourse with either 1, 5, or 50 different men (cf. Pinkerton & Abramson, 1993a, 1998). As indicated in the figure, the percentage of time that condoms are used—up to about 80%—is nearly proportional to the resultant reduction in the risk of HIV transmission, which suggests that even occasional condom use can be a highly effective safer sex strategy (Pinkerton & Abramson, 1996a). Obviously, for maximal effectiveness, condoms should be used for every act of intercourse.

Condom promotion interventions, which typically focus on multiple behavioral goals besides increasing condom use, include both "traditional" interventions, such as small-group counseling sessions that emphasize cognitive-behavioral strategies for reducing risk and community-level interventions that attempt to alter community norms regarding condom use and safer sex practices, as well as more novel strategies, such as condom social marketing, in which condoms are made available at reduced cost to at-risk individuals, or methods to increase condom acceptability, such as the video tape described by O'Leary (this volume) for male partners of at-risk women.

Several cost-effectiveness and cost-utility analyses have been conducted to evaluate the economic efficiency of small-group interventions based on sound cognitive-behavioral principles (Holtgrave & Kelly, 1996, 1997; Johnson-Masotti, Pinkerton, Kelly, & Stevenson, in press; Pinkerton, Holtgrave, & Jemmott, under review; Pinkerton, Holtgrave, & Valdiserri, 1997), and of community-level interventions that may include such elements as individualized risk assessment, social activities for member of the community, and training popular members of the community to endorse safer sex messages to their peers (Kahn, Kegeles, Hays, & Beltzer, under review; Pinkerton, Holtgrave, DiFranceisco, Stevenson, & Kelly, 1998a,b; Tao & Remafedi, 1997). For the most part, these interventions have been shown to be highly cost-effective, or even cost saving (Holtgrave & Pinkerton, 1998; Pinkerton, Kahn, & Holtgrave, under review).

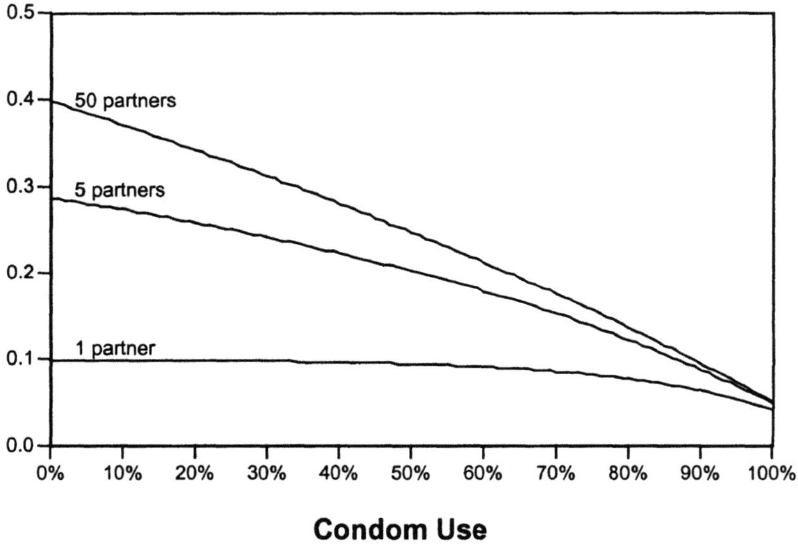

Figure 1. Probability of HIV transmission as a function of condom use for a woman who has 250 acts of receptive vaginal intercourse (infectivity = .001) and 250 acts of receptive anal intercourse (infectivity = .02) with either 1, 5, or 50 different men, assuming that condoms are 90% effective, and that 10%

Recently, Bedimo and colleagues (under review) performed a cost-utility analysis of Louisiana's condom social marketing program, which distributed free condoms through public health clinics, community mental health centers, substance abuse treatment centers, and more than 1000 businesses in communities with high rates of sexually transmitted diseases and HIV (Cohen, Farley, Bedimo-Etame, Scribner, Ward, Kendall, & Rice, 1999). The results of this analysis suggest that the program averted nearly 170 infections at a cost of approximately $3 million. The lifetime medical care cost of treating 170 cases of HIV disease is more than 10 times the amount the intervention cost, hence, the program is cost saving. Moses and colleagues (1991) assessed the cost-effectiveness of a sexually transmitted disease control program that focused on increasing condom use among a population of 1000 female commercial sex workers in Nairobi, Kenya. The program provided free condoms to the women and offered health education counseling to promote condom use. Moses and colleagues estimated that the program prevented between 6000 and 10,000 new cases of HIV infection each year at an annual cost of approximately $77,000. The cost per infection averted is therefore between $8 and $12, which is much less than the cost of HIV/AIDS medical care, estimates of which range between $100 and $1600 in Zaire and Tanzania (Over, Bertozzi, Chin, N'galy, & Nyamuryekung'e, 1988).

A mathematical modeling study by Pinkerton and colleagues (Pinkerton, Abramson, & Holtgrave, 1999) provides additional evidence that condoms can be highly cost-effective. The authors used a probabilistic model similar to the one described in the preceding section to estimate the potential societal savings in HIV-related medical care due to increased condom use. The analysis considered several condom use scenarios, including multiple uses with a single partner and multiple uses with multiple partners, for each of three populations: low-risk heterosexuals, high-risk heterosexuals, and men who have sex with men. The medical care savings exceeded the estimated cost of producing and distributing condoms in all but one of the scenarios. For multiple condom uses, the per-condom savings ranged from about 50¢ for low-risk heterosexuals to over $500 for multi-partnered men who have sex with men.

4.2 Alternative Strategies for Reducing HIV Infectivity

Members of this class of interventions follow the condom-promotion paradigm by attempting to reduce the infectivity of HIV. Alternatives to the male condom include the female condom, other barrier methods (including the diaphragm and the contraceptive sponge), and various forms of vaginal microbicides (including spermicides) that may be effective in preventing the transmission of HIV. Importantly, these methods can be used by women without necessarily requiring the full cooperation of her male sex partners (Cecil, Perry, Seal, & Pinkerton, 1998; Gollub & Stein, 1993; Moore, this volume; Stein, 1990, 1993, 1995; Stockbridge, Gollub, Stein, & El-Sadr, 1996). (The present discussion will focus on the use of these methods by women. However, men too can use microbicides and the "female condom" for protection during anal intercourse.)

Although there are no studies that evaluated the cost-effectiveness of the female condom, other barrier methods, or microbicidal strategies for preventing HIV transmission, the two fundamental questions are the same here as for the male condom. Namely, how much does the method cost on a per-act basis, and how effective is it in reducing the infectivity parameter? As mentioned above, the male condom is 90 to 95% effective at preventing HIV transmission, in practice (Pinkerton & Abramson, 1997). Wholesale, condoms cost less than a dime each (Murphy, 1990). The cost per condom distributed in the Louisiana condom social marketing program was about 17¢, including program-related overhead (Bedimo et al., under review). Similarly, the cost per condom distributed by 10 condom social marketing programs in various international settings ranged from 2¢ to 30¢ (Söderlund, Lavis, Broomberg, & Mills, 1993; World Bank, 1997).

The female condom is much more expensive than the male condom (Trussell et al., 1995). The female condom retails for more than $3 apiece (Elias & Coggins, 1996) and has an estimated wholesale cost in excess of $1 (Anonymous, 1993). Even if they were made available for half this cost, they would still be substantially more expensive than male condoms. The available evidence suggests that the contraceptive effectiveness of female and male condoms is similar (Elias & Coggins, 1996; Farr, Gabelnick, Sturgen, & Dorflinger, 1994; Trussell, Sturgen, Strickler, & Dominik, 1994). Its effectiveness against HIV and other STDs has not been established directly. Model-based estimates suggest that the female condom could reduce the per-act probability of HIV transmission by between 94 and 97% (Trussell, Sturgen, Strickler, & Dominik, 1994). These effectiveness estimates are similar to those obtained for male condoms (Pinkerton & Abramson, 1997). Direct comparisons of the effectiveness of male and female condoms have not been undertaken, however, and care should be exercised in interpreting the results of available studies. In sum, although more research on this important issue is needed, it appears that the HIV prevention effectiveness of female condom is likely to be similar to that of the male condom.

There is even greater uncertainty regarding the costs and HIV prevention effectiveness of microbicides. Although no microbicide is presently marketed as an HIV preventive, a number of promising candidates are undergoing clinical testing (Stephenson, 1999). The best-studied microbicide is the spermicide nonoxynol-9. Clinical trials that have investigated the effectiveness of nonoxynol-9 to reduce transmission of HIV and other STDs report conflicting results (Feldblum & Weir, 1994; Kreiss, Ngugi, Holmes, Ndinya-Achola, Waiyaki, Roberts, et al., 1992; Roddy, Schulz, Cates, 1998; Roddy, Zekeng, Ryan, Tamoufé, Weir, & Wong, 1998). Although disappointment over the failure of nonoxynol-9 to demonstrate a convincing prophylactic effect in clinical trials may have temporarily slowed research (Potts, 1994), interest in developing a vaginal microbicide to be used against HIV again appears to be high (Young, 1997).

Small increments in the effectiveness of male or female condoms, barrier methods, or vaginal microbicides, could have substantial HIV risk reduction benefits, as shown in Figure 2. This figure illustrates by how much a woman who engages in 250 acts each of vaginal and anal intercourse could reduce her probability of acquiring HIV if she used protection for every act of intercourse, rather than never, as a function of the effectiveness (percent reduction in infectivity) of her method of protection. For instance, consistent use of a 90% effective method would reduce her risk of becoming infected by between 59 and 87%, depending on the number of partners, whereas she could reduce her risk by between 77 and 93% by using a 95% effective method. Obviously, these estimates depend on the particular risk behaviors in which she engages. Nevertheless, they highlight the fact that a 5% increase in effectiveness yields better than a 15% reduction in risk. Therefore, techniques to increase the effectiveness of these methods of HIV prevention should be vigorously pursued (Pinkerton & Abramson, 1995), whether through improvements to the products themselves, including enhanced manufacturing and quality control procedures, or through better education in their proper use (Pinkerton, Abramson, & Holtgrave, 1999).

If, and it is important to stress the hypothetical, if female condoms, other barrier methods, and microbicides are viewed as alternatives to the male condom, then from an economic standpoint these alternatives should be recommended in preference to the male condom only if their cost-effectiveness ratio is superior to that of the male condom. However, female condoms are presently more expensive on a per-act basis than the male condom, and probably no more effective. Because small increments in the effectiveness of these methods can lead to large reductions in the risk of transmission, as indicated in Figure 2, cost is not nearly as important a consideration as effectiveness. In other words, the greater expense of female condoms could easily be offset if they were even slightly more effective than male condoms. The limited evidence that is currently available, however, suggests that the male condom is more cost-effective than the female condom, while the cost-effectiveness of other barrier methods and vaginal microbicides remains uncertain.

Importantly, if male condoms, female condoms, microbicides, and so forth are not strict alternatives, then recommendations regarding their use should not be based on economic considerations. Viewed as methods that women can use to protect themselves with limited assent of their partners, female-controlled methods are not strict alternatives to the male condom—indeed, they might be used simultaneously with male condoms to enhance protection. Consequently, to the extent that choices must be made between them, these choices probably should be made on other than economic grounds.

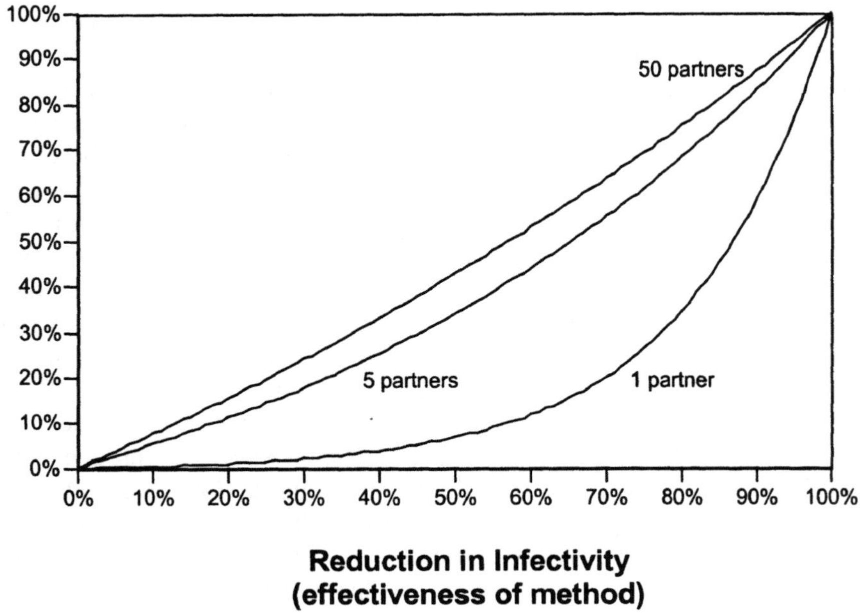

Figure 2. Reduction in the probability of HIV transmission as a function of reductions in the infectivity of the virus produced by an effective preventive method, such as condoms or microbicides. This analysis assumes that the method either is used consistently (i.e., for all acts of intercourse) or not at all. The sexual behavior assumptions are the same as in Figure 1.

4.3 "Alternative" Behavioral Strategies for Reducing HIV Risk

There are a number of behavioral strategies for reducing HIV risk besides the use of condoms, spermicides, and so forth. Persons who believe that they are at risk of HIV may be able to reduce their risk by having less sex (perhaps becoming abstinent), having sex with fewer partners, having sex only with partners they believe are not infected, and substituting less risky sexual activities for riskier ones (see Wolitski & Branson, this volume).

One of the most obvious strategies for reducing risk is to limit the number of sexual partners (m in Equation 2). The fewer partners someone has, the fewer chances he or she has to come into contact with an infected person. The impact of this strategy is evident in Figure 1, which compares the transmission risk for a woman who has either 1, 5, or 50 sex partners, each of whom has a 10% chance of being infected (notably, on average, 5 of the 50 partners would be expected to be infected). From this figure it is clear that large reductions in the number of partners can have a large effect on risk, particularly when the frequency of condom use is low and the risk of encountering an infected partner is high. An even more striking feature of the curves in Figure 1 is that they seem to converge as the frequency of condom use approaches 100%. Indeed, in the scenario depicted there, the risk for someone who has 50 partners but who always uses condoms is actually less than the risk for someone who has only 1 partner but never uses condoms (Pinkerton & Abramson, 1993a, 1998; Reiss & Leik, 1989). Thus, if reducing the number of partners makes someone feel safe enough that they stop using condoms as frequently, the net result could be an unfortunate increase in HIV risk (Abramson & Pinkerton, 1995).

A related strategy is to try to pick only uninfected partners (Hearst & Hulley, 1988), thereby reducing the probability that the partner is infected (π in Equation 2). The potential impact of this strategy is evident from a quick glance at Equation 2: the probability that someone will acquire HIV as a result of having sex with any one of his or her m partners equals the probability that the partner is infected times the probability that transmission would occur, given that the partner is infected.

Figure 3 illustrates the importance of π in determining the overall risk of HIV transmission. As expected, the probability of transmission rises quickly as the probability of selecting an infected partner grows. Notice, however, that consistent condom use substantially lessens the impact of this factor. Thus, for example, the risk from having protected sex with 50 different partners, 25 of whom are infected on average, is equal to the risk arising from unprotected sex with 50 partners, only 2 or 3 of who are (expected to be) infected. (These estimates, of course, pertain only to the specific example considered here and illustrated in Figure 3.) The main problem with the "know your partners" strategy is that it is very difficult to be certain, a priori, whether a prospective sex partner is infected or not. Although limiting the number of sexual encounters with anonymous partners obviously reduces one's risk of acquiring HIV, prudence suggests that condoms should be used with every partner of unknown HIV-status.

But, if there is good reason to believe that a particular partner is uninfected (so that π is very small), then it may be reasonable to dispense with condoms (Pinkerton & Abramson, 1992). This belief is the basis of the "negotiated safety" strategy that some gay couples—and presumably, some heterosexual couples—have embraced (Kippax, Crawford, Davis, Rodden, & Dowsett, 1993; Kippax, this volume). Negotiated safety requires that both partners be tested for HIV antibodies at least twice to ensure that neither is antibody-positive and that the seroconversion window period has elapsed. The couple then agrees either to remain mutually monogamous or to practice safe sex in all outside sexual relationships. Within the primary relationship, the couple may choose to forgo condoms, occasionally or entirely. In terms of the parameters of Equation 2, negotiated safety entails reducing π in order to tolerate greater infectivity (α). The danger here is obvious: if one or both partners are not safe in their extradyadic sexual activities, or if there is a "breakthrough infection" despite their precautions, then both partners are at risk. Nevertheless, on the face of it, negotiated safety would appear to confer substantial safety to the couple, provided they remain within the parameters of the agreement (Kippax, Noble, Prestage, Crawford, Campbell, Baxter, & Cooper, 1997). Further research examining the effectiveness and cost-effectiveness of this strategy is clearly warranted.

Someone might also attempt to reduce his or her HIV risk by becoming abstinent or, more generally, by having less sex. This strategy corresponds to reducing $\underline{n}$ or $\underline{k}$ in Equation 2. Complete abstinence eliminates the risk of acquiring HIV, of course. As reviewed by Jemmott (this volume), abstinence or delaying the initiation of sexual activity has been advocated for adolescents despite limited evidence supporting the effectiveness of abstinence promotion programs for this population. Moreover, abstinence is not a viable option for many persons—especially adults—who may instead choose to engage in sex less frequently. Epidemiologically, this is a sensible strategy, provided that condom use patterns are not altered (Pinkerton, in press). For instance, the risk from 10 acts of protected sex with an infected person is approximately equal to that of one unprotected act; so, for every act of intercourse that shifts from being protected to being unprotected, 10 other acts of intercourse would need to be eliminated to keep the overall risk approximately constant.

Many people may find it difficult to limit the number of sexual activities they engage in, and may choose instead to substitute safer activities for riskier ones, thereby reducing the infectivity parameter (Ridge, Plummer, & Minichiello, 1994; Wolitski & Branson, this volume). For example, a man might choose to engage in insertive rather than receptive anal intercourse with his non-regular male partners. Although this appears to be a sound strategy, condom use remains important regardless of the role adopted in anal intercourse.

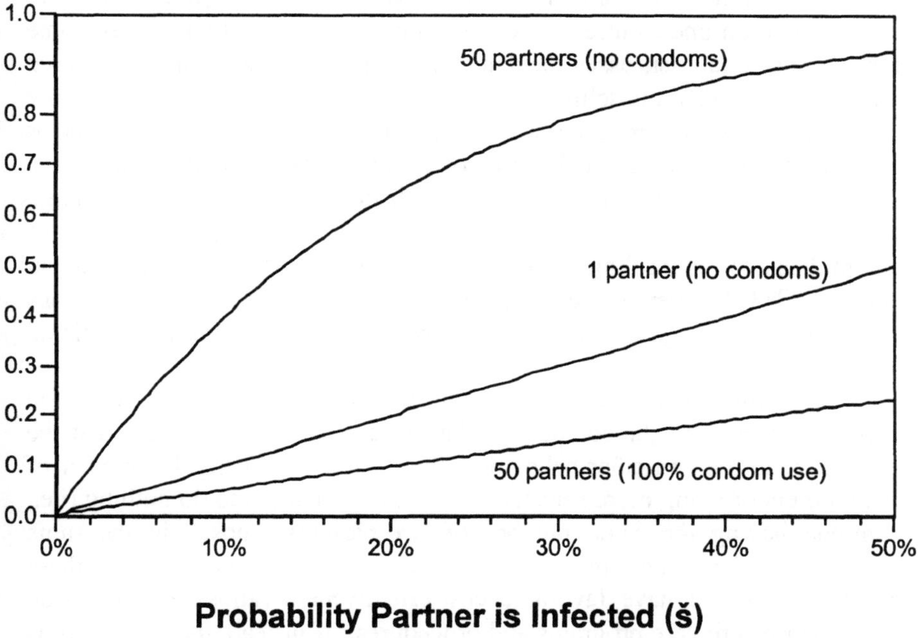

Figure 3. Probability of HIV transmission as a function of the probability that a partner is infected. The sexual behavior assumptions are the same as in Figure 1 except that three distinct scenarios are considered here: 50 partners with no condom use, 1 partner with no condom use, and 50 partners with consistent (100%) condom use.

The infectivity of condom-protected receptive anal intercourse is approximately .001, assuming that condoms are 95% effective, whereas the infectivity of insertive anal intercourse is about .0006 (Katz & Gerberding, 1997; Mastro & de Vincenzi, 1996). Thus, the risks from unprotected insertive intercourse and condom-protected receptive intercourse are similar. Other people might choose to substitute oral sex, mutual masturbation, or other forms of "outercourse" (Cobb, 1997) for penetrative activities. The infectivity associated with fellatio and cunnilingus are not well established, but these activities are believed to be much less risky than intercourse in any of its several variations. Mutual masturbation is nearly completely safe, provided that neither partner has cuts or sores that would permit viral entry.

What do these behavioral strategies cost, and are they cost-effective? At first glance it might appear that these strategies are free. Although this may be true in many instances—for example, someone might spontaneously decide to become abstinent—in other cases, these behavioral risk reduction techniques must be learned, whether through informal channels or through participation in more formal HIV risk reduction education activities. One of the main activities of community-based AIDS service organizations is to provide one-on-one "outreach" counseling, which usually includes some form of personal risk assessment and management plan. One of desired outcomes of this counseling process is the adoption of one or more behavioral changes to reduce risk. Thus, there may be societal costs, such as counseling costs, associated with behavioral risk reduction strategies. Additional societal costs could include such items as testing expenses (e.g., testing is an integral component of negotiated safety); the cost of comprehensive counseling and testing services has been estimated at between \$33 for persons testing antibody-negative to \$103 for persons testing antibody-negative (Farnham, Gorsky, Holtgrave, Jones, & Guinan, 1996).

The cost-effectiveness of behavioral approaches to risk reduction depends, in part, on the comparator that is selected. If it assumed that the alternative to the particular behavioral change (e.g., reducing the number of sex partners or being more selective in choosing them) is to do nothing (i.e., continue having the same number of sex partners, chosen in the same manner as before), then, in light of the their low cost, it is likely that these approaches would have favorable cost-effectiveness ratios in comparison with other health care programs and procedures. If instead, the alternative is to maintain the same number of partners or the same partner selection patterns, but to increase condom use, then the behavioral strategy might not seem cost-effective. As highlighted above, there are very few risk reduction strategies that are as effective as using condoms consistently. Because condoms are inexpensive also, the implication is that few risk reduction strategies will be as cost-effective as consistent condom use.

Although condoms are relatively inexpensive, they nevertheless still may not be affordable in some developing countries. In these situations, the correct comparator might not be condom use, but instead a "do-nothing" option, with zero cost and zero risk reduction effectiveness. Hence, behavioral risk management strategies, which might also include patronizing commercial sex workers less often or substituting non-penetrative activities for penetrative ones, could prove highly cost-effective. Further research in this area is clearly needed.

4.4 Biomedical Strategies for Reducing HIV Risk

Some biomedical therapies for HIV disease and other STDs have a beneficial "side effect"—they reduce the likelihood of HIV transmission or infection. For example, the highly active antiretroviral treatments that are used to limit the progression of HIV disease in infected persons may also cause them to be less infectious to their sexual partners, thereby reducing HIV transmission risks. Antiretroviral medications can also be used after potential exposure to decrease the likelihood that HIV will become established in the exposed person. Similarly, programs designed to control non-HIV STDs such as syphilis, chlamydia, and gonorrhea may have the added benefit of helping to reduce HIV incidence in the target community. Finally, pharmacological interventions such as serotonin update inhibitors for male sex offenders can reduce libido, with a possible benefit for HIV prevention efforts (Bradford & Kafka, this volume). The last of these will not be discussed further here because of the rather distant relationship between the goals of reducing recidivism among sex offenders and preventing the spread of HIV. We will also not discuss HIV vaccines because any such discussion of the cost-effectiveness of prophylactic vaccination would be highly speculative (see Edwards, Shachter, & Owens, 1998; Pinkerton & Abramson, 1993b).

A growing body of evidence suggests that the presence of non-HIV STDs can substantially increase vulnerability to HIV infection in uninfected persons and can increase the infectiousness of HIV-infected persons (Aral, this volume; Institute of Medicine, 1997). Consequently, efforts to detect and treat STDs can have a beneficial effect on HIV transmission rates by reducing the infectivity parameter (α in Equation 2). In one notable example, researchers in Mwanza, Tanzania trained primary health care workers to recognize and treat STD symptoms and provided STD-related medical equipment and supplies of appropriate medications (Grosskurth et al., 1995). A cost-effectiveness analysis of this intervention indicated that it reduced the incidence of HIV in the target communities by about 40% (Gilson et al., 1997). The annual cost of implementing this program, over and above the cost of existing efforts to control STDs, was $54,839, or about $218 per HIV infection averted. According to the authors of this study, in this sub-Saharan setting the lifetime cost of caring for someone with HIV is between $300 and $400. They concluded, therefore, that the intervention was cost saving.

Highlighting the link between HIV and other STDs, the recent Institute of Medicine report, The Hidden Epidemic, states that, "although the proportion of HIV infections that could be prevented in the United States by preventing other STDs has not been well defined...much—perhaps most—of the heterosexually transmitted HIV infection could be prevented by reducing other underlying STDs." The results of two recent modeling studies conducted by Chesson and colleagues suggest that syphilis was a co-factor in over 1000 cases of heterosexual HIV in 1996 (this represents about 3% of the total annual HIV incidence), and that each year, chlamydia, gonorrhea, and herpes are responsible for an additional 4050 cases of HIV infection among heterosexuals in the U.S. (Chesson & Pinkerton, under review; Chesson, Pinkerton, Rein, Kassler, & Irwin, 1999). They estimated that the total cost of syphilis-attributable HIV cases in 1996, including both direct costs (HIV treatment costs including antiretroviral therapy) and indirect costs (e.g., lost productivity) would exceed $750 million (Chesson, Pinkerton, Rein, Kassler, & Irwin, 1999). Even if the only benefit of a national syphilis elimination program were to prevent syphilis-attributable HIV infections, a program costing less than $833 million would likely pay for itself (Chesson, Pinkerton, Rein, Kassler, & Irwin, 1999). Similarly, the future medical care costs associated with treating HIV cases attributable to syphilis, chlamydia, gonorrhea, and herpes total nearly 1 billion dollars annually (Chesson & Pinkerton, under review). In combination, these studies demonstrate the substantial economic burden of STD-attributable HIV cases in the U.S.

Highly active antiretroviral therapies (HAART) can reduce plasma viral load levels by several "logs" (orders of magnitude), and may also reduce the quantity of infectious virus in genital secretions such as semen and cervico-vaginal fluids. This too could lower the infectivity parameter, allowing HAART to act as an HIV preventive (DeCock & Janssen, this volume). There is substantial uncertainty, however, regarding the precise relationship of reductions in plasma viral load and potential decreases in infectiousness. Evidence suggests that genital and plasma HIV arise from separate viral reservoirs (Byrn, Zhang, Eyre, McGowan, & Kiessling, 1997; Zhu et al., 1996), so that reductions in plasma viral load may not directly correlate with genital viral load (the available evidence is contradictory on this point). Nevertheless, it appears that plasma viral load is positively correlated with increased infectiousness (Fiore et al., 1997; Lee et al., 1996; Operskalski et al., 1997; Ragni, Faruki, & Kingsley, 1998) and that antiretroviral therapy can reduce infectiousness (Chirianni et al., 1992; Musicco et al., 1994).

If we assume that plasma viral load reductions are mirrored in infectiousness, then the one to two log reductions reported by many patients receiving HAART would correspond to a 90 to 99% reduction in infectivity (Pinkerton & Holtgrave, 1999b). If true, this would suggest that the risk of unprotected sex with someone on HAART would be similar or less than that associated with condom-protected sex with an infected person who is not receiving antiretroviral therapy. From an economic standpoint, the preventive benefits of HAART are essentially "free"; because patients are prescribed HAART for the health benefits it provides, any additional benefit in the form of reduced infectiousness is a bonus.

There is a sense in which the preventive benefits of HAART might not be free. Several recent studies have suggested that the availability of these therapies have lessened concern over HIV among some at-risk persons, which could lead some HIV-infected and at-risk individuals to become less vigilant in maintaining safer sex practices (Dilley, Woods, & McFarland, 1997; Kalichman, Nachimson, Cherry, & Williams, 1998; Kelly, Otto-Salaj, Sikkema, Pinkerton, & Bloom, 1998; Murphy, Miller, Appleby, Marks, & Mansergh, 1999). Again, it is possible that HAART does substantially decrease the probability of HIV transmission, and that this reduction would more than offset the increased infectiousness that would result if persons on effective antiretroviral regimens decided to forgo condoms entirely. In contrast, if the availability of HAART leads uninfected persons to take greater risks under the assumption that their sex partners, if infected, are nevertheless not infectious, then the "free" preventive benefits of HAART might in fact be accompanied by substantial societal and economic costs (Pinkerton & Holtgrave, 1999b). In any case, the potential epidemiological impact of HAART is limited. As many as half of all HIV transmission occurs during the very early phase of primary infection, prior to seroconversion, during which few HIV-infected persons are likely to be on effective antiretroviral therapy (Jacquez, Koopman, Simon, & Longini, 1994; Pinkerton & Abramson, 1996b).

Antiretroviral medications have also been used for "post-exposure prophylaxis," in which a combination of drugs is taken soon—ideally, within 24 to 92 hours—after a suspected exposure to HIV with the objective of preventing the virus from establishing a persistent infection. Typically, two or three antiretrovirals (usually zidovudine together with another nucleoside analog reverse transcriptase inhibitor and, optionally, a protease inhibitor) are taken for a 4-week period after the exposure. This approach was first implemented as a means to prevent occupational transmission to nurses, physicians (especially surgeons), laboratory workers, and others who might come into contact with potentially infectious substances (Centers for Disease Control, 1990, 1996; Gerberding, 1995; Henderson, 1991; Henderson & Gerberding, 1989). Although the data pertaining to the effectiveness of this method of prevention are quite limited, zidovudine prophylaxis was associated with a 79% to 81% reduction in the risk of seroconversion following percutaneous exposure to HIV-infected blood among occupationally-exposed health care workers who participated in a case control study in the U.S., U.K., and France (Cardo et al., 1997; Centers for Disease Control, 1995).

The effectiveness of regimens other than zidovudine (ZDV) monotherapy is not known, but all combinations used to date have included ZDV, and thus would be expected to be at least as effective as ZDV-monotherapy. A bigger unknown is how effective these regimens are against mucousal/sexual exposures to the virus, as opposed to the percutaneous exposures that are typical among occupational cases (Katz & Gerberding, 1997), or how effective they are when the initiation of therapy is delayed until days after the exposure, rather than mere hours. Despite these uncertainties, antiretroviral prophylaxis for persons with suspected sexual exposures is being offered in several large North American cities (France, 1999).

Antiretroviral post-exposure prophylaxis (PEP) is expensive. The estimated cost of therapy is approximately $1000 (Katz & Gerberding, 1998), including a 1-month supply of antiretroviral drugs, clinic visits, and laboratory work, but excluding potential costs such as time off from work due to complications of the therapy. But, of course, the lifetime cost of treating a person with HIV disease is much greater: $195,000 according to a recent analysis by Holtgrave and Pinkerton (1997). In essence, if PEP can prevent just one infection in 195 applications, then it would pay for itself in averted HIV/AIDS medical care costs. (And even if it did not actually save society money, it might still be cost-effective in comparison with other uses of societal health care resources.) Of course, whether or not PEP prevents someone from becoming infected is a function of variables other than simply the efficacy of PEP, such as the likelihood that the person was actually exposed and the probability that infection would have occurred in the absence of pharmacological intervention. As a consequence, the cost-effectiveness of PEP critically depends upon the circumstances surrounded the suspected exposure—in particular, the likelihood that the partner is infected (π) and the infectivity (α) of the specific sexual act. A cost-effectiveness study by Pinkerton and colleagues suggests that post-sex PEP would be cost-effective for a man or women who has had receptive anal intercourse with a partner of unknown HIV status (assuming that the probability that the partner is infected is greater than about one in five), or for a woman who has engaged in receptive vaginal intercourse with an HIV-infected heterosexual male, or, more generally, when it is extremely likely that the partner is infected (Pinkerton, Holtgrave, & Bloom, 1998). The use of PEP following insertive anal and vaginal intercourse does not appear to be cost-effective, even when it is known that the partner is infected (Pinkerton, Holtgrave, & Bloom, 1997, 1998).

4.5 Structural and Policy Approaches to Preventing HIV

Many HIV prevention interventions attempt to directly modify the behaviors implicated in HIV transmission, such as risky sex and drug use (especially injection). However, sex and substance abuse behaviors are influenced by many extrapersonal factors that reside at the environmental, structural, and superstructural levels. Environmental factors related to HIV transmission include poor living conditions, lack of social services, and underemployment (Sweat & Denison, 1998). An intervention that addresses these three illustrative environmental factors might entail the construction of a housing development close to available social services, including employment offices and job programs. (Although this chapter has mainly focused on sexual risk reduction, structural and policy interventions tend to be more broadly conceived and do not easily fit into the restricted framework adopted for the discussions above.)

Structural factors include laws and policies, both directly and indirectly focused on HIV/AIDS (Sweat & Denison, 1998). For example, some corporations in a European country had policies of performing HIV tests on job applicants and not hiring them if they were HIV seropositive. A media advocacy effort was launched to highlight this policy to the public and to pressure the firms to change their policies; this strategy was successful in modifying the discriminatory testing policies (Holtgrave, 1997). Policies that discourage women's economic independence, such as the personal property laws in many African nations, enhance women's dependence on male providers whom they may be reluctant to divorce or leave, even if their partners continue to place them at risk of HIV by insisting on engaging in unsafe sex. Changing these policies could help reduce the infection rate among monogamous African women.

Superstructural factors include macro-level political and social factors that lead to one group in society having unfair advantages in terms of resources and power (Sweat & Denison, 1998). Examples include sexism, racism, homophobia, and imperialism. Superstructural interventions are usually multifaceted, national-level social movements that address one or more of these factors. Clearly, the impact of these interventions extends well beyond HIV prevention.

Relatively few interventions that specifically address HIV-related environmental, structural and/or superstructural factors have been implemented. A few examples include: (a) changes in gay bath house policies in the mid- and late-1980s; (b) modifications in condom use policies in Thai brothels; and (c) Cuba's program of isolation and containment of HIV-infected persons (Sweat & Denison, 1998). Although there are data documenting the effectiveness of such interventions (particularly the program in Thai brothels), there is almost no cost-effectiveness literature on such interventions.

One notable example concerns the cost-effectiveness of changing syringe availability laws in the U.S. (Holtgrave, Pinkerton, Jones, Lurie, & Vlahov, 1998; Lurie, Gorsky, Jones, & Shomphe, 1998). In the early 1990s, Connecticut modified its laws concerning the purchase of drug injection equipment, such as syringes. The newer, more permissive law allowed persons to buy a small number of sterile syringes without requiring a written prescription from a physician. Subsequent analyses of this legislative change indicated that it led to a decrease in sharing among injection drug users (Groseclose et al., 1995; Valleroy et al., 1995; Vlahov, 1995; Wright-De Agüero, Weinstein, Jones, & Miles, 1998), which likely resulted in decreased HIV transmission rates. Holtgrave and colleagues (1998), extrapolating from the Connecticut experience, conducted a cost-effectiveness analysis of a hypothetical national HIV prevention program for injection drug users. This analysis, which presupposes changes in some states' syringe purchase and possession laws, modeled a national syringe provision program consisting mainly of increased pharmacy sales of sterile syringes, as well as limited needle and syringe exchange components. The results of this analysis indicated that, although the hybrid program would cost several hundred millions of dollars if implemented nationwide, it would avert enough HIV infections to be considered cost saving to society (Holtgrave et al., 1998).

Clearly much more cost-effectiveness research is needed in this area. However, such work will meet formidable methodological challenges. First, it is difficult to perform even basic cost analyses on these interventions because capturing all categories of resources consumed in, say, a national, multi-faceted social movement to confront homophobia would be a daunting task. Second, estimating the number of HIV infections prevented by such interventions is challenging because the effects of such interventions on the HIV epidemic can be quite real, yet diffuse and indirect. Developing a logic model linking a superstructural intervention and a reduction in HIV transmission in a specified geographic area would be a complicated undertaking. Third, interventions at "higher" levels that impact the HIV epidemic also have other important benefits, such as reductions in poverty or homophobia. Quantitatively capturing and estimating the magnitude of these additional benefits is a challenging undertaking.

5. DISCUSSION

This chapter provides an overview of the limited evidence available regarding the cost-effectiveness of non-traditional approaches to HIV prevention, such as the use of female condoms or vaginal microbicides, alternative behavioral strategies (including negotiated safety, reducing the number of sexual partners or being more careful in selecting partners, substituting safer behaviors for riskier ones, etc.), post-exposure prophylaxis, and the prevention and treatment of STDs, as well as a discussion of the cost-effectiveness of structural and policy interventions. This chapter also presents a framework for conducting economic evaluation analyses of HIV prevention strategies that focus on reducing sexual risks. As this review indicates, substantial research is needed to better quantify the economic efficiency of the range of available interventions.

Despite the dearth of cost and effectiveness information on many of the strategies discussed here, one tentative conclusion arises from the modeling examples presented above—namely, the importance of condoms, whether used alone or in combination with other prevention techniques. Condoms are very inexpensive and highly effective, and thus extremely cost-effective, at least in the developed world (Pinkerton, Abramson, & Holtgrave, 1999). Alternative HIV prevention strategies may be cost-ineffective if they inadvertently cause people to reduce their use of (male) condoms. This is especially true of potential alternatives to the male condom, such as female condoms or microbicides. In other instances, condoms can be combined with other prevention strategies to enhance risk reduction. For example, HIV-infected persons on HAART should continue to utilize condoms in all sexual encounters with HIV-negative persons or partners of unknown serostatus, despite the potential beneficial influence of HAART on infectiousness. Likewise, people who reduce the number of partners with whom they have sex would be well advised to continue to use condoms with all partners.

In some resource poor settings, even condoms may be too expensive. Alternative behavioral strategies, such as substituting non-penetrative sexual activities for penetrative ones, and biomedical approaches, such as STD prevention and treatment, could be especially important in these environments. Targeted condom use by commercial sex workers could also be a cost-effective strategy in countries where commercial sex is a significant transmission route. In many countries, legislative and policy changes would be required to support such efforts, by decriminalizing prostitution and introducing 100% condom use policies, for example.

Obviously, what is needed, the world over, is a highly effective preventive technique that is affordable by all countries. Many people hold high hopes that a prophylactic vaccine against HIV could provide an inexpensive means of preventing the spread of the virus. However, there are substantial scientific, social, and logistic barriers to the development and implementation of a global vaccination program (Pinkerton & Abramson, 1993b). Indeed, it is not certain that an effective and affordable vaccine can be developed. This, while vaccine research continues apace, greater efforts must be expended to improve existing preventive technologies, such as the male and female condom, microbicides, and biomedical strategies to reduce HIV transmission (Pinkerton & Abramson, 1995).

Prevention research traditionally focuses on enhancing effectiveness. However, to stem the growing HIV pandemic will require greater attention to the costs, as well as to the effectiveness, of HIV prevention techniques.

ACKNOWLEDGMENTS

The authors wish to thank Mary Turk, Allan Hauth, and Ralph Resenhoeft for research and bibliographic assistance. Preparation of this chapter was supported, in part, by grant P30-MH52776 awarded to the Center for AIDS Intervention Research and by grant R01-MH55440 awarded to the first author.

REFERENCES

Abramson, P.R. & Pinkerton, S.D. (1995). With Pleasure: Thoughts on the Nature of Human Sexuality. New York: Oxford University Press.

Anonymous (1993). The female condom. *Medical Letter on Drugs and Therapeutics*, 35, 123-124.

Bedimo, A.L., Pinkerton, S.D., Cohen, D.A., Gray, B., & Farley, T.A. (under review). Cost-effectiveness of a condom social marketing program. *Journal of the American Medical Association.*

Bloom, D.E. & Carliner, G. (1988). The economic impact of AIDS in the United States. Science, 239, 604-610.

Byrn, R.A., Zhang, D., Eyre, R., McGowan, K., & Kiessling, A.A. (1997). HIV-1 in semen: An isolated virus reservoir. *Lancet*, 350, 1141.

Cardo, D.M., Culver, D.H., Ciesielski C.A., Srivastava, P.U., Marcus, R., Abiteboul, D., Heptonstall, J., Ippolito, G., Lot, F., McKibben, P.S., Bell, D.M., and the Centers for Disease Control and Prevention Needlestick Surveillance Group (1997). A case-control study of HIV seroconversion in health care workers after percutaneous exposure. *New England Journal of Medicine*, 337, 1485-1490.

Cecil, H., Perry, M.J., Seal, D.W., & Pinkerton, S.D. (1998). The female condom: What we have learned thus far. *AIDS and Behavior*, 2, 241-256.

Centers for Disease Control (1990). Public Health Service statement on management of occupational exposure to human immunodeficiency virus, including considerations regarding post-exposure use. *Morbidity and Mortality Weekly Report*, 39 (no. RR-1).

Centers for Disease Control (1993). Supplemental guidance on HIV prevention community planning for noncompeting continuation of cooperative agreements for HIV prevention projects. Atlanta, GA: Centers for Disease Control.

Centers for Disease Control (1995). Case-control study of HIV seroconversion in health-care workers after percutaneous exposure to HIV-infected blood – France, United Kingdom, and United States, January 1988-August 1994. *Morbidity and Mortality Weekly Report*, 44, 929-933.

Centers for Disease Control (1996). Update: Provisional Public Health Service recommendations for chemoprophylaxis after occupational exposure to HIV. *Morbidity and Mortality Weekly Report*, 45, 468-472.

Chesson, H.W. & Pinkerton, S.D. (under review). STDs and the increased risk for HIV transmission: Implications for cost-effectiveness analyses of STD prevention interventions. *Journal of Acquired Immune Deficiency Syndromes*.

Chesson, H.W., Pinkerton, S.D., Rein, D., Kassler, W.J., & Irwin, K.L. (1999). New HIV cases attributable to syphilis in the United States: Estimates from a simplified transmission model. *AIDS*, 13, 1387-1396.

Chirianni, A., Perna, E., Liuzzi, G., D'Abbraccio, M., Bonadies, G., Paone, G., Foggia, M., Patricelli, V., & Piazza, M. (1992). Absence of anti-HIV seroconversion in heterosexual partners of HIV patients treated with zidovudine. International Conference on AIDS (abstract no. PoC 4530), June 19-24.

Clemmer, B. & Haddix, A.C. (1996). Cost-benefit analysis. In A.C. Haddix, S.M. Teutsch, P.A. Shaffer, D.O. Duñet (eds.), Prevention effectiveness: A guide to decision analysis and economic evaluation. New York: Oxford University Press; 85-102.

Cobb, J.C. (1997). Outercourse as a safe and sensible alternative to contraception. *American Journal of Public Health*, 87, 1380-1381.

Cohen, D.A., Farley, T.A., Bedimo-Etame, J.R., Scribner, R., Ward, W., Kendall, C., Rice, J. (1999). Implementation of a condom social marketing program in Louisiana, 1993 to 1996. *American Journal of Public Health*, 89, 204-208.

Dilley, J.W., Woods, W.J., & McFarland, W. (1997). Are advances in treatment changing views about high-risk sex? *New England Journal of Medicine*, 337, 501-502.

Drummond, M.F., Stoddart, G.L., & Torrance, G.W. (1987). Methods for the economic evaluation of health care programmes. New York: Oxford University Press.

Edwards, D.M., Shachter, R.D., & Owens, D.K. (1998). A dynamic HIV-transmission model for evaluating the costs and benefits of vaccine programs. *Interfaces*, 28, 144-166.

Elias, C.J. & Coggin, C. (1996). Female-controlled method to prevent sexual transmission of HIV. *AIDS*, 10 (suppl. 3), S43-S51.

Fabian, R. (1994). The qualy approach. In G. Tolley, D. Kenkel, & R. Fabian (eds.), Valuing Health for policy: An economic approach . Chicago: University of Chicago Press; 118-136.

Farnham, P.G., Gorsky, R.D., Holtgrave, D.R., Jones, W.K., & Guinan, M.E. (1996). Counseling and testing for HIV prevention: costs, effects, and cost effectiveness of more rapid screening tests. *Public Health Reports*, 111, 44-53.

Farr, G., Gabelnick, H., Sturgen, K., & Dorflinger, L. (1994). Contraceptive efficacy and acceptability of the female condom. *American Journal of Public Health*, 84, 1960-1964.

Feldblum, P.J. & Weir, S.S (1994). The protective effect of nonoxynol-9 against HIV infection. *American Journal of Public Health*, 84, 1032-1034

Fiore, J.R., Zhang, Y.J., Björndal, A., Di Stefano, M., Angarano, G., Pastore, G., & Fenyö, E.M. (1997). Biological correlates of HIV-1 heterosexual transmission. *AIDS*, 11, 1089-1094.

France, D. (1999). Emergency treatment to stop AIDS virus. New York Times, October 19.

Gerberding, J.L. (1995). Management of occupational exposures to blood-borne viruses. *New England Journal of Medicine*, 322, 444-451.

Gilson, L., Mkanje, R., Grosskurth, H., Mosha, F., Picard, J., Gavyole, A., Todd, J., Mayaud, P., Swai, R., Fransen, L., Mabey, D., Mills, A., & Hayes, R. (1997). Cost-effectiveness of improved treatment services for sexually transmitted diseases in preventing HIV-1 infection in Mwanza Region, Tanzania. *Lancet*, 350, 1805-1809.

Gold, M.R., Siegel, J.E., Russell, L.B., & Weinstein, M.C. (Eds.) (1996). Cost-effectiveness in health and medicine. New York: Oxford University Press.

Gollub, E.L., & Stein, Z.A. (1993). The new female condom–Item 1 on a women's AIDS prevention agenda. *American Journal of Public Health*, 83, 498-500.

Groseclose, S.L., Weinstein, B., Jones, T.S., Valleroy, L.A. Fehrs, L.J., & Kassler, W.J. (1995). Impact of increased legal access to needles and syringes on the practices of injecting-drug users and police officers--Connecticut, 1992-93. *Journal of Acquired Immune Deficiency Syndromes and Human Retrovirology*, 10, 82-89.

Grosskurth, H., Mosha, F., Todd, J., Mwijarubi, E., Klokke, A., & Senkoro, K., Mayaud, P., Changalucha, J., Nicoll, A., ka-Gina, G., Newell, J., Mugeye, K., Mabey, D., & Hayes, R. (1995). Impact of improved treatment of sexually transmitted diseases on HIV infection in rural Tanzania: randomised controlled trial. *Lancet*, 346, 530-536,1157-1160.

Haddix, A.C. & Shaffer, P.A. (1996). Cost-effectiveness analysis. In A.C. Haddix, S.M. Teutsch, P.A. Shaffer, D.O. Duñet (eds.), Prevention effectiveness: A guide to decision analysis and economic evaluation. New York: Oxford University Press; 103-129.

Hardy, A.M., Rausch, K., Echenberg, D., Morgan, W.M., & Curran, J.W. (1986). The economic impact of the first 10,000 cases of acquired immunodeficiency syndrome in the United States. *Journal of the American Medical Association*, 255, 209-211.

Hearst, N. & Hulley, S. B. (1988). Preventing the heterosexual spread of AIDS. *Journal of the American Medical Association*, 259, 2428-2432.

Henderson, D.K. (1991). Postexposure chemoprophylaxis for occupational exposure to human immunodeficiency virus type 1: Current status and prospects for the future. *American Journal of Medicine*, 91, 322S-319S.

Henderson, D.K. & Gerberding, J.L. (1989). Prophylactic zidovudine after occupational exposure to the human immunodeficiency virus: An interim analysis. *Journal of Infectious Diseases*, 160, 321-327.

Hodgson, T.A. (1994). Cost of illness in cost-effectiveness analysis: A review of the methodology. *Pharmacoeconomics*, 6, 536-552.

Holtgrave, D.R. (1994a). Cost analysis and HIV prevention programs. *American Psychologist*, 49, 1088-1089.

Holtgrave, D.R. (1994b). Setting priorities and community planning for HIV-prevention programs. *AIDS & Public Policy Journal*, 9, 145-150.

Holtgrave, D. R. (1997). Public health communication strategies for HIV prevention: past and emerging roles. *AIDS*, 11 (suppl. A), S183-S190.

Holtgrave, D.R. (1998). The cost-effectiveness of the components of a comprehensive HIV prevention program: A road map to the literature. In D.R. Holtgrave (ed.), Handbook of economic evaluation of HIV prevention programs. New York: Plenum Press; 127-134.

Holtgrave, D.R. & Kelly, J.A. (1996). Preventing HIV/AIDS among high-risk urban women: the cost-effectiveness of a behavioral group intervention. *American Journal of Public Health*, 86, 1442-1445.

Holtgrave, D.R., & Kelly, J.A. (1997). Cost-effectiveness of an HIV/AIDS prevention intervention for gay men. *AIDS and Behavior*, 1, 173-180.

Holtgrave, D.R., Leviton, L.C., Wagstaff, D., & Pinkerton, S.D. (1997). The cumulative probability of HIV infection: A summary risk measure for HIV prevention intervention studies. *AIDS and Behavior*, 1, 169-172.

Holtgrave, D.R. & Pinkerton, S.D. (1997). Updates of cost of illness and quality of life estimates for use in economic evaluations of HIV prevention programs. *Journal of Acquired Immune Deficiency Syndromes and Human Retrovirology*, 16, 54-62.

Holtgrave, D.R. & Pinkerton, S.D. (1998). The cost-effectiveness of small group and community-level interventions. In D.R. Holtgrave (ed.), Handbook of economic evaluation of HIV prevention programs. New York: Plenum Press; 119-126.

Holtgrave, D.R. & Pinkerton, S.D. (in press). The economics of HIV primary prevention. In J.L. Peterson & R.J. DiClemente (eds.), Handbook of HIV prevention. New York: Plenum.

Holtgrave, D. R., Pinkerton, S. D., Jones, S., Lurie, P., & Vlahov, D. (1998). Cost and cost-effectiveness of increasing access to sterile syringes and needles as an HIV prevention intervention in the United States. *Journal of Acquired Immune Deficiency Syndromes and Human Retrovirology*, 18 (suppl. 1), S133-S138.

Holtgrave, D.R., Qualls, N.L. & Graham, J.D. (1996). Economic evaluation of HIV prevention programs. *Annual Review of Public Health*, 17, 467-488.

Institute of Medicine (1997). The hidden epidemic: Confronting sexually transmitted diseases. Washington DC: National Academy Press.

Jacquez, J.A., Koopman, J.S., Simon, C.P., & Longini, I.M. (1994). Role of the primary infection in epidemic of HIV infection in gay cohorts. *Journal of Acquired Immune Deficiency Syndromes*, 7, 1169-1184.

Johnson-Masotti, A.P., Pinkerton, S.D., Kelly, J.A., & Stevenson, L.Y. (in press). Cost-effectiveness of an HIV risk reduction intervention for adults with severe mental illness. *AIDS Care*.

Kahn, J.G. & Haynes-Sanstad, K.C. (1997). The role of cost-effectiveness analysis in assessing HIV-prevention interventions. *AIDS & Public Policy Journal*, 12, 21-30.

Kahn, J.G., Kegeles, S.M., Hays, R., & Beltzer, N. (under review). The cost-effectiveness of the Mpowerment Project, a community-level intervention for young gay men.

Kalichman, S.C., Nachimson, D., Cherry, C., & Williams, E. (1998). AIDS treatment advances and behavioral prevention setbacks: preliminary assessment of reduced perceived threat of HIV-AIDS. *Health Psychology*, 17, 546-550.

Katz, M.H. & Gerberding, J.L. (1997). Postexposure treatment of people exposed to the human immunodeficiency virus through sexual contact or injection-drug use. *New England Medical Journal*, 336, 1098-1100.

Katz, M.H. & Gerberding, J.L. (1998). The care of persons with recent sexual exposure to HIV. *Annals of Internal Medicine*, 128, 306-312.

Kelly, J.A., Otto-Salaj, L.L., Sikkema, K.J., Pinkerton, S.D., & Bloom, F.R. (1998). Implications of HIV treatment advances for behavioral research on AIDS: Protease inhibitors and new challenges in HIV secondary prevention. *Health Psychology*, 17, 310-319.

Kippax, S., Noble, J., Prestage, G., Crawford, J.M., Campbell, D., Baxter, D., & Cooper, D. (1997). Sexual negotiation in the AIDS era: Negotiated safety revisited. *AIDS*, 11, 191-197.

Kippax, S., Crawford, J., Davis, M., Rodden, P., & Dowsett, G. (1993). Sustaining safe sex: a longitudinal study of a sample of homosexual men. *AIDS*, 7, 257-263.

Kreiss, J., Ngugi, E., Holmes, K., Ndinya-Achola, J., Waiyaki, P., Roberts, P.L., et al. (1992). Efficacy of nonoxynol 9 contraceptive sponge use in preventing heterosexual acquisition of HIV in Nairobi prostitutes. *Journal of the American Medical Association*, 268, 477-482.

Lee, T-H, Sakahara, N., Fiebig, E., Busch, M.P., O'Brien, T.R., & Herman, S.A. (1996). Correlation of HIV-1 RNA levels in plasma and heterosexual transmission of HIV-1 from infected transfusion recipients. *Journal of Acquired Immune Deficiency Syndromes and Human Retrovirology*, 12, 427-428.

Lurie, P., Gorsky, R., Jones, S., & Shomphe, L. (1998). An economic analysis of needle exchange and pharmacy-based programs to increase sterile syringe availability for injection drug users. *Journal of Acquired Immune Deficiency Syndromes and Human Retrovirology*, 18 (suppl. 1), S126-S132.

Mastro, T.D. & de Vincenzi, I. (1996). Probabilities of sexual HIV-1 transmission. *AIDS*, 10 (suppl. A), S75-S82.

Murphy, S.T., Miller, L.C., Appleby, P.R., Marks, G. & Mansergh, G. (1999). Antiretroviral drugs and sexual behavior in gay and bisexual men: When optimism enhances risk. Presented at the 1999 National HIV Prevention Conference, Atlanta, August 29-September 1, 1999.

Moses, S., Plummer, F.A., Ngugi, E.N., Nagelkerke, N.J.D., Anzala, A.O., & Ndinya-Achola, J.O. (1991). Controlling HIV in Africa: effectiveness and cost of an intervention in a high-frequency STD transmitter core group. *AIDS*, 5, 407-411.

Murphy, J.S. (1990). The condom industry in the United States. Jefferson, NC: McFarland.

Musicco, M., Lazzarin, A., Nicolosi, A., Gasparini, M., Costigliola, P., Arici, C., & Saracco, A. (1994). Antiretroviral treatment of men infected with human immunodeficiency virus type 1 reduces the incidence of heterosexual transmission. *Archives of Internal Medicine*, 154, 1971-1976.

Operskalski, E.A., Stram, D.O., Busch, M.P., Huang, W., Harris, M., Dietrich, S.L., Schiff, E.R., Donegan, E., & Mosley, J.W. (1997). Role of viral load in heterosexual transmission of human immunodeficiency virus type 1 by blood transfusion recipients. *American Journal of Epidemiology*, 146, 655-661.

Over, M., Bertozzi, S., Chin, J., N'galy, B., & Nyamuryekung'e, K. (1988). The direct and indirect costs of HIV infections in developing countries: The cases of Zaire and Tanzania. In A.F. Fleming, D.W. Fitzsimons, J. Mann, M. Carballo, & M.R. Bailey (eds.), The global impact of AIDS. New York: Alan R. Liss; 123-135.

Paltiel, A.D. & Stinnett, A.A. (1998). Resource allocation and the funding of HIV prevention. In D.R. Holtgrave (ed.), Handbook of economic evaluation of HIV prevention programs. New York: Plenum; 135-152.

Pinkerton, S.D. (in press). A relative risk-based, disease-specific definition of sexual abstinence failure rates. *Health Education and Behavior*.

Pinkerton, S.D. & Abramson, P.R. (1992). Is risky sex rational? *The Journal of Sex Research*, 29, 561-568.

Pinkerton, S.D. & Abramson, P.R. (1993a). Evaluating the risks: A Bernoulli process model of HIV infection and risk reduction. *Evaluation Review*, 17, 504-528.

Pinkerton, S.D. & Abramson, P.R. (1993b). HIV vaccines: A magic bullet in the fight against AIDS? *Evaluation Review*, 17, 579-602.

Pinkerton, S.D. & Abramson, P.R. (1995). The joys of diversification: Vaccines, condoms, and AIDS prevention. *AIDS & Public Policy Journal*, 10, 148-156.

Pinkerton, S.D. & Abramson, P.R. (1996a). Occasional condom use and HIV risk reduction. *Journal of Acquired Immune Deficiency Syndromes and Human Retrovirology*, 13, 456-460.

Pinkerton, S.D. & Abramson, P.R. (1996b). Implications of increased infectivity in early-stage HIV infection: Application of a Bernoulli-process model of HIV transmission. *Evaluation Review*, 20, 516-540.

Pinkerton, S.D. & Abramson, P.R. (1997). Effectiveness of condoms in preventing HIV transmission. *Social Science & Medicine*, 44, 1303-1312.

Pinkerton, S.D. & Abramson, P.R. (1998). The Bernoulli-process model of HIV transmission: Applications and implications. In D.R. Holtgrave (ed.), Handbook of economic evaluation of HIV prevention programs. New York: Plenum Press; 13-32.

Pinkerton, S.D., Abramson, P.R., & Holtgrave, D.R. (1999). What is a condom worth? *AIDS and Behavior*, 3, 301-312.

Pinkerton, S.D. & Holtgrave, D.R. (1998a). Assessing the cost-effectiveness of HIV prevention interventions: A primer. In D.R. Holtgrave (ed.), Handbook of economic evaluation of HIV prevention programs. New York: Plenum Press; 33-43.

Pinkerton, S.D. & Holtgrave, D.R. (1998b). A method for evaluating the economic efficiency of HIV behavioral risk reduction interventions. *AIDS and Behavior*, 2, 189-201.

Pinkerton, S.D. & Holtgrave, D.R. (1999a). Economic impact of delaying or preventing AIDS in persons with HIV. *American Journal of Managed Care*, 5, 289-298.

Pinkerton, S.D. & Holtgrave, D.R. (1999b). Combination antiretroviral therapies for HIV: Some economic considerations. In D.G. Ostrow & S.C. Kalichman (eds.), Psychosocial and public health impacts of New HIV therapies. New York: Kluwer Academic/Plenum; 83-112.

Pinkerton, S.D., Holtgrave, D.R., & Bloom, F.R. (1997). Postexposure treatment of HIV. *New England Journal of Medicine*, 337, 500-501.

Pinkerton, S.D., Holtgrave, D.R., & Bloom, F.R. (1998). Cost-effectiveness of post-exposure prophylaxis following sexual exposure to HIV. *AIDS*, 12, 1067-1078.

Pinkerton, S.D., Holtgrave, D.R., DiFranceisco, W.J., Stevenson, L.Y., & Kelly, J.A. (1998a). Cost-effectiveness of a community-level HIV risk reduction intervention. *American Journal of Public Health*, 88, 1239-1242.

Pinkerton, S.D., Holtgrave, D.R., DiFranceisco, W.J., Stevenson, L.Y., & Kelly, J.A. (1998b). Cost-effectiveness of a community-level HIV prevention intervention research trial. In D.R. Holtgrave (ed.), Handbook of economic evaluation of HIV prevention programs. New York: Plenum Press; 243-259.

Pinkerton, S.D., Holtgrave, D.R., DiFranceisco, W., Semaan, S., & Coyle, S.L. (under review). Cost-threshold analyses of the National AIDS Demonstration Research (NADR) HIV prevention interventions. *AIDS.*

Pinkerton, S.D., Holtgrave, D.R., & Jemmott, J.B. (under review). Economic analysis of an HIV risk reduction intervention for male African American adolescents. *Journal of Acquired Immune Deficiency Syndromes.*

Pinkerton, S.D., Holtgrave, D.R., Leviton, L.C., Wagstaff, D.A., & Abramson, P.R. (1998). Model-based evaluation of HIV prevention interventions. *Evaluation Review*, 22, 155-174.

Pinkerton, S.D., Holtgrave, D.R., Leviton, L.C., Wagstaff, D.A., Cecil, H., & Abramson, P.R. (1998). Toward a standard sexual behavior data set for HIV prevention evaluation. *American Journal of Health Behavior*, 22, 259-266.

Pinkerton, S.D., Holtgrave, D.R., & Valdiserri, R.O. (1997). Cost-effectiveness of HIV prevention skills training for men who have sex with men. *AIDS*, 11, 347-357.

Pinkerton, S.D., Holtgrave, D.R., Willingham, M., & Goldstein, E. (1998). Cost-effectiveness analysis and HIV prevention community planning. *AIDS & Public Policy Journal*, 13, 115-127.

Pinkerton, S.D., Kahn, J.G., & Holtgrave, D.R. (under review). The cost-effectiveness of community-level approaches to HIV prevention: A review. *Journal of Primary Prevention*.

Potts, M. (1994). The urgent need for a vaginal microbicide in the prevention of HIV transmission. *American Journal of Public Health*, 84, 890-891.

Ragni, M.V., Faruki, H., & Kingsley, L.A. (1998). Heterosexual HIV-1 transmission and viral load in hemophilic patients. *Journal of Acquired Immune Deficiency Syndromes*, 17, 42-45.

Rehle, T.M., Saidel, T.J., Hassig, S.E., Bouey, P.D., Gaillard, E.M., & Sokal, D.C. (1998). AVERT: a user-friendly model to estimate the impact of HIV/sexually transmitted disease prevention interventions on HIV transmission. *AIDS*, 12 (suppl. 2), S27-S35.

Reiss, I.L. and Leik, R.K. (1989). Evaluating strategies to avoid AIDS: Number of partners vs. use of condoms. *Journal of Sex Research*, 26, 411-433.

Rice, D.P. (1967). Estimating the cost of illness. *American Journal of Public Health*, 57, 424-440.

Rice, D.P. and Max, W. (1996). Appendix I: Productivity loss tables. In A.C. Haddix, S.M. Teutsch, P.A. Shaffer, and D.O. Duñet (Eds.), Prevention effectiveness: A guide to decision analysis and economic evaluation. New York: Oxford University Press; 187-192.

Ridge, D.T., Plummer, D.C., & Minichiello, V. (1994). Knowledge and practice of sexual safety in Melbourne gay men in the nineties. *Australian Journal of Public Health*, 18, 319-325.

Roddy, R.E., Schulz, F.F. Cates, W. Jr. (1998). Microbicides, meta-analysis, and the N-9 question: Where's the research? *Sexually Transmitted Diseases*, 25, 151-153.

Roddy, R.E., Zekeng, L., Ryan, K.A., Tamoufé, U., Weir, S.S., & Wong, E.L. (1998). A controlled trial of nonoxynol 9 film to reduce male-to-female transmission of sexually transmitted diseases. *New England Journal of Medicine*, 339, 504-510.

Scitovsky, A.A. & Rice, D.P. (1987). Estimates of the direct and indirect costs of acquired immunodeficiency syndrome in the United States, 1985, 1986, and 1991. *Public Health Reports*, 102, 5-17.

Schrappe, M. & Lauterbach, K. (1998). Systematic review on the cost-effectiveness of public health interventions for HIV prevention in industrialized countries. *AIDS*, 12 (suppl. A), S231-S238.

Söderlund, N., Lavis, J., Broomberg, J., & Mills, A. (1993). The costs of HIV prevention strategies in developing countries. *Bulletin of the World Health Organization*, 71, 595-604.

Stein, Z.A. (1990). HIV prevention: the need for methods women can use. *American Journal of Public Health*, 80, 460-462.

Stein, Z.A. (1993). HIV prevention: an update on the status of methods women can use. *American Journal of Public Health*, 83, 1379-1382.

Stein, Z.A. (1995). More on women and the prevention of HIV infection. *American Journal of Public Health*, 85, 1485-1488.

Stephenson, J. (1999). Report offers vision for microbicide development. *Journal of American Medical Association*, 281, 405.

Stockbridge, E.L., Gollub, E., Stein, Z., & El-Sadr, W. (1996). Power and the female condom. *Family Planning Perspectives*, 28, 78-79.

Sweat, M.D. & Denison, J. (1998). Changing public policy to prevent HIV transmission: The role of structural and environmental interventions. In D.R. Holtgrave (ed.), Handbook of economic evaluation of HIV prevention programs. New York: Plenum Press; 103-117.

Tao, G. & Remafedi, G. (1997). Economic evaluation of an HIV prevention intervention for gay and bisexual male adolescents. *Journal of Acquired Immune Deficiency Syndromes and Human Retrovirology*, 17, 83-90.

Trussell, J., Leveque, J.A., Koenig, J.D., London, R., Borden, S., Henneberry, J., LaGuardia, K.D., Stewart, F., Wilson, G., Wysocki, S., & Strauss, M. (1995). The economic value of contraception: A comparison of 15 methods. *American Journal of Public Health*, 85, 494-503.

Trussell, J., Sturgen, K., Strickler, J., & Dominik, R. (1994). Comparative contraceptive efficacy of the female condom and other barrier methods. *Family Planning Perspectives*, 26, 66-72.

Valdiserri, R.O., Aultman, T.V., & Curran, J.W. (1995). Community planning: A national strategy to improve HIV prevention programs. *Journal of Community Health*, 20, 87-100.

Valleroy, L.A., Weinstein, B., Jones, T.S., Groseclose, S.L., Rolfs, R.T., & Kassler, W.J. (1995). Impact of increased legal access to needles and syringes on community pharmacies' needle and syringe sales--Connecticut, 1992-1993. *Journal of Acquired Immune Deficiency Syndromes and Human Retrovirology*, 10, 73-81.

Vlahov, D. (1995). Deregulation of the sale and possession of syringes for HIV prevention among injection drug users. *Journal of Acquired Immune Deficiency Syndromes and Human Retrovirology*, 10, 71-72.

World Bank (1997). Confronting AIDS: Public priorities in a global epidemic. London: Oxford University Press.

Wright-De Agüero, L., Weinstein, B., Jones, T.S., & Miles, J. (1998). Impact of the change in Connecticut syringe prescription laws on pharmacy sales and pharmacy managers' practice. *Journal of Acquired Immune Deficiency Syndromes and Human Retrovirology*, 18(suppl 1), S102-110.

Young, B. (1997). The need for methods women can control for preventing HIV infection and other sexually transmitted diseases. California HIV/AIDS Update, 10(4).

Zhu, T., Wang, N., Carr, A., Nam, D.S., Moor-Jankowski, R., Cooper, D.A., & Ho, D.D. (1996). Genetic characterization of human immunodeficiency virus type 1 in blood and genetic secretions: Evidence for viral compartmentalization and selection during sexual transmission. *Journal of Virology*, 70, 3098-3107.

Chapter 8

"Gray Area Behaviors" and Partner Selection Strategies

Working Toward a Comprehensive Approach to Reducing the Sexual Transmission of HIV

Richard J. Wolitski and Bernard M. Branson
Division of HIV/AIDS Prevention, National Center for HIV, STD and TB Prevention, Centers for Disease Control and Prevention, Atlanta Georgia.

1. INTRODUCTION

Although we are now entering the third decade of the HIV/AIDS epidemic, a considerable amount of uncertainty remains regarding what have come to be known as "gray area behaviors." These are behaviors that fall somewhere in the middle on a continuum of practices ranging from those that are "safe" or "safer" to those that are "unsafe." The difficulty in formulating clear, accurate, and succinct messages about these behaviors has resulted in considerable confusion regarding these practices (and safer sex in general) in the minds of persons at-risk for HIV infection (Wenger, Kusseling, & Shapiro, 1995). This confusion on the part of community members, coupled with an over reliance on prevention messages that emphasize "use a condom every time," has contributed to the development of folk beliefs about HIV transmission that are based on research findings in some cases, but in other cases are largely the result of wishful thinking (Lowy & Ross, 1994). Despite their origin, these folk beliefs are often used to fill in gaps in scientific knowledge about the relative risk of specific sexual practices and serve as the foundation for the sexual decision making of an unknown proportion of at-risk men and women. In addition, confusion and frustration with what are perceived to be overly simplistic or inaccurate risk reduction messages have resulted in the beginnings of a backlash against prevention programs, which have been labeled the "condomocracy" by one commentator (Savage, 1999).

In this chapter we review the evidence regarding the relative risk of specific sexual practices that fall in the middle of the safe-unsafe continuum ("gray area behaviors") and examine the extent to which these behaviors are practiced within populations at increased risk for HIV infection. We also consider how substituting these behaviors for riskier sexual practices, along with partner selection strategies, play a role in sexual decision-making and risk for HIV infection. Finally, we present a model for estimating sexual risks that takes into account partner serostatus, the relative risk of specific sexual practices, and condom use. This model represents one attempt to integrate the available data into a tool for sexual decision-making that can be used to promote a more individualized approach to risk reduction that is based on the available epidemiological data.

2. ORAL SEX

There has been more debate and controversy surrounding the risk of HIV transmission via oral sex than any other sexual practice. To a large extent, this debate has been fueled by disagreement and confusion among prevention programs and health care providers about how to interpret the existing data and how to construct messages about oral sex (Gerbert, Herzig, & Volberding, 1997; Gerbert, Herzig, Volberding, & Stansell, 1999). Some providers of prevention messages classify unprotected oral sex as "possibly unsafe" or recommend the use of barrier protection during oral sex (Palacio, 1997; Gerbert, Herzig, & Volberding, 1997). While other providers consider oral sex to be "safe" or "safer" and promote messages that emphasize the lower risk of oral sex compared to riskier sexual practices such as unprotected anal sex (Nimmons & Meyer, 1995). Other agencies have adopted messages that reflect a harm reduction approach that focuses on reducing the risk of HIV and other sexually transmitted infections by using condoms, limiting exposure to ejaculate, or avoiding oral sex when there is evidence of oral infection or trauma (San Francisco Department of Public Health, 1996).

2.1 Risk Of HIV Transmission

There is considerable anecdotal evidence that HIV can be transmitted during oral sex. Case reports have documented the ability of HIV to be transmitted during receptive and insertive fellatio and while performing cunnilingus (for review see Rothenberg, Scarlett, del Rio, Reznik, & O'Daniels, 1998). These reports suggest that while trauma or disease of the oral mucosa may facilitate HIV transmission during receptive oral sex, infection may still occur without damage or disease of the oral cavity. Case reports also illustrate that the virus can be transmitted to an HIV-seronegative woman who performs cunnilingus on an HIV-seropositive woman (Marmor, et al., 1986; Monzon & Capellan, 1987).

Although these reports document that HIV can be transmitted during oral sex, they do not clarify the relative risk of oral sex compared to that of other sexual practices. In a review of the data regarding oral transmission of HIV, Rothenberg and colleagues (1998) found that prior to the mid 1990s, no study reported a significant association between oral sex and HIV infection. After that time, however, some studies began to find that receptive fellatio posed a small, but significant, risk for contracting HIV. Among studies of gay and bisexual men published in the mid-1990s, two studies reported a slight increase in risk of HIV infection that was attributable to receptive fellatio (Page-Shafer, Veugelers, Moss, Strathdee, Kaldor, & van Griensven, 1997; Samuel, Hessol, Shiboski, Engel, Speed, & Winkelstein, 1993) and two did not (Buchbinder, Douglas, McKirnan, Judson, Katz, & MacQueen, 1996; Ostrow, DiFranceisco, Chimiel, Wagstaff, & Wesch, 1995). Since these findings were published, a study of recently infected individuals has provided additional evidence regarding the relative risk of oral sex (Dillon, et al., 2000). Of 102 gay and bisexual men who were studied within 12 months of seroconversion, 19 cases (18%) were initially classified as potentially associated with oral sex. Following the initial patient assessment, additional interviews were conducted to solicit further information regarding sexual practices. When possible, separate interviews were also conducted with sex partners. Of the 19 initial cases, 8 (7.8% of the total sample) were ultimately determined by the investigators to be associated with oral sex. Of these 8 men, four reported having had protected anal intercourse, and four (3.9% of the total sample) reported no anal sex or only protected anal intercourse with an HIV-seronegative partner (whose HIV status was verified by the investigators).

Accurate estimates of the per-act risk of oral sex are difficult to obtain because it is a considerable challenge for researchers to recruit sufficient numbers of people who practice only certain sex acts. Vittinghoff and colleagues (1999) used data from a study of more than 2000 gay and bisexual men to estimate the per-contact risk of HIV infection associated with various sexual activities. The per-contact risk for unprotected receptive anal sex was 0.82 percent for a known HIV-seropositive partner and 0.27 percent for a partner whose status was unknown. The per-contact risk for unprotected receptive oral sex with an HIV-seropositive/unknown status partner was 0.04 percent, or approximately 7 to 20 times less than the risk associated with unprotected receptive anal intercourse. Other studies have estimated that the risk of receptive penile-oral sex is one-sixth to one-tenth the risk associated with receptive anal sex (Koopman, Simon, Jacquez, Haber, & Longini, 1992; Samuel, Hessol, Shiboski, Engel, Speed, & Winkelstein, 1993).

Some studies have found a significant association between insertive fellatio and HIV infection but this relationship probably reflects the fact that persons who engage in this practice are very likely to also engage in receptive fellatio (Rothenberg, Scarlett, del Rio, Reznik, & O'Daniels, 1998). Insertive fellatio and receiving cunnilingus are likely to present less risk for HIV infection compared to the risk associated with being the receptive partner during fellatio (Rothenberg, Scarlett, del Rio, Reznik, & O'Daniels, 1998). The risk of HIV transmission for all types of oral sex may be increased, however, by the presence of oral lesions, sexually transmitted infections, and oral trauma (Faruque, et al., 1996; Wallace et al., 1996; Rothenberg, Scarlett, del Rio, Reznik, & O'Daniels, 1998).

2.2 Prevalence Of The Behavior

Oral sex is widely practiced by heterosexual and homosexual couples. Among heterosexual men in the United States, 79% report having received fellatio and 77% report engaging in cunnilingus at least once during their lifetime. Fewer women report performing fellatio (68%) or receiving cunnilingus (73%; Lauman, Gagnon, Michael, & Michaels, 1994). These rates are lower than those reported for persons living in France and Finland but higher than those for persons living in Greece (Sandfort, Bos, Haavio-Mannila, & Sundet, 1998). For American and European heterosexual couples, oral sex takes place during a minority of sexual encounters and is usually followed by vaginal intercourse. For example, Lauman and colleagues (1994) reported that only 28% of men and 19% of women engaged in fellatio during their most recent sexual encounter. Similar findings have been reported for heterosexual men and women in France. Messiah and colleagues (1995) reported that approximately one-third of sexual encounters included oral sex and vaginal intercourse but that there were few encounters that included oral sex without vaginal intercourse. In contrast to heterosexuals, oral sex is practiced more often by homosexual couples and is more frequently performed to orgasm. For example, Samuels and colleagues (1993) provide data indicating that 88% of men who have sex with men (MSM) had engaged in oral sex during follow-up periods that ranged from 6-25 months; 25% of sexually active MSM had oral sex and did not report engaging in anal sex. Page-Shafer and colleagues (2000) found that only 8% of MSM seeking HIV testing in a San Francisco clinic had exclusively practiced oral sex. Of these, 94% reported engaging in receptive fellatio without a condom, and 22% reported oral exposure to ejaculate. Oral sex is also common among lesbians; more than 90% of women in one study reported engaging in cunnilingus with one or more partners (Morrow, 1995).

Relatively few data are available regarding the substitution of oral sex for higher risk sexual practices. Few low-income women attending a Missouri clinic (5%) reported engaging in oral sex as a specific HIV risk reduction strategy. There is some evidence indicating that gay and bisexual men have adopted oral sex and other lower risk behaviors as risk reduction strategies with at least the same frequency as consistent condom use during receptive anal sex (Ostrow & Di Franceisco, 1996).

2.3 Summary

Taken as a whole, these studies indicate that oral sex poses substantially less risk for HIV infection than does unprotected receptive anal sex. However, these studies also indicate that oral sex, particularly receptive fellatio, cannot be considered to be free of risk. Factors such as the presence of oral lesions, sexually transmitted infections, and trauma to the oral cavity may all increase the risk of infection during oral sex. Even though oral sex is less efficient at HIV transmission than other sex acts, if oral sex is practiced more frequently or with riskier partners (because it is believed to be safe), this practice would account for an increased proportion of HIV infections in the future. We agree with Rothenberg and colleagues (1998) that "it may be misleading to couch future recommendations [regarding oral sex] in terms such as 'safe' or 'safer', which are ambiguous and subjective at best, since risk is a function of both the estimate for transmission and the frequency of the event" (p. 2102). The challenge to prevention programs and researchers is to find ways of communicating the relative risks of oral sex that are easy to understand and allow individuals to make accurate judgements about their risk of infection so that they can make informed decisions about the level of risk that they are willing to accept.

3. WITHDRAWAL PRIOR TO EJACULATION

Vaginal and anal intercourse with withdrawal have generally been considered to be risky sexual activities due to the presence of HIV in pre-ejaculatory fluid (Ilaria, et al., 1992; Pudney, Oneta, Mayer, Seage, & Anderson, 1992) and concern about the ability of insertive partners to reliably pull out prior to ejaculation. There are few documented cases in which intercourse without ejaculation has been clearly associated with HIV transmission. In one case, a multi-drug resistant strain of HIV was transmitted to the receptive partner during an act of anal intercourse in which the insertive partner withdrew prior to ejaculation (Hecht et al., 1998)

3.1 Risk Of HIV Transmission

Theoretically, vaginal or anal sex without ejaculation might pose less risk than intercourse with ejaculation because the amount of virus is lower due to the smaller volume of fluid that passes between partners. Data from a European multicenter study on the heterosexual transmission of HIV provides some empirical evidence that withdrawal may reduce the risk of HIV infection. De Vincenzi (1994) reported that withdrawal prior to ejaculation significantly reduced the risk of HIV infection among 70 female partners of HIV-infected men who failed to consistently use condoms during vaginal and anal intercourse. Over a two-year period, none of 12 women whose partners "nearly always" practiced withdrawal seroconverted. Seroconversion occurred in 2 of 34 women whose partner withdrew during 50% or more of sexual contacts compared with 6 of 24 among women whose partners "never or rarely" practiced withdrawal. On the other hand, Kippax and colleagues (1998) found that positive beliefs about the safety of withdrawal were a significant independent predictor of seroconversion among gay and bisexual men. These investigators also conducted univariate analyses showing that seroconverters were more likely to have engaged in anal sex with withdrawal than were men who remained uninfected. Unfortunately, the study did not differentiate between men who only reported unprotected anal sex with withdrawal from those who reported anal sex with ejaculation, making it impossible to evaluate the relative risk of these two practices in this sample.

3.2 Prevelance of the Behavior

The family planning literature shows that withdrawal continues to be a popular contraceptive method even in developed countries where other methods are widely available (Rogow & Horowitz, 1995; Trussell & Kost,

1987). For example, withdrawal was the third most frequently used birth control method in a nationally representative sample of sexually experienced adolescents in the United States (Santelli, et al., 1997)–12% of young men and 13% of young women reported that they had used withdrawal as a birth control strategy at last intercourse.

Although these studies provide useful information about the extent to which withdrawal is practiced, they provide little information about its use as an HIV prevention strategy. In one five-city study (Wilson, et al., 1996), fewer HIV-seropositive women (10%) reported using withdrawal as a birth control strategy compared with HIV-seronegative women (23%). However, their use of this method as an HIV prevention strategy was not assessed. One study directly examined this issue among women receiving services through health programs for women, infants, and children. Of the 1,325 women who used one or more strategies to reduce HIV transmission, 9.4% reported they ended sex before their partner ejaculated as a risk reduction strategy (Crosby, Yarber, & Meyerson, 2000). Women with higher monthly incomes were less likely to use withdrawal compared to those with lower incomes. In addition, women who used condoms more frequently were more likely to report ending sex prior to ejaculation. In a European study of serodiscordant couples, 34% reported that they "never or rarely" practiced withdrawal (De Vincenzi, 1994). Gómez and colleagues (1999) found that one-in-ten HIV-seropositive male IDUs had practiced withdrawal with a primary female partner during the prior three months but approximately twice as many reported intercourse to ejaculation. A qualitative study of substance users in London suggests that withdrawal may be coupled with condom use in some instances (Quirk, Rhodes, & Stimson, 1998). The authors described two types of "unsafe protected sex" that may be thought of as modified withdrawal strategies: condom use for ejaculation only and condom use after limited unprotected sex.

There is evidence that some MSM may have adopted withdrawal as a risk reduction strategy. Patterns of sexual behavior among HIV-seropositive MSM suggest that some are using withdrawal as a risk reduction strategy (Gómez & the Seropositive Urban Men's Study, 1999). Among HIV-seropositive men with seronegative main partners, insertive anal intercourse with ejaculation was reported by 21% of men, and anal intercourse without ejaculation was reported by 36% of these men. The same pattern was observed for non-main seronegative partners as well as main and non-main partners whose serostatus was not known.

Data from the Sydney Men and Sexual Health Study indicate that withdrawal prior to ejaculation has increased among gay and bisexual men (Kippax, Song, Know, Crawford, Van De Ven, & Prestage, 1998). Of men who engage in anal intercourse, the percentage of those who practiced withdrawal during insertive anal intercourse increased from 38% to 50% over a ten-year period. An analysis of data from 1997 indicates that many men who practice withdrawal also engage in unprotected anal sex to ejaculation (Juliet, Know, Crawford, & Kippax, 2000). Only 8% of men with regular partners were classified as "true withdrawers." These men practiced withdrawal and did not report unprotected anal sex to ejaculation. Among men with non-main partners, 10% were true withdrawers. Men who practiced withdrawal held more positive beliefs regarding the safety of this practice compared to those who did not engage in withdrawal.

Gold and Skinner (1997) suggest that MSM who report unprotected anal sex may not be using withdrawal as a carefully reasoned risk reduction strategy. Instead, they may be using beliefs about the protective effects of withdrawal as a "last minute" rationalization or justification when they want to engage in unprotected anal sex. Beliefs regarding the protective effects of withdrawal were endorsed more frequently by the 734 men in this Australian study than were any other self-justifications for having unprotected anal sex. Gold and Skinner reason that the strength of these men's motivation to have unprotected sex leads them to view withdrawal as an acceptable risk reduction strategy in "the heat of the moment" even though they might otherwise consider this proposition to be based on incomplete information or faulty reasoning.

3.3 Summary

Regardless of the basis for decisions to practice withdrawal, some individuals have adopted this method as a strategy to reduce the risk of HIV transmission associated with unprotected intercourse. Relatively few persons report consistently using withdrawal as a risk reduction strategy—most report practicing withdrawal during some sexual encounters, and using condoms or engaging in unprotected intercourse to ejaculation during others. The protective effects of withdrawal and the ability of men to follow through with intentions to withdraw prior to ejaculation have not been adequately studied. Although evidence from a study of serodiscordant heterosexual couples indicates that withdrawal may be protective (compared to intercourse to ejaculation), the practice of withdrawal has been associated with seroconversion among homosexual men. It is not possible at this time to reliably estimate the reduction in risk associated with withdrawal, making it difficult to formulate clear prevention messages about the effectiveness of this method (or lack thereof) compared to the effectiveness of condom use and other risk reduction strategies. It is reasonable to encourage withdrawal in situations where intercourse would otherwise be performed to ejaculation without a condom. The potential danger, however, is that messages and beliefs regarding the efficacy of withdrawal may provide a justification for having unprotected intercourse and ultimately lead to increased risk of HIV infection.

4. SELECTIVE PRACTICE OF INSERTIVE VERSUS RECEPTIVE ANAL INTERCOURSE BASED ON HIV SEROSTATUS

The differential risk of HIV transmission to the receptive partner during anal intercourse have caused some gay and bisexual men to form the belief that insertive partners or "tops" are unlikely to get HIV and that the risk associated with unprotected insertive anal sex is an acceptable one (Lowy & Ross, 1994). Given this belief, some men may make differential decisions regarding the role that they are willing to perform during anal sex in light of their own and their partner's HIV status. For example, some HIV-seropositive men may be comfortable being the receptive partner during unprotected anal intercourse because they believe that this practice poses relatively little risk of HIV transmission to their partner.

4.1 Risk Of HIV Transmission

Epidemiologic studies provide some support for this belief about the relative risk of insertive anal intercourse but also provide evidence that this practice does present a risk of HIV infection to the insertive partner. Although unprotected insertive anal intercourse has been found in some studies to be a risk factor for HIV seroconversion, this association is usually not found when multivariate analyses that control for other risk factors are performed (e.g., Buchinder, et al., 1996;Caceres & van Griensven, 1994; Detels, et al., 1989; Ostrow, DiFranceisco, Chimiel, Wagstaff, & Wesch, 1995; Page-Safer, et al., 1997; Vittinghoff, et al., 1999). It is important to acknowledge, however, that these studies have documented cases in which insertive anal intercourse was the likely mode of transmission for a small number of men. A large multi-site study of 2,189 gay and bisexual men is one of the few to provide relative risk estimates for insertive anal intercourse and other sexual practices (Vittinghoff, et al., 1999). This study estimated that the per-contact risk for unprotected insertive anal intercourse with a partner who was HIV-seropositive or whose status was unknown was 0.06 percent (95% CI = 0.02, 0.19 percent). This rate was significantly lower than the per-contact risk estimate for unprotected receptive anal intercourse (0.27 percent, 95% CI = 0.06, 0.49 percent) but slightly higher than the per-contact risk estimate for receptive oral sex (0.04 percent, 95% CI = 0.01, 0.17 percent).

It is possible that a larger proportion of infections may be attributable to insertive anal intercourse at this time compared to earlier in the epidemic. Ostrow and colleagues (1995) found that insertive anal intercourse was not a significant risk factor for seroconversion among men interviewed between 1984-1988 (OR = 1.76, 95% CI = 0.98, 3.17) but that it was a significant risk factor among men interviewed between 1989 and 1992 (OR = 4.37, 95% CI = 1.59, 12.01). This difference was not significant, however, when other sexual practices and substance use were added to the model. Given these data, the authors concluded that there was not strong evidence supporting the hypothesis that insertive anal intercourse had become a more important risk factor for HIV seroconversion.

4.2 Prevalence Of The Behavior

Insertive anal intercourse is practiced by the majority of sexually active gay men, however, only a minority always adopt the insertive role. Samuel and colleagues (1993) provide data showing that 64% of participants from three San Francisco cohort studies had engaged in insertive anal intercourse during the follow-up period. Of these, 36% reported that they had only engaged in the insertive role. Some data indicate that men may make decisions about whether to engage in the insertive or the receptive role based on knowledge of their own and their partner's HIV status. For example, Gómez and colleagues (1999) have shown that HIV-seropositive MSM are less likely to adopt the insertive role (which poses the greatest risk to an uninfected partner) during unprotected anal intercourse with partners who are known to be HIV-seronegative (9% in the prior three months) than those who are HIV-seropositive (23%). Slightly more men reported engaging in unprotected receptive anal intercourse with HIV-seronegative (13%) and HIV-seropositive partners (26%), but it is unclear whether this reflects a conscious risk reduction strategy or merely a preference for receptive sex.

4.3 Summary

Insertive anal intercourse has been consistently found to pose substantially less risk than receptive anal intercourse. By choosing to engage in insertive anal intercourse rather than receptive anal intercourse, uninfected men may reduce their risk of HIV infection. Similarly, by choosing to engage in receptive anal intercourse, HIV-seropositive men may reduce the risk of HIV transmission to an uninfected partner. This is not to say that these practices are without risk. As with other lower risk practices, if the behavior is engaged in frequently and with serodiscordant partners, insertive anal intercourse would present a considerable risk for infection over a lifetime of sexual encounters.

The specific risk associated with insertive anal intercourse has not been adequately determined. Additional data are needed in order to more reliably estimate the relative risk of HIV acquisition associated with insertive anal intercourse, and new studies may need to be designed in order to address this gap in existing knowledge. One of the challenges associated with evaluating the specific risk of insertive anal intercourse has been that relatively few persons engage only in this practice. As is the case with oral sex, this makes it difficult to accurately estimate the risk associated with this behavior without differentially recruiting persons who have limited sexual repertoires.

While unprotected insertive anal intercourse cannot be considered to be risk-free for an uninfected person, this practice would probably reduce risk if it were adopted as a substitute for receptive anal intercourse. An inherent difficulty in this strategy, however, is the fact that this sexual act requires one partner to adopt the insertive role and the other, the receptive role. In any given occasion of anal intercourse, one partner is at greater risk for HIV infection relative to the risk of the other partner. Thus, successful adoption of insertive anal intercourse as a risk reduction strategy necessitates accurate knowledge of one's own seronegative status and knowledge of the sexual partner's serostatus. Regardless of the relative risk of HIV transmission, both partners remain at risk of contracting other sexually transmitted diseases that may facilitate the transmission and acquisition of HIV infection (Doll & Ostrow, 1999; Fleming & Wasserheit, 1999).

5. PARTNER SELECTION STRATEGIES

Sexual transmission of HIV requires intimate contact with an infected partner. For those who are uninfected, behavioral strategies that prevent or limit exposure to HIV-seropositive partners will reduce the risk of HIV infection. This risk is reduced to zero for persons who abstain from sexual contact with others and those who are in a mutually monogamous relationship with an uninfected partner. Those who are not in a mutually monogamous relationship can reduce their risk by selecting sex partners who are also uninfected. The success of these strategies depends largely upon individuals' accurate knowledge of their own HIV status, their partners' knowledge of their own status, the ability of both to accurately disclose their status to each other, and the willingness of men and women to select partners based on HIV status.

5.1 Knowledge And Disclosure Of HIV Status

Of the 800,000 to 900,000 persons living with HIV infection in the United States, the Centers for Disease Control and Prevention estimates that 175,000 to 275,000 of them do not know that they have HIV (Janssen, 2001). It is likely that some of these persons suspect that they are infected, but many may incorrectly believe that they are not infected because of assumptions about the risk of their own behavior, ignorance, or the results of a prior HIV antibody test. Differences between self-perceived and actual HIV status have been found among young gay and bisexual men. Hays and colleagues (1997) reported that 4% of young gay and bisexual men who had previously tested HIV-seronegative, and 9% of those who did not know their HIV status, were seropositive when tested for exposure to HIV. One-in-four of the young men who tested seropositive did not know that they were infected.

Many men and women who know that they are HIV-seropositive are often reluctant to disclose their status to all of their sex partners, particularly those who are non-main or casual partners (Marks, Burris, & Peterman, 1999; Wolitski, Rietmeijer, Goldbaum, & Wilson, 1998). One study reported that 40% of patients attending an HIV clinic had failed to disclose their HIV status to at least one sex partner (Stein, et al., 1998), and another found that 29% had not disclosed to any current partners (Wenger, Kusseling, Beck & Shapiro, 1995). Disclosure is typically a mutual process and may be triggered by a partner's disclosure of his or her own HIV status, a partner's inquiry, or by the perceived HIV status of the partner.

Just as some persons living with HIV are reluctant to disclose that they are seropositive, many uninfected persons do not ask potential sex partners about their risk history or HIV status. A study of gay and bisexual men found that only 23% of American and 24% of Danish men always asked potential sex partners about their HIV status (Wiktor, et al., 1990). Crosby and colleagues (2000) interviewed women about the strategies they use to protect themselves from HIV–more women reported asking their partner about his sexual history (41%) than directly asking if he has HIV (14%). Together, these data indicate that reluctance to be tested for HIV, unwillingness to ask potential sex partners about their HIV status, and failure to disclose information about HIV status act as barriers to the successful use of partner selection strategies.

5.2 Use Of Partner Selection Strategies

Despite barriers to the widespread use of partner-based risk reduction strategies, there is evidence that HIV status plays some role in partner selection. The majority of HIV-seronegative gay and bisexual men (83%) prefer romantic partners who are also uninfected but most HIV-seropositive men (63%) have no preference with regard to the serostatus of romantic partners (Hoff, McKusick, Hilliard, & Coates, 1992). Hamars and colleagues (1997) found that from 1986 to 1993, HIV status was increasingly mentioned in personal ads seeking sex partners. Overall, HIV was mentioned in only 2% of advertisements but was higher for men seeking male partners (8%). When asked how they select sexual partners, only 7% of African American and 15% of European American women reported that they limit partners to those who are not infected or are at low risk for HIV, however, almost none (1% of African Americans and 2% of European Americans) indicated that they chose partners without concern for AIDS (Hobfoll, Jackson, Lavin, Britton, & Shepherd, 1993).

Even when men and women do not select partners based on HIV status, they often take their partner's HIV status into account when deciding the types of sex they want to engage in. HIV-seropositive gay and bisexual men are more likely to have unprotected anal intercourse with partners who are also HIV-seropositive than with those who are HIV-seronegative (Gómez and the Seropositive Urban Men's Study Team, 1999; Hoff et al., 1997; Wiktor, et al., 1990). Men who are HIV-seronegative are more likely to have unprotected anal intercourse with uninfected partners than with HIV-seropositive partners (Hoff et al., 1997; Wiktor, et al., 1990). Similarly, HIV-seropositive male injection drug users are more likely to have had unprotected vaginal intercourse with women who are seropositive than with those who are uninfected or whose serostatus is not known (Gómez and the Seropositive Urban Men's Study Team, 1999). In addition to information about HIV status, persons in serodiscordant relationships may also rely on knowledge about the serosositive partner's viral load and current HIV treatments. Beliefs about the protective effects of HIV treatment and undetectable viral load may cause some people, especially gay men, to be more willing to have unprotected sex with a partner whose serostatus is different than their own (Kalichman, Nachimson, Cherry, & Williams, 1998; Miller, et al., 2000; Remien & Smith, 2000; Remien, Halkitis, O'Leary, & Hays, 1998).

In situations where a partner's HIV status is not known, the perceived HIV status or "safety" of the partner may affect condom use and sexual practices. A growing number of studies has shown that men and women make judgments about a partners' HIV status (or risk of transmitting HIV) based on partner characteristics (e.g., education, profession, appearance, preference for insertive anal sex), their relationship with the partner, or the context within which sexual activity occurs (Clark, Miller, Harrison, Kay, & Moore, 1996; Gold & Skinner, 1996; Gold, Skinner, & Hinchy, 1999; Fisher

& Fisher, 1996; Suarez & Miller; 2001; Williams, et al., 1992). In general, these studies indicate that HIV-seronegative persons are often motivated to perceive people whom they are sexually attracted to in a positive light (particularly primary partners) and to discount the possibility that the partner is infected. The same cues that HIV-seronegative persons use to infer serostatus may be interpreted by those who are HIV-seropositive as an indication that the partner is already infected. For example, an HIV-seronegative person may take a partner's willingness to have unprotected intercourse as an indication that he is also uninfected, whereas an HIV-seropositive person may interpret this situation as indicating that the partner is not concerned about contracting HIV because he or she is already carries the virus.

5.3 Effectiveness Of Partner Selection Strategies

In theory, partner-based strategies have the potential to be highly effective, however, little effort has been directed toward assessing the feasibility and effectiveness of these approaches. We are unaware of any studies that have specifically examined the use of of partner selection strategies to reduce the risk of HIV infection. Research on negotiated safety, a strategy in which HIV-seronegative men in a committed relationship agree to have unprotected sex only with each other, provides relevant information about establishing and communicating serostatus within existing relationships but does not address the initial selection of seroconcordant partners (see Kippax, this volume). It is troubling that there has been relatively little evaluation of partner selection as a risk reduction strategy given the large amount of evidence that clearly indicates the dangers associated with selecting partners who are at increased risk for HIV infection (e.g., Buchbinder et al., 1996; Petersen, Doll, White, Johnson, & Williams, 1993). The importance of partner selection is self-evident when partners are chosen from subgroups that are defined by HIV status or behaviors that put them at risk for HIV infection (such as injection drug use). The influence of partner selection may be more difficult to discern when the pool of potential partners is defined by characteristics of individuals and social networks that are less directly linked to HIV prevalence. Age is one such factor. Studies have found that young women and men who have sex with older men (who are more likely to be infected than their younger counterparts) are at greater risk for infection than are those who choose partners closer to their own age (Blower, Service, & Osmond, 1997; Westover, et al., 1996).

5.4 Summary

For an uninfected person, accurately selecting partners who are also uninfected would constitute an effective strategy for avoiding HIV infection. The real-world effectiveness of this strategy has not been studied and is potentially jeopardized by a number of factors. In order to work, partner selection strategies depend upon persons' accurate knowledge of their own and their partner's HIV status. Although the majority of persons living with HIV know that they are infected, a substantial proportion do not. Persons who have been tested for HIV are often reluctant to ask about HIV or share their test results when starting a new relationship. Despite these potential barriers, many people do consider HIV status when forming new sexual relationships. The quality of the information that many people use to make judgments about HIV status is questionable and may be the result of faulty inferences based on physical characteristics or motivation to see the partner in a favorable light. The potential pitfalls and lack of data make it extremely difficult to formulate specific recommendations regarding the widespread promotion of these strategies at this time.

6. INTEGRATIVE MODEL OF SEXUAL RISK

Estimating the effectiveness of these alternatives for reducing risk poses a considerable challenge: the question is multidimensional. Studies of the efficacy of a particular prevention strategy usually assume that all other factors remain unchanged. However, many factors interact when people make choices about behaviors to reduce risk. For example, although some people may adopt safer behaviors with all partners, it is perhaps more common for them to practice safer sex with partners they perceive to be risky and risky sex with those who are perceived to be safe (Peterman et al, 2000). Paradoxically, STD or HIV infections could conceivably increase after adoption of protective behaviors such as condom use, because a perception of safety may lead to sex with larger numbers of partners, with riskier partners, or both. Similarly, a protective behavior that is less efficacious but used consistently because it is easy to adopt can have greater overall effectiveness than some other, safer behavior that is difficult to sustain.

For an uninfected person, every sexual encounter presents a potential risk of acquiring HIV. Individuals develop their personal strategy for avoiding HIV infection by balancing choices associated with different risks (infection) and those associated with different benefits (the pleasure of unencumbered sex). Ideally, these choices would be based on accurate perception of the risks from different combinations of behaviors. In practice, however, the perceived hierarchy of risks from different activities often does not match the data from epidemiological studies (Lowy and Ross, 1994).

As discussed in this chapter, the risk of acquiring HIV sexually depends on the choice of specific sex acts and the choice of partner, as well as condom use. A model has been developed that quantifies the magnitude of risks and benefits resulting from each of these choices, taking into account differences in HIV prevalence (Varghese et al, 2000). The model used the available information on the sensitivity of HIV tests, the effectiveness of condom use, and the risk for HIV infection associated with different sex acts to estimate the per-act relative risk of acquiring HIV for different sexual activities, depending on knowledge of the partner's HIV status and condom use (see Table 1). The conclusion of this analysis seems intuitively obvious: choosing a partner based on knowledge of the partner's HIV infection status has the greatest influence on the risk of HIV acquisition. Having sex with a partner who recently tested negative for HIV reduces risk 47-fold compared with a partner whose HIV status is unknown. However, this relative risk also depends on the HIV prevalence among potential partners. The likelihood of infection in a partner of unknown HIV status is much higher for groups with 10% HIV prevalence (as in some communities of MSM) than for a person from communities with 1% HIV prevalence (that observed among many heterosexuals attending STD clinics.) For various sex acts, the reduction in relative risk for HIV infection differs widely. Choosing to perform receptive fellatio instead of receptive anal sex reduces risk 50-fold. A 13-fold reduction in risk results from choosing to perform insertive fellatio instead of insertive anal sex. Using a condom results in a 20-fold reduction in risk for any sex act.

By multiplying the relative risks for each choice (partner, sex act, and condom use), the overall relative risk of HIV acquisition during various sexual encounters can be calculated. The overall relative risk is lowest for a person who chooses a partner who recently tested negative (relative risk = 1), has insertive fellatio (risk = 1) and uses a condom (risk = 1): overall relative risk = 1. With the same partner, insertive vaginal sex (relative risk = 10) using a condom (risk = 1) increases the overall relative risk to 10, but vaginal sex (risk = 10) without a condom (risk = 20) increases the overall relative risk to 200. The relative risk is highest when a person has receptive anal sex (100) without a condom (20) with a partner who is HIV positive (4700), an overall relative risk of 9,400,000.

These relative risks for HIV acquisition can be converted to absolute risks by using the observed rate of HIV transmission from infected males to uninfected females during vaginal sex without a condom: 0.1% (Leynaert et al, 1998). By either multiplying or dividing this number by the corresponding relative-risk estimates, absolute risk estimates can be calculated for other combinations of activities (see Figure 1). Thus, the absolute per-act risk of acquiring HIV from receptive anal sex with an HIV positive partner is 5 per 1000. Where HIV prevalence is 10%, the per-act absolute risk of HIV for a man who has receptive anal sex without a condom with a male partner of unknown serostatus is 5 per 10,000. For this individual, adoption of one risk-reduction behavior reduces the absolute per-act risk to a range between 1 and 2.5 per 100,000. Although a per-act risk of 2 per 100,000 seems tiny, it constitutes a high cumulative risk. Having sex once a day at this risk of infection, more than 7% of people would become infected within 10 years.

This model offers several insights, despite its sometime daunting mathematics. First, it provides a means to rank the relative effectiveness of different prevention strategies, alone and in combinations. Second, the figure illustrates that, for many persons, adopting a single risk reduction strategy is not sufficient to prevent HIV infection during a lifetime of sexual activity. Many heterosexuals and others in communities with low prevalence can reduce their cumulative risk of HIV infection to negligible levels with a single risk reduction step. However, because of high HIV prevalence among potential partners, many gay men and injection drug users would need to adopt at least two safer sexual behaviors to achieve a comparable reduction in absolute risk.

Quantifying risks provides an important context both for improved partner selection strategies and for so-called "gray-area" behaviors. Although previous work has suggested that serologic screening, counseling, condom use, and safer sex acts are ways to reduce the risk of HIV acquisition, most of these studies did not quantify risks or compare choices (Peterman and Curran 1986; Friedland and Klein 1987; Goedert 1987; Francis and Chin 1987; Hearst and Hulley 1988). Estimates indicate that two-thirds of persons with HIV are aware of their infection (Sweeney et al, 1997). For persons who are uninfected, it has become clear that discussing HIV status and choosing a partner who has recently tested negative can be one of the most effective ways to reduce risk. All risk of sexually acquired HIV can be eliminated only by eliminating all sexual contact. Short of that, any sexual contact brings some risk of infection, and several steps are necessary to sufficiently reduce the cumulative risk over a lifetime of sexual activity. Behaviors such as those discussed in this chapter and elsewhere in this volume can help to both improve the acceptability and complement the effectiveness of risk reduction strategies comprised of several components. Hopefully, they will also provide opportunities for individuals to choose a combination of risk reduction behaviors that they will be able to sustain.

Table 1. Relative risk (RR) estimates for choice of partner, sex act, and condom use

	RR of HIV Acquisition	
Choice of Partner	**1% HIV Prevalence**	**10% HIV Prevalence**
Recent negative HIV test	1	10
Unknown serostatus	47	471
HIV Positive	4706	4706
Choice of Sex Act		
Insertive fellatio	1	1
Receptive fellatio	2	2
Insertive vaginal	10	10
Receptive vaginal	20	20
Receptive anal	100	100
Choice of Condom Use		
Yes	1	1
No	20	20

7. IMPLICATIONS FOR RESEARCH AND PREVENTION EFFORTS

Beliefs about gray area behaviors and the selection of sexual partners influence the sexual decision making processes of many people. Unfortunately, prevention programs have sometimes provided mixed messages regarding these strategies or, in some cases, have largely ignored them. There is a need to implement studies that are designed to clarify the relative risks and benefits of these practices and to evaluate how messages about these strategies can best be integrated into prevention programs. Failure to meet the information needs of community members may result in continued confusion about these practices and may lead some people to discount the relevance of prevention messages. Given that some community members have already adopted these strategies there is an urgent need to improve the quality of scientific knowledge regarding the potential role of gray area behaviors, partner selection, and other potentially feasible methods for reducing HIV risk (Wolitski, Halkitis, Parsons, & Gomez, in press). In

Figure 1: Changes in risk for HIV infection based on choices of partner, sex act, and condom use

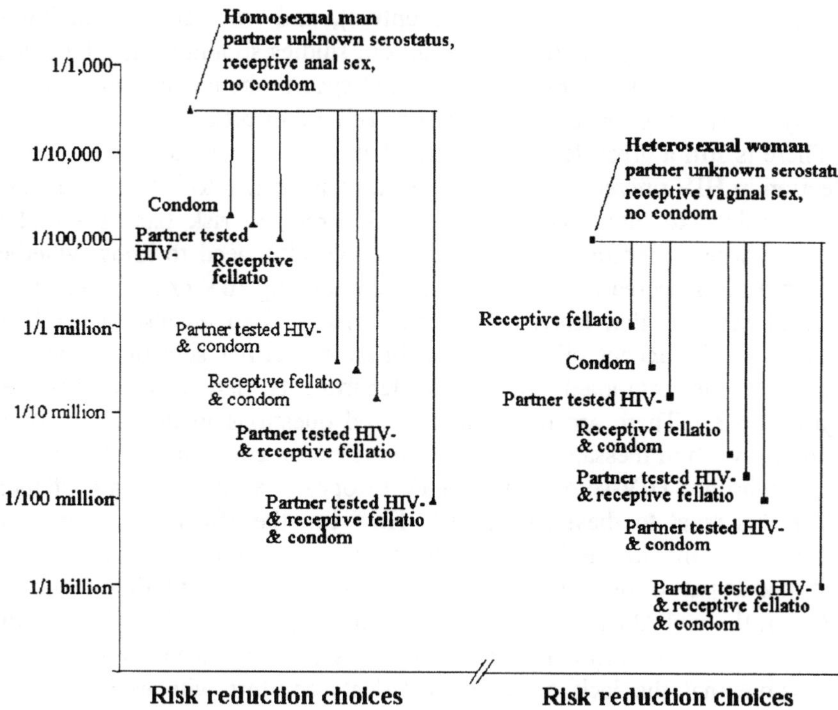

addition there is also a pressing need to better understand how this information can be communicated in a manner that is understandable and leads to a further reduction in HIV infections.

There are considerable gaps in our existing knowledge regarding the relative risks and potential benefits of gray area behaviors. Improved behavioral surveillance is needed to clarify the extent to which gray area behaviors are being practiced within at-risk communities. On-going longitudinal studies are needed to document factors that are currently associated with HIV seroconversion as the relative importance of specific sexual practices may change as higher risk behaviors are practiced less (or more) frequently. Prior estimates of the relative risk of specific sexual practices may need to be reconsidered if it is found that highly active antiretroviral therapies effectively reduce HIV transmission at the community level (see Paxton and Janssen, this volume). In addition to these new or expanded efforts, there are many opportunities for researchers to capture information about a broader range of sexual practices in epidemiological and behavioral research that is planned or already underway. Studies of sexual behavior should include the serostatus of the respondent, the serostatus of sex partners, the respondent's role in specific sexual practices (i.e., insertive or receptive), and whether these activities were performed to ejaculation. In addition, studies should assess the extent to which persons have consciously adopted specific behaviors (and avoided others) as a strategy for reducing their risk of HIV infection.

There is still a great deal to be learned about the potential role of partner selection in HIV prevention efforts. Research is needed to better understand how people take into account actual and perceived risk factors for HIV infection when selecting sexual partners. We also need to know whether these strategies decrease the likelihood of contracting HIV or promote a false sense of security that leads to increased risk. There is also a need for research on the acceptability and feasibility of partner selection strategies that could be promoted by health departments and community-based organizations. There are many unanswered questions in this area: What should prevention messages about partner selection communicate? How will people who are HIV-seronegative, HIV-seropositive, and unaware of their HIV status react to these messages? How can the effectiveness of these messages be maximized? These questions all deserve to be carefully examined as part of our efforts to reduce individuals' risk of HIV infection.

Given the well-documented role of partner selection in the spread of the HIV epidemic, it is surprising that so much research still needs to be done. It is possible that the lack of research reflects comfort with easily defined measures of risk (e.g., frequency of unprotected anal intercourse) that can be asked globally rather than with reference to specific sexual partners or types of partners. It may also reflect concern about the ability of at-risk persons to reliably identify low-risk partners or fear that increased attention to the selection of partners based on HIV status could result in a system of "viral apartheid" in which people living with HIV are not only viewed as less desirable sexual partners but as less desirable human beings. In evaluating the potential role of partner selection strategies, public health officials and researchers must remain sensitive to the possibility that such efforts may contribute to the marginalization of HIV-seropositive people and actively work against this possibility to ensure that HIV prevention efforts do not inadvertently add to the stigma already experienced by those living with HIV.

The fact that multiple factors determine the risk for HIV infection during a single sexual encounter suggests a need for a more multifaceted approach to reducing sexual transmission. This approach needs to recognize that partner selection, specific sexual practices, condom use, and other factors (e.g., STDs, viral load) all work together to place individuals at risk for infection (see O'Leary, Peterman, & Aral, this volume). Given the complexity involved, it is likely that such an approach will require that prevention efforts be carefully tailored to the needs of clearly defined at-risk communities and take into account the needs and preferences of at-risk individuals. For some persons, consistent condom use may represent the most acceptable and effective strategy. For others, selecting partners based on serostatus or substituting lower-risk practices for higher-risk practices may work best. The complexity of the issues involved and the potential confusion that may result from presenting individuals with too many choices emphasizes the need for additional research on the construction of hierarchical prevention messages and algorithms to estimate the relative risk of various methods that are used individually or in combination with other methods. It is critical that this research be undertaken given the possibility that providing more prevention options could undermine prevention efforts and ultimately result in an increase in HIV infections rather than a decrease. For example, women who received information about condoms and other risk reduction strategies in one study perceived condoms to be less effective and were less willing to use them compared to women who only received information about condoms (Miller, Murphy, Clarke, & Moore, 1998).

More than twenty years has passed since the first AIDS cases were identified in 1981. During this period, prevention programs and grass roots organizations have been highly successful in communicating basic information about HIV transmission and risk reduction to at-risk populations and the general community. However, their messages have not always reflected the full-range of risk reduction options that are available and may have inadvertently contributed to confusion about the risk of some sexual activities. It is critical that these messages be reevaluated in light of scientific advances, shifts in the course of the epidemic, and the increased sophistication of message recipients. Failure to do so may cause some men and women to become frustrated with prevention efforts that attempt to simplify or ignore the full complexity of their sexual relationships and their personal decision making processes.

ACKNOWLEDGEMENTS

The authors would like to thank Ron Stall, Troy Suarez, Ann O'Leary, Steve Jones, and Ida Onorato for their comments as well as Laura Whalen for her assistance with identifying and obtaining some of the references.

REFERENCES

Blower, S. M., Service, S. K., & Osmond, D. (1997). Calculating the odds of HIV infection due to sexual partner selection [letter]. *AIDS and Behavior*, 1, 273-274.

Buchbinder, S. P., Douglas, J. M., McKirnan, D. J., Judson, F. N., Katz, M. H., & MacQueen, K. M. (1996). Feasibility of human immunodeficiency virus vaccine trials in homosexual men in the United States: risk behavior, seroincidence, and willingness to participate. *Journal of Infectious Disease*, 174, 954-961.

Clark, L. F., Miller, K. S., Harrison, J. S., Kay, K. L., & Moore, J. (1996). The role of attraction in partner assessments and heterosexual risk for HIV. In S. Oskamp, S. C. Thompson (Eds), Understanding and preventing HIV risk behavior: safer sex and drug use (pp. 80-99). Thousand Oaks, CA: Sage.

Crosby, R. A., Yarber, W. L., & Meyerson, B. (2000). Prevention strategies other than male condoms employed by low-income women to prevent HIV infection. *Public Health Nursing*, 17, 53-60.

Detels, R., English, P., Visscher, B. R., Jacobson, L., Kingsley, L. A., Chmiel, J. S., Dudley, J. P., Eldred, L. J., & Ginzburg, H. M. (1989). Seroconversion, sexual activity, and condom use among 2915 seronegative men followed for up to 2 years. *Journal of Acquired Immune Deficiency Syndromes*, 2, 77-83.

DeVincenzi, I., for the European Study Group on Heterosexual Transmission of HIV. (1994). A longitudinal study of human immunodeficiency virus transmission by heterosexual partners. *New England Journal of Medicine*, 331, 341-346.

Dillon, B., Hecht, F., Swanson, M., Goupil-Sormany, I., Grant, R., Chesney, M., & Kahn, J. (2000, January). *Primary HIV infection associated with oral transmission.* Paper presented at the 7th Conference on Retroviruses and Opportunistic Infections, Chicago, IL.

Doll, L. S., & Ostrow, D. G. (1999). Homosexual and bisexual behavior. K. K. Holmes, P. Mardh, P. F. Sparling, S. M. Lemon, Stamm W. E., P. Piot, J. N. Wasserheit (Eds), Sexually Transmitted Diseases (pp. 151-162). New York: MacGraw-Hill.

Faruque, S., Edlin, B. R., McCoy, C. B., Word, C. O., Larsen, S. A., Schmid, S., Von Bargen, J. D., & Serrano, Y. (1996). Crack cocaine smoking and oral sores in three inner-city neighborhoods. *Journal of Acquired Immune Deficiency Syndrome*, 13, 87-92.

Fisher, J. D., & Fisher, W. A. (1996). The infromation-motivation-behavioral skills model of AIDS risk behavior change: empirical support and application. S. Oskamp, & S. C. Thompson (Eds), Understanding and preventing HIV risk behavior: safer sex and drug use (pp. 100-127). Thousand Oaks, CA: Sage.

Fleming, D. T., & Wasserheit, J. N. (1999). From epidemiological synergy to public health policy and practice: the contribution of other sexually transmitted diseases to sexual transmission of HIV infection. *Journal of Sexually Transmitted Infections*, 75, 3-17.

Francis, D. P., & Chin, J. (1987). The prevention of acquired immunodeficiency syndrome in the United States. An objective strategy for medicine, public health, business, and the community. *JAMA*, 257, 1357-1366.

Friedland, G. H., & Klein, R. S. (1987). Transmission of the human immunodeficiency virus. *New England Journal of Medicine*, 317, 1125-1135.

Gerbert, B., Herzig, K., & Volberding, P. (1997). Counseling patients about HIV risk from oral sex. *Journal of General Internal Medicine*, 12, 698-704.

Gerbert, B., Herzig, K., & Volberding, P.(1999). Perceptions of health care professionals and patients about the risk of HIV transmission through oral sex: a qualitative study. *Patient Education and Counseling*, 38, 49-60.

Goedert, J. J. (1987). What is safe sex? Suggested standards linked to testing for HIV. *New England Journal of Medicine*, 316, 1339-1342.

Gold, R. S., & Skinner, M. J. (1996). Judging a book by its cover: gay men's use of perceptible characteristics to infer antibody status. *International Journal of STD and AIDS*, 7, 39-43.

Gold, R. S., & Skinner, M. J. (1997). Unprotected anal intercourse in gay men: the resolution to withdraw before ejaculating. *Psychological Reports*, 81, 496-498.

Gold, R. S., Skinner, M. J., & Hinchy, J. (1999). Gay men's stereotypes about who is HIV infected: a further study. *International Journal of STD and AIDS*, 10, 600-605.

Gómez, C. A., & the Seropositive Urban Men's Study Team. (1999, August). *Sexual HIV transmission risk behaviors among HIV-seropositive (HIV+) injection drug users and HIV+ men who have sex with men: implications for interventions*. Paper presented at the National HIV Prevention Conference , Atlanta, GA.

Hamers, F. F., Bueller, H. A., & Peterman, T. A. (1997). Communication of HIV serostatus between potential sex partners in personal ads. *AIDS Education and Prevention*, 9(1), 42-48.

Hays, R. B., Paul, J., Ekstrand, M., Kegeles, S. M., Stall, R., & Coates, T. J. (1997). Actual versus perceived HIV status, sexual behaviors and predictors of unprotected sex among young gay and bisexual men who identify as HIV-negative, HIV-positive and untested. *AIDS*, 11, 1495-1502.

Hearst, N., & Hulley, S. B. (1988). Preventing the heterosexual spread of AIDS: are we giving our patients the best advice? *JAMA*, 259, 2428-2432.

Hecht, F. M., Grant, R. M., Petropoulos, C. J., Dillon, B., Chesney, M. A., Tian, H., Hellman, N. S., Bandrapalli, N. I., Digilio, L., Branson, B., & Kahn, J. O. (1998). Sexual transmission of an HIV-1 variant resistant to multiple reverse-transcriptase and protease inhibitors. *New England Journal of Medicine*, 339, 307-311.

Hobfoll, S. E., Jackson, A. P., Lavin, J., Britton, P. J., & Shepherd, J. B. (1993). Safer sex knowledge, behavior, and attitudes of inner-city women. *Health Psychology*, 12, 481-488.

Hoff, C. C., Stall, R., Paul, J., Acree, M., Daigle, D., Phillips, K., Kegeles, S., Jinich, S., Ekstrand, M., & Coates, T. J. (1997). Differences in sexual behavior among HIV discordant and concordant gay men in primary relationships. *Journal of Acquired Immune Deficiency Syndromes and Human Retrovirology*, 14,72-78.

Ilaria, G., Jacobs, J. L., Polsky, B., Koll, B., Baron, P., MacLow, C., & Armstrong, D. (1992). Detection of HIV-1 DNA sequences in pre-ejaculatory fluid [letter]. *Lancet*, 340, 1469.

Janssen, R. (2001, February). *Serostatus approach to fighting the HIV epidemic (SAFE): a new prevention strategy to reduce transmission.* Paper presented at the 8th Conference on Retroviruses and Opportunistic Infections, Chicago, IL.

Kalichman, S. C., Nachimson, D., Cherry, C., & Williams, E. (1998). AIDS treatment advances and behavioral prevention setbacks: preliminary assessment of reduced perceived threat of HIV-AIDS. *Health Psychology*, 17, 546-550.

Kippax, S., Campbell, D., Van de Ven, P., Crawford, J., Prestage, G., Knowx, S., Culpin, A., Kaldor, J., & Kinder, P. (1998). Cultures of sexual adventurism as markers of HIV seroconversion: a case control study in a cohort of Sydney gay men. *AIDS Care*, 10, 677-688.

Kippax, S., Song, A., Knox, S., Crawford, J., Van de Ven, P., & Prestage, G. (1998, July). *Changes in anal sexual practices among gay men 1986-1997: a rational response to HIV?* Paper presented at the XII International Conference on AIDS, Geneva, Switzerland.

Koopman, J. S., Simon, C. P., Jacquez, J. A., Haber, M., & Longini, M. (1992, July). *HIV transmission probabilities for oral and anal sex by stage of infection.* Poster presented at the VIII International Conference on AIDS, Amsterdam, the Netherlands.

Laumann, E. O., Gagnon, J. H., Michael, R. T., & Michaels, S. (1994). The social organization of sexuality: sexual practices in the United States. Chicago: University of Chicago Press.

Leynaert, B., Downs, A. M., & de Vincenzi, I. (1998). Heterosexual transmission of HIV: variability of infectivity throught the course of infection. *American Journal of Epidemiology*, 148, 88-96.

Lowry, E., & Ross, M. W. (1994). 'It'll never happen to me': gay men's beliefs, perceptions and folk constructions of sexual risk. *AIDS Education and Prevention* , 6, 467-482.

Marks, G., Ruiz, M. S., Richardson, J. L., Reed, D., Mason, H. R., Sotelo, M., Turner, P. A. (1994). Anal intercourse and disclosure of HIV infection among seropositive gay and bisexual men. *Journal of Acquired Immune Deficiency Syndromes*, 7, 866-869.

Marks, G., Burris, S., & Peterman, T. A. (1999). Reducing sexual transmission of HIV from those who know they are infected: the need for personal and collective responsibility. *AIDS*, 13, 297-306.

Marmor, M., Weiss, L. R., Lynden, M., & et al. (1986). Possible female-to-female transmission of human immunodeficiency virus [letter]. *Annuls of Internal Medicine*, 105, 969.

Mastro, T. D., & deVincenzi, I. (1996). Probabilities of sexual HIV-1 transmission. *AIDS*, 10 (Suppl A), S75-S82.

Messiah, A., Blin, P., Fiche, V., & the ACSF Group. (1995). Sexual repertoires of heterosexuals: implications for HIV/sexually transmitted disease risk and prevention. *AIDS*, 9, 1357-1365.

Miller, L., Murphy, S. T., Clarke, L., & Moore, J. (1998, July). *Increasing options or condom substition? Impact of hierarchical messages on women's evaluations of HIV prevention methods.* Paper presented at the XII International Conference on AIDS, Geneva, Switzerland.

Miller, M., Meyer, L., Boufassa, F., Persoz, A., Sarr, A., Robain, M., Spira, A., & the SEROCO Study Group. (2000). Sexual behavior changes and protease inhibitor therapy. *AIDS*, 14, F33-F39.

Monzon, O. T., & Capellan, J. M. B. (1987). Female-to-female transmission of HIV [letter]. *Lancet*, ii, 40-41.

Nimmons, D., & Meyer, I. (1995). Oral sex and HIV risk among gay men. New York: Gay Men's Health Crisis.

Ostrow, D. G., & DiFranceisco, W. (1996, July). *Why some gay men choose condoms and other switch to "safer" sex.* Paper presented at the XI International Conference on AIDS, Vancouver, Canada.

Ostrow, D. G., DiFranceisco, W. J., Chimiel, J. S., Wagstaff, D. A., & Wesch, J. (1995). A case-control study of human immunodeficiency virus type 1 seroconversion and risk-related behaviors in the Chicago MACS/CCS cohort, 1984-1992. *American Journal of Epidemiology*, 142, 875-883.

Page-Schafer, K., Veugelers, P. J., Moss, A. R., Strathdee, S., Kaldor, J. M., & van Griensven, G. J. (1997). Sexual risk behavior and risk factors for HIV-1 seroconversion in homosexual men participating in the Tricontinental Seroconverter Study, 1982-1994. American Journal of Epidemiology, 146, 531-542. [Published erratum: *American Journal of Epidemiology*, 146, 1076.]

Peterman, T. A., & Curran, J. W. (1986). Sexual transmission of human immunodeficiency virus. *JAMA*, 256, 2222-2226.

Peterman, T. A., Lin, L. S., Newman, D. R., Bolan, G., Zenilman, J., Douglas, J. M., Rogers, J., & Malotte, C. K. (2000). Does measured behavior reflect STD risk? *Sexually Transmitted Diseases*, 27, 446-451.

Petersen, L. R., Doll, L. S., White, C. R., Johnson, E., & Williams, A. (1993). Heterosexually acquired human immunodeficiency virus infection and the United States blood supply: considerations for screening of potential blood donors. *Transfusion*, 33, 552-557.

Pudney, J., Oneta, M., Mayer, K., Seage, G. I., & Anderson, D. (1992). Pre-ejaculatory fluid as potential vector for sexual transmission of HIV-1 [letter]. *Lancet*, 340, 1470.

Quirk, A., Rhodes, T., & Stimson, G. V. (1998). 'Unsafe protected sex': qualitative insights on measures of sexual risk. *AIDS Care*, 10, 105-114.

Remien, R. H., Halkitis, P. N., O'Leary, A., & Hays, R. (1998, June). *Perceptions, attitudes, and sexual risk among HIV-positive men with undetectable plasma viral loads.* Poster presented at the XII International Conference on AIDS, Geneva, Switzerland.

Remien, R. H., & Smith, R. A. (2000). HIV prevention in the era of HAART: implications for providers. *AIDS Reader*, 10, 247-251.

Richters, J. (1994). Coitus interruptus: could it reduce the risk of HIV transmission? *Reproductive Health Matters*, 3, 105-107.

Richters, J., Knox, S., Crawford, J., & Kippax, S. (2000). Condom use and 'withdrawal': exploring gay men's practice of anal intercourse. *International Journal of STD and AIDS*, 11, 96-104.

Rogow, D., & Horowitz, S. (1995). Withdrawal: a review of the literature and an agenda for research. *Studies in Family Planning*, 26, 140-153.

Rothenberg, R. B., Scarlett, M., del Rio, C., Reznik, D., & O'Daniels, C. (1998). Oral transmission of HIV. *AIDS*, 12, 2095-2105.

Samuel, M. C., Hessol, N., Shiboski, S., Engel, R. R., Speed, T. P., & Winkelstein, W. Jr. (1993). Factors associated with human immunodeficiency virus seroconversion in homosexual men in three San Francisco cohort studies, 1984-1989. *Journal of Acquired Immune Deficiency Syndromes*, 6, 303-312.

San Francisco Department of Public Health. (1996). Oral sex: using your head. San Francisco: Author.

Sandfort, T., Bos, H., Haavio-Mannila, E., & Sundet, J. M. (1998). Sexual practices and their social profiles. M. Hubert, N. Bajos, & T. Sandfort (Eds). Sexual behaviour and HIV/AIDS in Europe (pp. 106-164). London: UCL Press.

Santelli, J. S., Warren, C. W., Lowry, R., Sogolow, E., Collins, J., Kann, L., Kaufmann, R. B., & Celentano, D. D. (1997). The use of condoms with other contraceptive methods among young men and women. *Family Planning Perspectives*, 29, 261-267.

Sarius, F., Edlin, B. R., McCoy, C. B., Word, C. O., Larsen, S. A., Scott, S. D., VonBargen, J. C., & Serrano, Y. (1996). Crack cocaine smoking and oral sores in three inner-city neighborhoods. *Journal of Acquired Immune Deficiency Syndromes*, 13, 87-92.

Savage, D. (1999, July). Bucking the condomocracy. *OUT*, 34.

Stein, M. D., Freedberg, K. A., Sullivan, L. M., Savetsky, J., Levenson, S. M., Hingson, R., & Samet, J. H. (1998). Sexual ethics: disclosure of HIV-positive status to partners. *Archives of Internal Medicine*, 158, 253-257.

Suarez, T., & Miller, J. (2001). Negotiating risks in context: a perspective on unprotected anal intercourse and barebacking among men who have sex with men. *Archives of Sexual Behavior*, 30, 287-300 .

Sweeney, P. A., Fleming, P. L., Karon, J. M., & Ward, J. M. (1997, September). A minimum estimate of the number of living HIV infected persons. Interscience Conference on Antimicrobial Agents and Chemotherapy, Toronto, Canada.

Trussell, J., & Vaughan, B. (1999). Contraceptive failure, method-related discontinuation and resumption of use: results from the 1995 National Survey of Family Growth. *Family Planning Perspectives*, 31, 64-72.

Varghese, B., Maher, J. E., Peterman, T. A., Branson, B. M., & Steketee, R. W. (in press). Reducing the risk of sexual HIV transmission: Quantifying the per-act risk for HIV infection based on choice of partner, sex act and condom use. *Sexually Transmitted Diseases*.

Vittinghoff, E., Douglas, J., Judson, F., McKirnan, D., MacQueen, K., & Buchbinder, S. P. (1999). Per-contact risk of human immunodeficiency virus transmission between male sexual partners. *American Journal of Epidemiology*, 150(3), 306-311.

Wallace, J. I., Weiner, A., Steinberg, A., & Hoffman, B. (1992, July). *Fellatio is a significant risk behavior for acquiring AIDS among New York City streetwalking prostitutes*. Poster presented at the VIII International Conference on AIDS, Amsterdam, the Netherlands.

Wenger, N. S., Kusseling, F. S., Shapiro, M. F. (1995). Misunderstanding of 'safer sex' by heterosexually active adults. *Public Health Reports*, 110, 618-621.

Westover, B. J., Miller, K., Clark, L., Levin, M., Gray-Ray, P., Velez, C., & Webber, M. (1996, July). *Sexual involvement with older men: HIV-related risk factors for adolescent women*. Paper presented at the XI International Conference on AIDS, Vancouver, British Columbia.

Wiktor, S. Z., Biggar, R. J., Melbye, M., Ebbesen, P., Colclough, G., DiGioia, R., Sanchez, W. C., Grossman, R. J., & Goedert, J. J. (1990). Effect of knowledge of human immunodeficiency virus infection status on sexual activity amng homosexual men. *Journal of Acquired Immune Deficiency Syndromes*, 3, 62-68.

Williams, S. S., Kimble, D. L., Covell, N. H., Weiss, L. H., Newton, K. J., Fisher, J. D., & Fisher, W. A. (1992). College students use implicit personality theory instead of safer sex. *Journal of Applied Social Psychology*, 22(12), 921-933.

Williams, S. S., & Semanchuk, L. T. (1999). Perceptions of safer sex negotiation among HIV- and HIV+ women at heterosexual risk: a focus group analysis. *International Quarterly of Community Health Education*, 19, 119-131.

Wilson, T., Barkan, S., Gurtman, A., Massad, S., Nubent, B., Padian, N., Richardson, J., & Riester, K. (1996, July). *The sexual and contraceptive behavior of women infected with HIV*. Paper presented at the XI International Conference on AIDS, Vancouver, British Columbia.

Winkelstein, W., Lyman, D. M., Padian, N., Grant, R., Samuel, M., Wiley, J. A., Anderson, R. E., Lang, W., Riggs, J., & Levy, J. A. (1987). Sexual practices and risk of infection by the human immunodeficiency virus: the San Francisco Men's Health Study. *JAMA*, 257, 321-325 .

Wolitski, R. J., Halkitis, P. N., Parsons, J. T., & Gómez, C.A. (in press). HIV-seropositive gay and bisexual men's awareness and use of alternative barrier methods for preventing HIV transmission. *AIDS Education and Prevention*.

Wolitski, R. J., Reitmeijer, C. A. M., Goldbaum, G. M., & Wilson, R. M. (1998). HIV serostatus disclosure among gay and bisexual men in four American cities: general patterns and relation to sexual practices. *AIDS Care*, 10, 599-610.

Chapter 9

Selective Serotonin Reuptake Inhibitors as a Treatment for Sexual Compulsivity

Troy Suarez and Ann O'Leary
Division of HIV/AIDS Prevention, National Center for HIV, STD and TB Prevention, Centers for Disease Control and Prevention, Atlanta Georgia

And

Jon Morgenstern, Andrea Allen, and Eric Hollander
Department of Psychiatry
Mount Sinai School of Medicine
New York City, NY

1. INTRODUCTION

Since the discovery of the sexually transmitted virus HIV as the cause of AIDS and related illnesses twenty years ago, prevention efforts have encouraged the adoption of safe sexual behaviors. Abstinence, condom use and mutual monogamy are ways to prevent HIV transmission. Having unprotected sex with multiple partners–particularly among populations with elevated HIV prevalence–carries substantial risk for HIV infection and transmission. While many individuals have changed their sexual practices in order to avoid exposure to HIV, many others have not. It is important to identify subgroups of individuals less likely to respond to conventional HIV prevention messages and interventions, and to develop prevention approaches more likely to be effective with each particular subgroup. One psychosocial factor that is associated with HIV-risk behavior is sexual compulsivity (SC). Because self-identification of SC is far more common among men than women (reviewed in Black, 2000), and since gay men are at greatly elevated risk of sexually acquired HIV infection and transmission, the importance of SC to HIV prevention in the U.S. is particularly pronounced among this population. For this reason, the present discussion will be focused on men who have sex with men (MSM).

In this chapter we begin with a discussion of SC, its manifestations, and diagnostic issues. We then review the literature on SC and HIV risk behavior among gay men. Following this we will describe the existing evidence for the effectiveness of selective serotonin reuptake inhibitor (SSRI) medications in reducing obsessive-compulsive behavioral disorders and sexual disorders. We will argue that, despite significant social barriers to implementation, the promise of SSRI medications as a method of reducing unwanted sexually compulsive behaviors and thereby preventing HIV transmission among individuals with SC is sufficient to warrant research on this topic. Finally, we will describe an ongoing research study evaluating SSRI treatment for SC among MSM.

2. WHAT IS SEXUAL COMPULSIVITY?

2.1 Classification And Diagnosis Of Sexual Compulsivity

Sexual compulsivity (SC) is characterized by sexual fantasies and behaviors that increase in frequency and intensity so as to interfere with personal, interpersonal, or vocational pursuits (Kafka, 1994). Those with SC tend to report persistent preoccupations with sexual thoughts, strong urges for sex, and feelings of losing control. During the last two decades there has been a growing interest in understanding and treating compulsive sexual behavior (CSB). Numerous articles and books have been published on the topic including ones on clinical descriptions (e.g., Coleman, 1987), studies of comorbidity (e.g., Kafka & Prentky, 1998), psychosocial interventions (e.g., Carnes, 2000), and pharmacological treatments (Kafka, 1994). Despite advances in knowledge about SC, there continues to be substantial controversy about its definition and nature. As a result, there are no accepted diagnostic schemes or criteria that can be used to define or assess the disorder. In addition, few empirical studies have been undertaken to assess the reliability and validity of competing nosological paradigms. In this section, we consider existing views on the classification of CSB and offer suggestions for future empirical studies.

2.2 Nosologic Controversies

It is generally agreed that compulsive sexual behaviors can be divided into paraphilic and non-paraphilic types (Kafka, 1994). Paraphilias refer to recurrent, intense sexually arousing fantasies and behaviors that are defined as socially deviant. These include activities involving 1) nonhuman objects, 2) the suffering or humiliation of oneself or ones sexual partner, or 3) children or other nonconsenting persons" (APA, 1994, p .522). Although not formally classified as impulse control disorders or obsessive-compulsive disorders, paraphilias are often described as having an impulsive, obsessive or compulsive quality to them (Bradford 1991, 1994, 1996; Carnes, 1990, 1991; Coleman, 1990, 1992; Kafka, 1995, 2000a; Stein et al., 1992). Kafka and colleagues (1992, 1995, 1999, 2000a) suggested the diagnostic category of paraphilia-related disorder (PRD), arguing that hypersexual disorders, e.g., protracted promiscuity, compulsive masturbation, and substance use to enhance sexual pleasure, differ from paraphilias in that they represent exaggerated expressions of socially acceptable behaviors (Kafka and Prentky, 1992). Paraphilia-related sexual disorders refer to recurrent, intense sexually arousing fantasies, urges, and behaviors that are socially sanctioned, but lead to a loss of control over behavior and repeated negative consequences, for greater than 6 month's duration, so as to preclude or significantly interfere with the capacity for reciprocal affectionate activity" (Kafka & Prentky, 1992, p 351). Prevalence for PRD in the general population approaches 6% (Black et al., 1997; Schaffer & Zimmerman, 1990); however, rates may be higher among MSM given the incidence of other addictive disorders and patterns of sexual behaviors in this group. Protracted promiscuity is one of the most common PRD, affecting 50%-75% of clinically recorded patients (Black et al., 1997; Kafka & Prentky, 1992; Kafka & Prentky, 1994; Kafka & Hennen, 1999). Protracted promiscuity is "a persistent pattern of sexual conquests involving a succession of people who exist only as things to be used" (APA, 1980). Paraphilic and non-paraphilic disorders appear in DSM-III-R, but non-paraphilic disorders were deleted in DSM-IV. Controversies about the definition and nature of sexual compulsivity focus primarily on non-paraphilic disorders.

The earliest and most prominent model for defining and explaining SC is the addiction paradigm. Carnes (1983; 1991; 2000) has been one of the strongest proponents of this position. According to Carnes, CSB is best described as sex addiction and is characterized by a progressive loss of control over the frequency and type of sexual activity leading to severe negative consequences. Carnes views on the progression of sex addiction are similar to concepts used in alcoholism. Carnes has identified different stages of progression and indicated that, if left unchecked, sex addition eventually leads to sexual offending. Carnes also notes that in sex addiction, similar to substance abuse, there is a pathological relationship to a mood-altering experience. Similarly, Carnes views the pathological processes involved in SC as potentially explained by psychobiological theories of addiction.

Goodman (1992) articulated a similar view of sex addiction based on the DSM tradition defining substance dependence. He noted that SC was characterized by the hallmark attributes of dependence. These include: loss of control, continuation despite negative consequences, and the capacity of SC to produce pleasurable effects and to be used as a means to avoid painful internal states. Both Goodman and Carnes have presented diagnostic criteria that can be used to assess sex addiction closely modeled on DSM-III-R substance dependence. For example, criteria include tolerance and withdrawal. In addition, in many instances, the criteria are very close in wording to DSM-III-R dependence criteria with the word sex or sexual impulse replacing substance.

Although the addiction paradigm has led to little empirical research, it has been a useful heuristic for clarifying some of the complex issues involved in classifying SC and in generating alternative conceptualizations of the disorder. The addiction paradigm has been criticized from three perspectives. First, several authors have noted that when used outside of the scientific literature the term addiction can take on overly broad and vague meanings (Coleman, 1990; Saulnier, 1996). For example, Griffin-Shelly (1991) defined sexual addiction as "an enslavement to an activity, person, or thing that is characterized by imbalance, lack of control, loss of power, distortion of values, inflexible centralness to the person's life, unhealthiness, pathology, chronicity, progression, and potential fatality" (Shelly, 1991, pgs 7-8). When defined broadly the term addiction adds little or nothing to clarifying the true nature of the disorder. Moreover, applying the term of addiction to SC can lead to oversimplification of the complex psychosocial determinants of this disorder with negative implications for treatment. For example, Coleman (1990) notes that there is a historical tendency to use a twelve-step program of spiritual recovery as a cornerstone of treating SC.

Second, authors have argued that support for classifying SC as an addiction is lacking and that other classification models have a better fit. Historically, substance dependence has involved physiological manifestations of tolerance and withdrawal. These are clearly absent in SC. Similarly, substance dependence has been characterized as a chronic, relapsing condition. However, there is no empirical support for the notion of progression in SC or for a rapid reinstatement of dependence once the problem has been resolved (Gold & Heffner, 1998). For these reasons, Barth and Kinder (1987) argue that SC should be classified as an impulse control disorder.

Coleman (1991) has argued that SC is not an addiction, but a symptom of an underlying obsessive-compulsive disorder (OCD) in which anxiety-drive behavior happens to be sexual in nature. Coleman notes that complaints of SC patients fit many of the criteria of OCD. For example, patients with SC are preoccupied with thoughts about sex and display compulsions to engage in sexual behaviors that are time-consuming and interfere with daily functioning. Moreover, protracted promiscuity appears to be driven more by anxiety reduction than sexual desire. In fact, most sexual compulsives report mood change immediately following the behavior in a similar fashion that people with OCD report anxiety reduction or mood change immediately following the ritualized behavior (Black et al., 1997; Coleman, 1990, 1992). Coleman acknowledges that according to DSM-IV, activities that are pleasurable cannot be classified within the realm of OCD. However, he argues that individuals with CSB rarely report pleasure from their sexual behavior and experience thoughts around sex as intrusive and senseless. Indeed, preliminary data from the CDC funded Seropositive Urban Men's Study (SUMS), a study of sexually active HIV-positive MSM from New York City and San Francisco also supports the theory of SC (O'Leary, Parsons, Purcell, & Macari, 2000). SUMS data demonstrates that SC men find less satisfaction with sex than with non-SC men, suggesting that pleasure may not be a primary determinant of sexually compulsive behavior.

Third, a number of authors have argued that the addiction paradigm, especially as operationalized by criteria of Goodman and Carnes, makes it difficult, if not impossible, to clearly demarcate normal from pathological sexual activity. For example, Levine and Troiden (1988) argue that sex addiction defines excessive sexual behavior that does not fit normative standards as pathological. Although it has been argued that sex addiction should not be equated with hypersexuality or nympomania (Orford, 1978), the criteria offered by Carnes and Goodman would likely diagnose most cases of excessive sexual activity, even in the absence of subjective distress or impairment, as pathological.

Moser (1993) argues that sex addiction criteria adapted from DSM substance dependence would lead to the diagnosis of clearly normal sexual behavior as sex addiction. For example, he notes that married couples could be diagnosed as sex addicts because they would meet the criteria of being preoccupied with sexual activities and spending more time engaging in sex than intended. Moser adds that it is not clear whether more precise wording of the criteria would resolve this problem or whether the entire concept of applying an addiction paradigm to sexual behavior is problematic.

For reasons noted above several authors have developed alternative diagnostic criteria that include impairment as a necessary condition for diagnosis. Black (2000) proposed criteria for SC that include a maladaptive preoccupation with sexual cognitions or behaviors coupled with impairment or significant distress. Kafka (1994, pg. 39) defines non-paraphilic SC as "sexually arousing fantasies, urges, or activities involving culturally sanctioned sexual interests and behaviors that increase in frequency and intensity (for at least 6 months duration) so as to interfere with the capacity for reciprocal affectionate sexual activity".

Most men with SC also have other PRD, paraphilias, anxiety disorders, depression, and substance abuse problems (Black et al., 1997; Carnes, 1990; Carnes, 1991; Kafka, 1991; Kafka & Prentky, 1992; Kafka & Prentky, 1994). More than 66% of SC compulsive men currently report depression, anxiety and/or alcohol and substance abuse disorders (Black et al., 1997). Lifetime prevalence of these disorders approaches 75% in men with PRD (Kafka & Prentky, 1994). Nearly 30% report childhood sexual and/or physical abuse. Common comorbid paraphilias and PRD include compulsive masturbation, voyeurism, and dependence on pornography (Black et al., 1997; Kafka & Prentky, 1994). Other clinical symptoms associates with paraphilias are low self-esteem, social anxiety, social skills impairment, guilt, and additional expressions of socially deviant impulse control problems (Black et al., 1997; Kafka, 1997).

2.3 Research Directions in Nosology

In their summary of the SC literature Gold and Heffner (1998) state that the field has reached a point where further advances cannot be made without empirical research. The positions reviewed above suggest a number of promising directions for empirical scrutiny. First, operational criteria presented by Carnes and Goodman should be revised to address obvious threshold and reliability problems. Furthermore, dependence criteria should not mimic DSM-III-R language, but should be formulated based on the conceptual underpinnings of the DSM dependence criteria: the alcohol dependence syndrome of Edwards and Gross (1976). Diagnostic studies should test whether SC fits the critical features of the dependence syndrome. For example, do criteria cohere, form a continuun of severity, and are they independent of more mild manifestations of sexual impulsive behaviors (Zeidonis & Kosten, 1992)?

In addition, alternative conceptualizations of SC should be assessed. For example, do impairment criteria yield more valid diagnostic groups than addiction criteria? Similarly, do individuals with SC report a loss of pleasure around sex and experience thoughts about sex as senseless and intrusive? If so, this would support an OCD conceptualization. Finally, studies should examine the course and onset of SC symptoms to determine whether the disorder is progressive and characterized by repeated relapse episodes. Empirical studies addressing these questions would help to substantially advance current understanding of SC and lead to more reliable and valid definitions of the disorder.

Finally, research should identify factors that may be unique to MSM. There is reason to speculate that the descriptive features of SC might differ in MSM, because sociocultural factors such as norms about sexual expression are thought to influence the prevalance and nature of SC (Laumann et al., 1994). Interestisngly, there is indication that SC is associated with childhood sexual abuse (Carnes & Delmonico, 1996), the latter being significantly associated with sexual risk behavior among MSM (O'Leary, Purcell, Remien & Gomez, 2001; Paul, Catania, Pollack, & Stall, 2001).

2.4 The Biology Of SC

Regardless of the adopted theory, SC appears to have a strong biological etiology (Bradford & Greenberg, 1996; Kafka, 1995, 1997a; Greenberg & Bradford, 1997; Stein et al., 1992). Kafka's (1997a) monoamine theory of hypersexuality suggests that dysregulations in the biological amines serotonin, dopamine, and norepinephrine are responsible for SC. Because monoamines are involved in appetitive dimensions of male sexual behavior, alteration of monoamine transmission can have substantial effects on sexual functioning (Bradford & Greenberg, 1996; Kafka, 1995, 1997; Greenberg & Bradford, 1997; Stein et al., 1992). Monoamines also appear to modulate comorbid disorders generally seen in SC, including impulsivity, anxiety, depression, and compulsivity (Bradford & Greenberg, 1996; Kafka, 1997; Greenberg & Bradford, 1997). The most significant finding is that SSRIs can ameliorate paraphilic and paraphilic-related arousal and behavior while leaving intimate sexual functioning in tact (Bradford & Greenberg, 1996; Kafka, 1994, 1995, 1997; Kafka & Prentky, 1992, 1994; Greenberg & Bradford, 1997; Stein et al., 1992).

Although SC has been associated with increases in both central norepinephrine and dopamine, and decreases in central serotonin, the role of catecholamines in SC has been far less researched than that of serotonin (Kafka, 1995). With respect to dopamine, there is some evidence that neuroleptics also have the potential to reduce sexually compulsive behavior; however, these medications should not be considered for nonpsychotic individuals due to nonspecificity of effect and frequent adverse side effects (Kafka, 1995). Whereas dopaminergic antagonists inhibit sexual behavior, dopamine and norepinephrine agonists, such as psychostimulants may disinhibit sexual behavior (Schaffer, 1994).

3. SC AND HIV RISK BEHAVIOR AMONG MSM

Although many MSM have reduced their sexual risk behaviors, some continue to engage in unprotected sex. Recent investigations of risk behaviors among cohorts of HIV seropositive (HIV+) and seronegative (HIV-) MSM have shown that approximately 25-30% of both groups continue to report unprotected anal intercourse (UAI) (Dilley, McFarland, Sullivan, & Discepola, 1998; Halkitis & Parsons, 1999; Kalichman, Greenberg, & Abel, 1997). It has been argued that prevention efforts targeting MSM are still urgently needed (Kelly, 1997; Wolitski, Valdiserri, Denning, & Levine, 2001). One recommended strategy is to identify distinct subpopulations who, are at greatest risk for HIV infection or transmission and develop interventions specifically designed for these subgroups. The underlying premise of this strategy is to both tailor and target interventions to the 25-30% of MSM most in need.

As discussed above, a defining characteristic of SC is loss of control over sexual behavior (Black et al., 1997; Kafka & Prentky, 1994). This loss of control can lead directly to risky sexual behavior. Further, Quadland and Shattls (1987) suggest that individuals who are preoccupied with sex may be inclined to engage in high-risk behaviors despite the threat of HIV infections. Sometimes men with SC feel so out of control that they will engage in higher-risk behavior and then feel guilty afterwards. This guilt might then serve as a point from which a vicious cycle begins—sexual behavior occurs to ease the guilt, but the behavior causes more guilt, which leads to more sex (Kafka, 2000a; Suarez & Kauth, 2001; Suarez & Miller, 2001). Wolfe (2000) in his book 'Men Like Us' suggests that worrying about HIV, yet regularly having risky sex anyway is diagnostic of SC in MSM.

We do not know the full extent of the prevalence of SC among MSM, as no studies to date have systematically investigated this problem with large samples of MSM. Black's (2000) review of SC suggests that 5-6% of the general population suffers from SC. Through our work with community-based organizations (CBOs) servicing the needs of MSM in New York City in 1999, we were surprised to find that 26 weekly Sexual Compulsives Anonymous (SCA) self-help groups met at the NYC Lesbian and Gay Community Services Center. This indicates that, at least in HIV epicenters (possibly due to concerns about HIV infection and transmission), many individuals seek help for this problem.

Although, logically, it would appear that sexually compulsive males would be at higher risk for transmission or infection of HIV, very few studies have investigated this relationship. In those studies where SC has been measured, it was measured mostly in MSM populations; however, it is likely that the same findings apply to those with SC in general rather than just to MSM. It appears that men with SC are at higher risk for many reasons (Benotsch, Kalichman, & Kelly, 1999; Exner at al., 1997; Kalichman & Rompa, 1995; Kalichman, Greenberg, & Abel, 1997; Quadland, 1985; Quadland & Shattls, 1987).

One risk factor for acquiring HIV is the absolute number of sexual partners that an individual has (McKusick, Conant, & Coates, 1985; Solomon & DeJong, 1986). With more partners, the likelihood that at least an occasional slip can lead to infection or transmission increases. Further, for those individuals engaging in anal intercourse even with condoms, the more frequently the behavior occurs, the greater the probability of encountering condom manufacturing defects that can lead to breakage or user failure (Pinkerton & Abramson, 1996, Pinkerton, Abramson, & Turk, 1998). Of course, there are a significant number of individuals who do not use condoms and continually place themselves or their sex partners at risk for infection with HIV and other sexually transmitted diseases.

Men with SC have far greater numbers of partners and are less safe with the partners that they do have (Benotsch, Kalichman, & Kelly, 1999; Kalichman & Rompa, 1995; Kalichman, Greenberg, & Abel, 1997; Quadland, 1985). Kalichman, Greenberg, and Abel (1997) interviewed 223 HIV-positive men participating in substance abuse groups and HIV prevention programs. Across the groups, participants higher in SC reported multiple UAI episodes. Likewise, Benotsch, Kalichman, and Kelly (1999) reported that of 112 HIV-positive MSM, those men who scored higher on SC reported engaging in more frequent UAI with more partners. This group also rated higher-risk activities as more pleasurable than lower-risk activities. Finally, data from the CDC funded Seropositive Urban Men's Study (SUMS) found that those scoring higher on Kalichman's SC scale also reported more sexual partners in the past 3 months, greater frequency of looking for sexual partners in public cruising areas and parks, and more unprotected anal sex with HIV-negative or serostatus unknown sex partners.

The relationship between SC and risk behavior is not limited to HIV-positive men. Quadland (1985) reported that sexual compulsives differed from controls in both the frequency and type of sexual behavior. They engaged in higher-risk behavior with more partners. Similarly, Kalichman and Rompa (1995) found that SC predicted UAI and fewer intentions to reduce risk for HIV infection among HIV-negative gay men. Of the 156 men of varying HIV status interviewed by Exner and Colleagues (1997), those who reported difficulty controlling their behavior reported more occasions of receiving ejaculate anally. Additionally, these men reported greater number of one-time sex partners and a greater likelihood of substance abuse during sex.

As stated earlier, substance abuse is highly prevalent among men with paraphilia-related disorders in general. Studies also evidence a high rate of substance use, e.g., poppers, alcohol, and speed among sexually compulsive males during sexual behavior (Benotsch et al., 1999; Exner et al., 1997). One diagnostic feature of PRD is the dependence on substances to enhance sexual pleasure (Kafka, 2000a). Substance use itself is highly predictive of HIV risk behavior as the use of substances can cloud judgment and lead to risk behavior (see McKirnan, Ostrow, & Hope, 1996).

These studies provide strong evidence that men with SC may be at substantial risk for HIV infection or transmission. Not only do men with SC engage in higher-risk behavior, but they also have high number of sexual partners. Moreover, these men report frequent substance use during sexual behavior that can lead to risky behavior even when intending to engage in safer sexusl behaviors. Clearly, MSM with SC are an important population with respect to HIV infection and transmission.

Despite intending to engage in safer sex, many people are motivated to reevaluate their commitment and down-regulate their safer sex adherence as the sexual encounter unfolds (Suarez, Kelly, Pinkerton et al., 2001; Suarez & Miller, 2001). These "justifications" include the assumption of seroconcordant partner status (Gold, 2000; Suarez, Kelly, Pinkerton et al., 2001; Suarez & Miller, 2001). Both HIV-positive and HIV-negative men display this bias. This allows men to rationalize their risk behavior so as to reduce guilt surrounding risk behaviors (Suarez et al., 2001). By assuming serconcordance and using other "justifications" for unsafe sex, both HIV-negative and HIV-positive men with SC may play a significant part in propagating the epidemic (Kalichman & Rompa, 1995; Kalichman, Greenberg, & Abel, 1997).

4. CLINICAL PSYCHIATRIC USES OF SSRI DRUGS

4.1 SSRI use in Depression

SSRIs have become the medication treatment of choice for depression, replacing the older tricyclic antidepressants (TCAs) even though, among general outpatient populations, there are no differences in efficacy among the classes of antidepressants. Overall, approximately 60% to 80% of patients with major depression have a clinically meaningful response to a single trial of antidepressant medication if given in an adequate dose for at least 6 weeks, and some of the others have a partial response (Hollander & Wong, 2000). Approximately 10% to 15% of patients generally dropout of medication treatment in the first three weeks (American Psychiatric Association, 1993).

Along with newer generation antidepressants and those that inhibit both serotonin and norepinephrine (SNRIs), SSRIs have a more favorable side-effect profile than older antidepressants such as TCAs and monoaminoxidase inhibitors (MAOIs). The TCAs and MAOIs need to be started at lower levels and titrated more slowly to effective doses in order to minimize patients' experience of adverse side effects. In contrast, since they induce fewer and less severe side effects, the SSRIs, SNRIs and newer generation antidepressants can be started at an effective dose for depression. In addition, the TCAs and MAOIs pose a much more serious danger in overdose and misuse than the SSRIs.

Antidepressant effects for all these medications usually develop slowly over time, therefore an adequate evaluation of the efficacy of a particular medication requires a trial of approximately 6 weeks. For those who do not respond adequately to the initial medication, a switch to another medication or the addition of another medication (especially if there was a partial response) is advisable. It is important to realize that many patients who are termed refractory have not received an adequate trial in terms of the dose or the length of treatment.

4.2 SSRI Use in Obsessive-Compulsive Spectrum Disorders

SC is characterized by intrusive sexual thoughts and repetitive sexual behaviors that cause distress and interfere with other important areas of the person's life. Not only do these thoughts and behaviors resemble the obsessive thoughts and compulsive behaviors found in obsessive-compulsive disorder, but the disorders have other similarities as well. Indeed, SC is one of a number of disorders with intrusive thoughts or repetitive behaviors as a central symptom; these are now considered part of an obsessive-compulsive spectrum based on this symptom similarity and other features they share with one another, such as etiology, associated features (age at onset, clinical course, family history and comorbidity), and treatment response (Hollander, 1993). These distinct but related disorders are found in several diagnostic categories, including somatoform disorders (hypochondriasis, body dysmorphic disorder [BDD]), eating disorders (anorexia nervosa, bulimia nervosa, binge eating), sexual disorders (paraphilias, SC), other impulse control disorders (pathological gambling, kleptomania, trichotillomania), and impulsive personality disorders (borderline, antisocial), among others (Hollander, 1998; Hollander & Rosen, 2000).

OC spectrum disorders all involve repetitive behavior and an inability to effectively inhibit the behavior that causes distress and impairment;

however, these disorders vary in the extent to which they are characterized by compulsivity versus impulsivity. The spectrum can be conceptualized as a continuum ranging from the more compulsive disorders, such as hypochondriasis, OCD and BDD, to the more impulsive subgroup that is of particular interest here, including sexual compulsivity, pathological gambling, compulsive shopping, and kleptomania (Hollander & Rosen, 2000). As one can see, the compulsive end of the spectrum can also be thought of as risk averse, disorders which involve an overestimation of the likelihood of future harm; the impulsive end can be considered risk seeking, involving acting without realistic consideration of future harm. As discussed earlier, SC seems to involve a disorder of impulse control that, at least at the time of the impulsive activity, can be characterized by an underestimation of the negative consequences of impulsivity along with the inability to control the behavior. This is a key to the increased risk of HIV among this population.

Phenomenologically, the compulsive and impulsive disorders seem to differ in that for compulsive disorders, the repetitive behavior is anxiety reducing but not pleasurable, in contrast, for the impulsive disorders, the repetitive behavior is has some pleasurable aspects, however, this distinction is not always pronounced especially as, over time, pleasure seems to be lost or at least greatly outweighed by distress. Notably, these impulsive disorders are also often discussed as addictions and self-help treatment programs modeled on Alcoholics Anonymous have arisen to treat them. These disorders differ from traditional addictions most notably in that they do not involve the intake of psychoactive substances but they have many similarities to addictions.

It is well established that serotonin reuptake inhibitors (SRIs: SSRIs and the tricyclic clomipramine) are effective in treating OCD albeit at higher doses and for longer trials than found necessary for depression (Hollander et al., 2000); substantial evidence is accumulating to support the efficacy of SRIs in treating the OC spectrum disorders as well (Hollander, 1998; Hollander & Allen, 2001). There is evidence that SRIs are effective in treating disorders throughout the OC spectrum.

Early reports of BDD treatment suggested a response to SRIs such as clomipramine, fluoxetine, and fluvoxamine (Hollander et al. 1989b; Hollander et al. 1993a; Phillips et al 1993) in contrast to other pharmacological agents such as neuroleptics, trazodone, lithium, benzodiazapines, tricyclics (other than clomipramine) and anticonvulsants, all of which were found to be generally ineffective (Phillips et al 1993; Hollander et al 1993a). In a study of BDD patients with skin picking behavior, Phillips and Taub (1995) reported significant improvement in 49% of patients receiving SRIs while only 10% improved with other psychotropic medications. Hollander et al. (1999), conducted a double-blind, 16 week crossover study of 29 patients with BDD comparing clomipramine, an SRI, and desipramine, a norepinephrine reuptake inhibitor. Clomipramine was superior to desipramine in the acute treatment of both specific symptoms and overall severity of BDD. In an open label trial of fluvoxamine in 30 patients, Phillips et al. (1998) found 63% of patients responded to treatment. Thus, based on current information, an SRI would be the first line treatment for BDD with the same dosage and length of trial used for OCD.

SRIs are also considered the first line treatments for trichotillomania, however, research results are less consistent, less robust, and less well maintained than those found for OCD and body dysmorphic disorder (Hollander & Allen, 2001). Research has included studies of: clomipramine (Swedo et al. 1989a, 1989b, 1993; Pollard et al. 1991); fluoxetine (Streichenwein and Thornby, 1995; Pigott et al. 1992); fluvoxamine (Christenson and Crow 1996; Stanley et al. 1997); venlafaxine (Ninan et al. 1998); and citalopram (Stein et al. 1997b). SRIs appear to be helpful in some patients with trichotillomania, both in terms of reducing anxiety and subjective tension and in reducing, and in some cases eliminating, the compulsive hair pulling. However, the effect may not be maintained with continued treatment. Overall, research suggests trichotillomania shows a more minimal response for all treatment modalities compared to OCD and body dysmorphic disorder, including a weaker response to serotonin reuptake inhibitors. It may also be helpful to conceptualize trichotillomania as a tic-like disorder, and as such, addition of low-dose atypical neuroleptics may be helpful in ameliorating the hair pulling.

Importantly, there is evidence that SRIs are effective in the treatment of pathological gambling. This disorder may be the spectrum disorders most similar to SC since it appears to have a very similar phenomenology, as well as the similarities in course, comorbidities and neurobiology that are found across the spectrum.

Clomipramine was effective in reducing gambling urges and behavior in a double-blind single case study (Hollander et al., 1992) and a single-blind fluvoxamine, placebo-controlled study of 10 pathological gamblers in which seven of the 10 patients responded to fluvoxamine; all of these patients were abstinent at the end of the 8-week period (Hollander et al., 1998). Of the three who failed to respond, two had an additional diagnosis of cyclothymia and fluvoxamine appeared to exacerbate their gambling and mood symptoms, highlighting the importance of identifying those patients with comorbid bipolar spectrum disorders as these may have a significant impact on medication strategies. In addition, a 16-week double-blind placebo controlled fluvoxamine trial replicated the finding that fluvoxamine is significantly superior to placebo in decreasing gambling urges and behavior (Hollander et al., 2000). Randomized placebo-controlled and maintenance trials are required to confirm these findings and to determine whether improvement persists. Yet, at this preliminary stage, these agents appear to be potentially useful in treating this disabling disorder, and this adds further support to the importance of investigating the efficacy of SRIs in the treatment of SC and other impulsive spectrum disorders.

4.3 SSRIs Use in Sexual Disorders

Most SSRIs such as Prozac, Zoloft, and Luvox have demonstrated efficacy in reducing the spectrum of paraphilic and paraphpilia-related disorders (Bradford & Greenberg, 1996; Kafka, 1994, 1995, 1997; Kafka & Prentky, 1992, 1994; Greenberg & Bradford, 1997; Stein et al., 1992). [A review of the biological mechanism of action for SSRIs with respect to sexual behavior is beyond the scope of this chapter. For more extensive reviews, consult Bradford and Greenberg (1996), Kafka (1997a), and Greenberg and Bradford (1997).] Initial investigations of the use of SSRIs with paraphilias arose because of their well-known sexual side effects; however, recent research suggests that sexual side effects are independent of reduced symptomatology (Greenberg & Bradford, 1997; Kafka & Prentky, 1992, Kafka, 1997). Although aberrant sexual behaviors are reduced with these treatments, conventional sexual functioning can be enhanced in many individuals with paraphilias after a relatively short period of treatment with SSRIs (Greenberg & Bradford, 1997). Some patients report decreased libido, anorgasmia, and impotence after treatment with SSRIs; however, titrating the dose can frequently reduce these effects. This effect is important in that the goal of treatment is not only the suppression of deviant sexual interests but also the replacement of these interests with normative sexual interests (Bradford, 1998).

The use of SSRIs in treating sex offenders is well established (Bradford & Greenberg, 1996; Coleman, Dwyer, Abel et al., 2000; Federoff, 1993; Greenberg & Bradford, 1997; Kafka, 1994; Kafka & Prentky, 1992). Other aberrant sexual behaviors where these medications have been successfully used include sexual masochism (Kafka, 1994; Kafka & Prentky, 1992; Masand, 1993), transvestic Fetish (Kafka, 1994; Masand, 1993), voyeurism (Azhar & Varma, 1995; Emmanuel, 1991; Perilstein, Lipper, & Friedman, 1991), fetish (Kafka, 1994; Lorefice, 1991), exhibitionism (Kafka, 1994; Kafka & Prentky, 1992; Perilstein, Lipper, & Friedman, 1991), compulsive masturbation (Kafka, 1994; Kafka & Prentky, 1992), pornography dependence (Kafka, 1994; Kafka & Prentky, 1992) and SC (Aguirre, 1999; Kafka, 1994; Kafka, 2000b; Kafka & Prentky, 1992). In most studies, patients have reported reductions in total time consumed by deviant fantasies, paraphilic masturbation and overt sexual behaviors, and decreased penile tumescence (when assessed) to sexually arousing unconventional stimuli (Bradford, 1995; Bradford & Greenberg, 1996; Greenberg & Bradford, 1997; Kafka, 1994; Kafka 2000a, 2000b).

Selective serotonin reuptake inhibitors (SSRIs) have even been used to treat SC, albeit without control conditions. Nevertheless, results appear promising. Kafka and Prentky (1992) reported significant reductions in SC behavioral and cognitive symptoms among paraphilic men treated with a 12-week open trial of fluoxetine (Prozac). Kafka (1994) reported similar promising results in a later study with sertraline (Zoloft) or fluoxetine. Greenberg et al. (1996) reported findings in a retrospective study of 58 paraphilics treated with either fluoxetine, fluvoxamine, or sertraline. Their findings indicated a significant reduction in SC symptoms, and concluded there were no significant differences in efficacies among the three SSRIs. Black (2000) cites other studies that reached a similar conclusion. There are a number of hypotheses about the mechanisms of action of SSRIs on SC (Kafka, 1997). However, as mentioned above, existing evidence suggests that the effect is not related to SSRIs adverse effects on sexual functions such as ejaculatory dysfuction (cf. Greenberg & Bradford, 1997). In addition, Kafka & Prentky (1992) reported that treatment response to SSRI was independent of depression scores. These authors have concluded that a double blind placebo controlled study of SSRIs to treat paraphilias and other SC-related problems is warranted. However, to date no trial has been reported. There are no known studies examining the effects of SSRIs on SC in MSM.

5. HIV PREVENTION FOR SEXUALLY COMPULSIVE MALES

Existing behavioral interventions may not be suitable for people with SC, as SC tends to result in a more rigid pattern of sex behavior that is resistant to change (Kalichman & Rompa, 1995). Further, interventions for those with SC may require intensive clinical treatment and long-term follow-up (Kalichman, Greenberg, & Abel, 1997). Anecdotes suggest that gay men with SC report extreme difficulty engaging in safer sex behaviors due to high levels of impulsivity around sex activities, poor planning, generally poor social/behavioral coping skills, and history of trauma leading to poor self-care behaviors. Moreover, many men with SC may lack the long-term commitment necessary to maintain behavioral changes.

From a psychotherapeutic point of view, cognitive-behavioral therapy (CBT) would seem the most appropriate approach. CBT builds individualized skills for self-control through a process of identifying antecedents to the target behavior (unprotected sex) and learning to manage them through problem solving, practice, goal setting and self-reward. While many HIV risk behavior change interventions contain skills-building exercises loosely based on CBT procedures (e.g., NIMH Multisite HIV Prevention Trial Group, 1998), intensive, individualized self-management skill building is limited because of the group format and lack of time. Further, in this work it is generally assumed that the at-risk participants will not be willing or able to complete daily self-monitoring records, and little intensive effort is made to identify person-specific antecedents. Interestingly, we were unable to find a single published report of a controlled CBT therapeutic trial for the treatment of sexual compulsivity.

For those men who lack long-term commitment, but are motivated to reduce their SC and HIV risk behavior, SSRIs may be an alternative, or ancillary, approach. By reducing the number of sexual contacts and allowing for a sense of control over sexual behaviors, SSRIs may be useful in reducing HIV transmission or infection risk behavior in willing individuals.

6. SOCIAL BARRIERS TO THE USE OF SSRIS TO REDUCE MSM SEXUAL ACTIVITY

Gay men suffer discrimination, stigmatization and rejection on the basis of their sexuality, often beginning at an early age. Thus, efforts to influence gay male sexual behavior even when driven by a desire to reduce the HIV epidemic, has often pushed sensitive buttons. Programs designed to curtail the sexual activity of gay men have been met with ambivalence and even hostility–for example, around the closing of bathhouses in San Francisco at the beginning of the epidemic (see Shilts, 1987). Thus, the suggestion that gay men should take drugs to limit their sexual activity is likely to mobilize strong opposition in some quarters of the gay community. It is important to note that we are advocating that these agents be tested as a strategy for men *who are seeking help because they are concerned about their sexual behavior* because it is interfering with their life functioning, or as it might be related to concern about STD/HIV infection or transmission. We would advocate strongly against the use of SSRIs to treat sexual behavior that is dystonic due to internalized homophobia.

7. DESCRIPTION OF OUR ONGOING STUDY OF SSRI TREATMENT FOR SEXUALLY COMPULSIVE MSM

Several of the authors of the present chapter (all but Suarez) are currently collaborating on a study of sexually compulsive MSM in New York City. One component of this study will be a preliminary double-blind trial of the SSRI citalopram to reduce HIV risk behavior in a sample of help-seeking men who meet stringent criteria for SC. In addition, we hope that our research will shed additional light on the nature of SC and the optimum methods for diagnosing and assessing it, as well as on the subjective realities of the men who suffer from the disorder.

REFERENCES

Aguirre, B. (1999). Fluoxetine and compulsive sexual behavior. *Journal of the Academy of Child and Adolescent Psychiatry, 38*(8), 943.

Allen, A. & Hollander, E. (2000). Body Dysmorphic Disorder. *Psychiatric Clinics of North America*, 23:617-628.

APA. (1980). *Diagnostic and statistical manual of mental disorders, third edition (DSM-III).* American Psychiatric Association: Washington DC.

APA (1994). Diagnostic and Statistical Manual of Mental Disorders – IV (DSM-IV). American Psychiatric Association: Washington, DC.

Azhar, M.Z., Varma, S.L. (1995). Response to clomipramine in sexual addiction. *European Psychiatry, 10,* 263-265.

Barth, R.J., & Kinder, B.N. (1987). The mislabeling of sexual impulsivity. *Journal of Sex and Marital Therapy 13(1),* 15-23.

Benotsch, E.G., Kalichman, S.C., & Kelly, J.A. (1999). Sexual compulsivity and substance use in HIV-seropositive men who have sex with men: Prevalence and predictors of high-risk behaviors. *Addictive Behaviors, 24,* 857-868.

Black, D. W. (2000). The epidemiology and phenomenology of compulsive sexual behavior. *CNS Spectrums, 5,* 26-35.

Black, D.W., Kehrberg, L.L.D., Flumerfelt, D.L., & Schlosser, S.S. (1997). Characteristics of 36 subjects reporting compulsive sexual behavior. *American Journal of Psychiatry, 154,* 243-249.

Bradford, J.M.W. (1991). The role of serotonin reuptake inhibitors in forensic psychiatry. Congress of European College of Neuropsychopharmacology: The Role of Serotonin in Psychiatric Illness, IVth ECNP Monte Carlo, Monaco, 9th October, published abstract.

Bradford, J.M.W. (1994). Can Pedophilia Be treated? *The Harvard Mental Health Letter 10(8).*

Bradford, J.M.W. (1995). Pharmacological Treatment of the Paraphilias. In J.M. Oldham & M.B. Riba (Eds.), *Review of Psychiatry,* pp.755-778. American Psychiatric Association: Washington DC.

Bradford, J.M.W. (1998). Treatment of men with paraphilia. New England Journal of Medicine, 338, 464-465.

Bradford, J.M.W., & Greenberg, D.M. (1996). Pharmacological treatment of deviant sexual behavior. *Annual Review of Sex Research, 7*, 283-306.

Carnes, P. (1983). *The Sexual Addiction.* Minneapolis, MN: CompCare Publications.

Carnes, P. (1990). Sexual addiction. In A. Horton, BL Johnson, et al. (Eds.), The Incest Perpetrator: A family member no one wants to treat. Sage publications: Newbury Park, CA.

Carnes, P. (1991). Don't Call It Love: Recovery from sexual addiction. Bantam Books: New York, NY.

Carnes, P. (2000). Open Hearts: Renewing Relationships with Recovery, Romance and Reality. Arizona: Gentle Path Press.

Carnes, P., Delmonico, D. (1996). Childhood Abuse and Multiple Addictions: Research findings in a sample of self-identified sexual addicts. *Sexual Addiction & Compulsivity: The Journal of Treatment and Prevention,* 3(3), 258.

Christenson, G.A. & Crow, S.J. (1996). The characterization and treatment of trichotillomania. *Journal of Clinical Psychiatry*, 57 (suppl 8):42-47, discussion 48-.9

Coleman, E. (1987). Sexual compulsivity: definition, etiology, and treatment considerations. *Journal of Chemical Dependency Treatment, 1*, 189-204.

Coleman, E. (1990). The obsessive-compulsive model for describing compulsive sexual behavior. American Journal of Preventive Psychiatry and Neurology, 2(3), 914.

Coleman, E. (1991). Compulsive sexual behavior: New concepts and treatments. *Journal of Psychology & Human Sexuality, 4*,37-52.

Coleman E. (1992). Is your patient suffering from compulsive sexual behavior? *Psychiatric Annals, 22(6)*, 320-25.

Coleman, E., Dwyer, S., Abel, G. et al. (2000). Standards of care for the treatment of adult sex offenders. *Journal of Psychology & Human Sexuality, 11*, 11-17.

Dilley, J.W., McFarland, W., Sullivan, P., & Discepola, M. (1998). Psychosocial correlates of unprotected anal sex in a cohort of gay men attending an HIV-negative support group. AIDS Education and Prevention, 10(4), 317-26.

Edwards, G., & Gross, M.M. (1976). Alcohol dependence: provisional description of a clinical syndrome. *British Medical Journal, 1;*1(6017), 1058-61.

Emmanuel, N.P., Lydiard, R.B., Friedman, L.J. (1991). Fluoxetine treatment of voyeurism [Letter]. *American Journal of Psychiatry, 148*, 950.

Exner, T.M., Bahlburg, H.F. & Ehrhardt, A.A. (1992). Sexual self control as a mediator of high risk sexual behavior in a New York City cohort of HIV+ and HIV- gay men. *Journal of Sex Research, 29*, 389-406.

Fedoroff, P. (1993). Serotonergic Drug Treatment of Deviant Sexual Interests. *Annals of Sex Research, 6*, 105-121.

Gold, R. S. (2000). AIDS education for gay men: Towards a more cognitive approach. *AIDS Care, 12*, 267-272.

Gold, S.N., & Heffner, C.L. (1998). Sexual addiction: many conceptions, minimal data. Clinical Psychology Review, 18(3), 367-81.

Goodman, A. (1992). Sexual addiction: designation and treatment. *Journal of Sex and Marital Therapy, 18*, 303-314.

Greenberg, D.M. & Bradford, J.M.W. (1997). Treatment of the paraphilic disorders: A review of the role of the selective serotonin reuptake inhibitors. *Sexual Abuse: A Journal of Research and Treatment, 9*, 349-360.

Greenberg, D.M., Bradford, J.M.W., Curry, S., O'Rourke, A. (1996). A comparison of treatment of paraphilias with three serotonin reuptake inhibitors: A retrospective study. *Bulletin of the American Academy of Psychiatry and Law, 24*, 525-532.

Griffin-Shelley, E. (1991). *Sex and Love Addiction, Treatment, and Recovery.* Praeger Publishers. New York.

Halkitis, P.N. & Parsons, J.T. (1999). Oral sex and HIV risk reduction: Perceived risk, behaviors, and strategies among young HIV negative men. *Journal of Psychology & Human Sexuality, 11*(4),27-51.

Hollander E. (ed.) (1993). *Obsessive-Compulsive Related Disorders.* American Psychiatric Press, Inc. Washington,D.C.

Hollander E. (1998). Treatment of obsessive-compulsive spectrum disorders with SSRIs. *British Journal of Psychiatry*, 173 (supplement 35):7-12.

Hollander, E. & Allen, A. (2001). Serotonergic drugs and the treatment of disorders related to obsessive-compulsive disorder. In: Pato MT & Zohar J (eds.) *Current Treatments of Obsessive-Compulsive Disorder*, 2nd Edition. Washington, DC, American Psychiatric Publishing, Inc.

Hollander E, Allen A, Kwon J, Aronowitz B, Schmeidler J, Wong C. & Simeon D. (1999). Clomipramine vs. desipramine crossover trial in body dysmorphic disorder: selective efficacy of a serotonin reuptake inhibitor in imagined ugliness. *Archives of General Psychiatry*, 56:1999-

Hollander E, Cohen LJ, & Simeon D. (1993) Obsessive-compulsive spectrum disorders: Body dysmorphic disorder. *Psychiatric Annals*, 23:359-364.

Hollander E., DeCaria C.M., Finkell JN, Begaz T., Wong C.M. Cartwright C. (2000). A randomized double-blind fluvoxamine/placebo crossover trial in pathological gambling. *Biological Psychiatry*, 47:813-817.

Hollander E., DeCaria C.M., Mari E., Wong C.M., Mosovich S., Grossman R. & Begaz T., (1998). Short-term single-blind fluvoxamine treatment of pathological gambling. *American Journal of Psychiatry*, 155, 1781-1783.

Hollander E., DeCaria C., Nitescu A., Gulley R., Suckow R.F., Cooper T.B., Gorman J.G., Klein D.F. & Liebowitz M.R., (1992). Serotonergic function in obsessive-compulsive disorder: Behavioral and neuroendocrine responses to oral m-CPP and fenfluramine in patients and healthy volunteers. *Archives of General Psychiatry*, 49, 21-28.

Hollander E, Fay M, Cohen B, et al, (1988) Serotonergic and noradrenergic function in obsessive-compulsive disorder: behavioral findings. *American Journal of Psychiatry* 145:1015-1017.

Hollander E, Hwang M, Mullen LS, et al. (1993). Clinical and research issues in depersonalization syndrome [letter]. *Psychosomatics*, 34:193-4.

Hollander E, Kaplan A, Allen A, Cartwright C. (2000). Pharmacotherapy for obsessive-compulsive disorder. *Psychiatric Clinics of North America*, 23:643-656.

Hollander. E., Liebowitz, M.R., Winchel, R., Klumker, A., & Klein, D.F. (1989). Treatment of body-dysmorphic disorder with serotonin reuptake blockers. *American Journal of Psychiatry, 146*(6), 768-70.

Hollander, E. & Rosen, J. (2000). Impulsivity. *Journal of Psychopharmacology*, 14 (supplement 1):39-44.

Hollander E, Wong CM. (2000) *Contemporary Diagnosis and Management of Common Psychiatric Disorders*, (pages 51-57). Newtown, Pennsylvania: Handbooks in Health Care.

Kafka, M.P. (1991). Successful antidepressant treatment of nonparaphilic sexual addictions and paraphilias in men. *Journal of Clinical Psychiatry, 52*, 60-65.

Kafka, M.P. (1994). Sertraline pharmacotherapy for paraphilias and paraphilia-related disorders: An open trial. *Annals of Clinical Psychiatry, 6*, 189-195.

Kafka, M.P. (1995). Current concepts in the drug treatment of paraphilia and paraphilia-related disorders. *Practical Therapeutics, 3*, 9-21.

Kafka, M.P. (1997). A monoamine hypothesis for the pathophysiology of paraphilic disorders. *Archives of Sexual Behavior, 26*, 343-358.

Kafka, M.P. (1997). Hypersexual desire in males: An operational definition and clinical implications for males with paraphilias and paraphilia-related disorders. *Archives of Sexual Behavior, 26*, 505-526.

Kafka, M.P. (2000a). The paraphilia-related disorders: Nonparaphilic hypersexuality and sexual compulsivity/addiction. In S. Lieblum and R.C. Rosen (Eds.) *Principles of Practice of Sex Therapy* (pp. 471-503), New York: Guilford..

Kafka, M.P. (2000b). Psychopharmacological treatments for nonparaphilic compulsive sexual behaviors. *CNS Spectrums, 5*, 49-59.

Kafka, M.P., & Hennen, J. (1999). The paraphilia-related disorders: An empirical investigation of nonparaphilic hypersexuality disorders in outpatient males. *Journal of Sex and Marital Therapy, 25*, 305-319.

Kafka, M.P., Prentky, R. (1992a). A comparative study of nonparaphilic sexual addictions and paraphilias in men. *Journal of Clinical Psychiatry, 53*, 345-350.

Kafka, M.P., Prentky, R. (1992b). Fluoxetine treatment of nonparaphilic sexual addictions and paraphilias in men. *Journal of Clinical Psychiatry, 53*, 351-358.

Kafka, M.P., Prentky, R. (1994). Preliminary observations of the DSM-III-R Axis I comorbidity in men with paraphilias and paraphilia-related disorders. *Journal of Clinical Psychiatry, 55*, 481-487.

Kafka, M.P., Prentky, R. (1997). Compulsive sexual behavior characteristics. *American Journal of Psychiatry, 154*, 1632.

Kafka, M.P., & Prentky, R.A. (1998). Attention-deficit/hyperactivity disorder in males with paraphilias and paraphilia-related disorders: a comorbidity study. *Journal of Clinical Psychiatry, 59*(7), 388-96.

Kalichman, S.C., & Rompa, D. (1995). Sexual sensation seeking and sexual compulsivity scales: Reliability, validity, and predicting HIV risk behavior. *Journal of Personality Assessment, 65*, 586-601.

Kalichman, S.C., Greenberg, J., & Abel, G.G. (1997). HIV-seropositive men who engage in high-risk sexual behaviour: psychological characteristics and implications for prevention. *AIDS Care, 9*, 441-450.

Kelly, J.A. (1997). HIV risk reduction intervention for persons with serious mental illness. Clinical Psychology Review, 17, 293- 309.

Laumann, E., Michael, R. and Gagnon, J. (1994) *The Social Organization of Sexuality.* University of Chicago Press, Chicago.

Levine, M. P. & Troiden, R. R. (1988). The myth of sexual compulsivity. *Journal of Sex Research, 25*, 347-363.

Lorefice, L.S. (1991). Fluoxetine treatment of a fetish. *J Clinical Psychiatry, 52(*1), 41.

Masand, P.S. (1993). Successful treatment of sexual masochism and transvestic fetishism associated with depression with fluoxetine hydrochloride. *Depression, 1*, 50-52.

McKirnan, D. J., Ostrow, D. G., and Hope, B. (1996). Sex, drugs and escape: a psychological model of HIV-risk sexual behaviors. *AIDS Care, 8*, 665–669.

McKuisck, L., Conant, M., & Coates, T.J. (1985). The AIDS epidemic: A model for developing intervention strategies for reducing high-risk behavior in gay men. *Sexually Transmitted Disease, 12*, 229-234.

Moser, C. (1993). A response to Aviel Goodman's "Sexual addiction: designation and treatment". Journal of Sex and Marital Therapy, 19(3), 220-4.

The NIMH Multisite HIV Prevention Trial Group (1998). The NIMH Multisite HIV Prevention Trial: Reducing sexual HIV risk behavior. *Science, 280,* 1889-1894.

Ninan PT, Knight B, Kirk L, et al (1998). A controlled trial of venlafaxine in trichotillomania: interim phase 1 results. *Psychopharmacology Bulletin*, 34:221-224

O'Leary, A., Parsons, J., Purcell, D. H, & Macari, S. (2000, March). Combining Quantitative and Qualitative Methods to Understand Compulsive Risky Sexual Behavior among HIV-Seropositive Gay and Bisexual Men. Society for Applied Anthropology, San Francisco.

O'Leary, A., Purcell, D., Remien, R. H., & Gomez, C. (2001, under review). Childhood sexual abuse and sexual transmission risk among HIV-seropositive men who have sex with men.

Orford, J. (1978) Hypersexuality: implications for a theory of dependence. *British Journal of* Addiction to Alcohol Other Drugs, 73(3), 299-10.

Paul, J. P., Catania, J., Pollack, L., & Stall, R. (2001). Understanding childhood sexual abuse as a predictor of sexual risk-taking among men who have sex with men: The Urban Men's Health Study. *Child abuse and Neglect, 25*, 557-584.

Perilstein, R.D., Lippers, S., & Friedman, L.J. (1991). Three cases of paraphilias responsive to fluoxetine treatment. Journal of Clinical Psychiatry, 52(4), 169-170.

Phillips KA, Dwight MM, McElroy SL. (1998). Efficacy and safety of fluvoxamine in body dysmorphic disorder. *Journal of Clinical Psychiatry*, 59:165-171.

Phillips KA, McElroy SL, Keck PE, Jr, et al. (1993) Body dysmorphic disorder: 30 cases of imagined ugliness. *American Journal Psychiatry*, 150:302-8.

Phillips KA, Taub SL. (1995). Skin picking as a symptom of body dysmorphic disorder. *Psychopharmacology Bulletin* 31:279-88.

Pigott TA, L'Heueux F, Grady TA, et al: (1992). Controlled comparison of clomipramine and fluoxetine in trichotillomania. In: Abstracts of Panels and Posters of the 31st Annual Meeting of the American College of Neuropsychopharmacology; San Juan Puerto Rico. 157, December.

Pinkerton, S.D., & Abramson, P.R. (1996). Occasional condom use and HIV risk reduction. Journal of Acquired Immune Deficiency Syndrome, 13, 456-460.

Pinkerton, S.D., & Abramson, P.R., & Turk, M.E. (1998). Updated estimates of condom effectiveness. Journal of the Association of Nurses in AIDS Care, 9(6), 88-89.

Pollard CA, Ibe IO, Krojanker DN, et al: (1991). Clomipramine treatment of trichotillomania: a follow-up report on four cases. *Journal Clinical Psychiatry*, 52:128-130.

Quadland, M.C. (1985). Compulsive sexual behavior: Definition of a problem and an approach to treatment. Journal of Sex and Marital Therapy, 11(2), 121-132.

Quadland, M.C., & Shattls, W.D. (1987). AIDS, sexuality, and sexual control. Journal of Homosexuality, 14(1-2), 277-298.

Saulnier, C.F. (1996). African-American women in an alcohol intervention group: addressing personal and political problems. *Substance Use and Misuse, 31*(10), 1259-78.

Schaffer, H.J. (1994). Considering two models of excessive sexual behaviors: Addiction and obsessive compulsive disorder. *Sexual Addiction & Compulsivity, 1*, 6-18.

Shilts, R., 1987. *And The Band Played On.* St. Martin's Press, N.Y.

Solomon, M.Z., & DeJong, W. (1986). Recent sexually transmitted disease prevention efforts and their implications for AIDS health education. *Health Education Quarterly, 13*, 301-316.

Stein, D.J., Hollander, E., Anthony, D.T., et al. (1992). Serotonergic medications for sexual obsessions, sexual addictions, and paraphilias. *Journal of Clinical Psychiatry, 53*, 267-271.

Stein DJ, Bouwer C, Maud CM. (1997) Use of the selective serotonin reuptake inhibitor citalopram in treatment of trichotillomaina. *European Archives of Psychiatry and Clinical Neuroscience*, 247:234-6.

Stanley MA, Breckenridge JK, Swann AC et al. (1997) Fluvoxamine treatment of trichotillomania. *Journal of Clinical Psychopharmacology*, 17:278-83.

Streichenwein SM, Thornby JI. (1995). A long-term, double-blind, placebo-controlled crossover trial of the efficacy of fluoxetine for trichotillomania. *American Journal of Psychiatry*, 152:1192-1196.

Suarez, T. & Kauth, M.R. (2001). Assessing basic HIV transmission risk and the contextual factors associated with HIV risk behavior in men who have sex with men. *Journal of Clinical Psychology/In Session: Psychotherapy in Practice, 57*(5), 1-15.

Suarez, T. & Miller, J.G. (2001) Negotiating risks in contexts: A perspective on barebacking and unprotected anal intercourse among men who have sex with men – Where do we go from here. *Archives of Sexual Behavior, 30*(3), 287-300.

Suarez, T., Kelly, J.A., Pinkerton, S.D., Stevenson, Y.L., Hayat, M.J., Smith, M.D., Ertl, T. (2001). The Influence of a Partner's HIV Serostatus and Viral Load on Perceptions of Sexual Risk Behavior in a Community Sample of Gay and Bisexual Men. Manuscript under review.

Swedo SE, Lenane MC, Leonard HL. (1993) Long-term treatment of trichotillomania (hair pulling) (letter). *New England Journal of Medicine*, 329:141-142.

Swedo SE, Leonard HL, Rapoport JL, et al. (1989) A double-blind comparison of clomipramine and desipramine in the treatment of trichotillomania (hair pulling). *New England Journal of Medicine*, 321:497-501.

Swedo SE, Rapoport JL, Leonard H, et al. (1989). Obsessive-compulsive disorder in children and adolescents: clinical phenomenology of 70 consecutive cases. *Archives of General Psychiatry*, 46:335-341.

Wolfe, D. (2000). *Men Like Us: The GMHC complete guide for gay men's sexual, physical, and emotional well-being.* Random House: New York, NY.

Wolitski, R. J., Valdiserri, R. O., Denning, P. H., & Levine, W. C. (2001). Are we headed for a resurgence of the HIV epidemic among men who have sex with men? *American Journal of Public Health, 91*, 883-888.

Ziedonis, D.M. & Kosten, T.R. (1992) Behavioral Pathology. *Annual Review of Addictions Research and Treatment*, 15, 109-123.

Chapter 10

Prevention Triage: Optimizing Multiple HIV Intervention Strategies

Ann O'Leary and Thomas Peterman
Division of HIV/AIDS Prevention, National Center for HIV, STD and TB Prevention, Centers for Disease Control and Prevention, Atlanta Georgia

And

Sevgi O. Aral Ph.D.
Division of STD Prevention, National Center for HIV, STD and TB Prevention, Centers for Disease Control and Prevention, Atlanta Georgia

1. THE OPENING OF OPTIONS AND PREVENTION TRIAGE

As this chapter is being written, almost exactly twenty years after HIV/AIDS was first noted as *pneumocystis carinii* pneumonia in five gay men, the epidemic is exploding across much of the world. It is a "generalized" epidemic–affecting the general population, not just specific risk groups–in many countries in sub-Saharan Africa, and threatens to replicate this pattern throughout much of Asia, Latin America, and Eastern Europe. It is clear that our prevention efforts to date have not solved the problem, although this is at least as much due to lack of political and financial will as to limitations in our restricted set of prevention strategies. Even in U.S. communities where condoms are widely available free of charge, the epidemic continues to spread. This book has reviewed numerous approaches to the control of this disease, arguing that condom use cannot be treated as if it were a "magic bullet" solution to the problem. Only a highly effective vaccine, should one become available, can hope to become a single strategy with the potential for eliminating HIV and AIDS from the world.

For the majority of public health problems, a single solution has been sought. Antibiotics are effective treatments for bacterial infection, and vaccines prevent viral disease. Motorcycle helmets prevent motorcycle deaths. Condoms are an appealing single solution: they are effective when used properly; they are inexpensive and simple to use. However, as discussed in the opening chapter, numerous conditions militate against their use. The point of this book has been to illustrate the many different types of approaches that can contribute to HIV prevention efforts. With multiple strategies available, a new research agenda is in order. First, more research is needed to establish the effectiveness of the strategies described here. Second, we must study how to frame messages and target them to the appropriate subgroups to achieve the greatest prevention effects.

The chapters in this volume describe numerous strategies that can potentially be used to reduce the probability of transmission of HIV. Some, such as policy interventions and universal STD treatment, do not require individuals to select their preferred HIV prevention strategy. However, for many approaches described here, more than one prevention strategy may be available to an individual. Individuals must then decide on which strategy or strategies they will rely–or someone must guide them to those most likely to be effective for the person in their situation. Individuals may choose to use more than one strategy–indeed, most of the approaches described in this book are perfectly compatible with condom use, and with each other. However, even for individuals with similar risk and demographic characteristics, different strategies may be preferable. For example, for some gay men in long-term relationships negotiated safety may be the optimal strategy, while for others with multiple casual partners encountered under the influence of drugs, avoidance of anal sex may be the most effective one. And personal characteristics and target population exigencies may dictate the superiority of one method over another. STD control might be very effective in impoverished nations with high STD incidence rates, while abstinence may be optimal for adolescents who have not yet become sexually active. Condom promotion may be less effective than psychopharmacologic treatment among those suffering from sexual compulsivity.

If our prevention armamentarium includes multiple, complex options, achieving the best fit between the individual and the strategy or strategies employed will be necessary. Only when the proper fit is achieved will the strategy be most effective for the individual and most cost-effective for society. The term "prevention triage" is meant to convey a process of matching at-risk populations or groups (for example, defined on the basis of psychosocial, behavioral, or geographic factors) to the intervention messages and strategies most likely to produce the greatest reduction in risk of HIV transmission or infection in that context.

Behavioral interventions that have been rigorously evaluated have overwhelmingly sought to increase condom use (comprehensively reviewed in Peterson and DiClemente, 2000). Some have also advocated reducing number of partners, although this has been achieved in very few studies. The research team of John and Loretta Jemmott and colleagues has conducted limited testing of abstinence interventions. But condom recommendations have been the primary message in practically every tested intervention.

It is interesting to note that the near-singular reliance on condom use has not always been our public health strategy for combating the HIV/AIDS epidemic. The earliest Morbidity and Mortality Weekly Reports (MMWR) issued by the CDC-- of *pneumocystis pneumonia* in five homosexual men in June 1981 (Centers for Disease Control, 1981a; Centers for Disease Control, 1998b), and of Kaposi's sarcoma and generalized lymphadenopathy (Centers for Disease Control, 1981b; Centers for Disease Control, 1982)–did not contain a recommendation for condom use, as the cause was not known to be infectious or sexually transmitted. By March of 1983, the Public Health Service published its first set of recommendations for the prevention of AIDS (Centers for Disease Control, 1983); it is interesting to note that partner selection figured among them: "Sexual contact should be avoided with persons known or suspected to have AIDS. Members of high risk groups should be aware that multiple sexual partners increase the probability of developing AIDS" –but condom use did not. In fact, condoms were mentioned for the first time in 1985 (Centers for Disease Control, 1985). The final paragraph states:"Consistent use of condoms should assist in preventing infection with HTLV-III/LAV, but their efficacy in reducing transmission has not yet been proven." Additional recommendations to reduce sexual transmission were published in March 1986 (Centers for Disease Control, 1986); in addition to condoms, mutual monogamy was emphasized. In 1994 (Centers for Disease Control, 1994), delay of onset of sexual activity was recommended for youths, and mutual monogamy was again suggested, in addition to condom use.

Thus, although tested behavioral interventions have almost always emphasized condom use, the public health community has been giving multiple messages all along. It has nearly always been stated that the best strategy is to have an uninfected partner, though there has always been some concern about the ability to determine if a partner was infected--first because the test was new, then some persons appeared to have HIV despite a negative HIV test, and all along there has been the question of the veracity of a potential partner's self report. Having an uninfected partner suggests some sort of joint antibody testing and agreeing either to monogamy or condom use with secondary partners–"negotiated safety"–but no intervention delivering this message has yet been evaluated.

In fact, with some exceptions (STD control; abstinence), the strategies described in the preceding chapters have not been tested. Few structural interventions have been rigorously evaluated, partly because it is difficult to do so. The use of pharmacotherapy to treat sexual compulsivity is currently being evaluated in the first double-blind controlled trial. Results from studies of STD control to prevent HIV have been mixed, although it makes sense logically that STD lesions should facilitate HIV transmission. Similarly, it makes sense that some partner selection strategies (particularly ones based on serostatus) and other gray-area behaviors such as withdrawal prior to ejaculation should reduce risk, but the research has not been conducted to document this. Given the evidence that viral load levels affect infectivity, effective treatment should also make a difference–but, again, hard evidence does not exist. Of the approaches described in this book, only abstinence and female condom use are widely accepted as being effective.

However, let us assume that research will continue, and that we will be provided with an increasing number of prevention options. The process of matching populations or groups to strategies will then become a necessary activity. One very basic question in need of research concerns the degree to which individuals should choose among multiple options, versus being provided with a more limited set by the public health community. If the latter sounds paternalistic to readers, please bear in mind that the ensuing discussion is directed toward the goal of achieving maximal reduction in the HIV epidemic, with other considerations (freedom of choice, empowerment) secondary to that goal. The present discussion pertains to prevention intervention development specifically, rather than to broad-based public health messages.

2. SHOULD WE PROVIDE MULTIPLE CHOICES IN INTERVENTIONS?

2.1 Advantages

One advantage to individual choice among available options is that individuals know better than anyone else the details of their life circumstances. To give an example, in a study described in O'Leary (1999), data regarding the feasibility of negotiated safety were collected from 353 Latina women in New York City. They were asked to rate their self-efficacy to convince their partner to use condoms with them, and to convince their partners to use condoms with others (self-efficacy was higher for the latter). Then they were asked how much they would trust their partner to adhere to the negotiated safety agreement. Here, there was wide variation, with 42% women reporting that they would trust their partners, but 30% reporting low levels of trust. Assuming their estimates to be accurate, one would not want to see the latter women engaging in negotiated safety agreements. One would want these women to make a different choice, based on information only available to them.

Indeed, the optimal prevention strategy for one person may be unavailable to others. However, the optimal strategy may be complex, and avoided due to concern about adherence to a complex strategy. For example, research on the prevention of HIV transmission to infants via breastfeeding (e.g., Coutsoudis and colleagues, 1999) has focused on breastfeeding—consistent or mixed with other feeding forms, both of which carry risk of transmission—and infant formula, which carries an almost equivalent risk of infant death, due to diarrheal disease, in developing contexts, as well as HIV stigma (Nduati and colleagues, 2000). The fairly obvious solution that the child is breastfed by a seronegative wet-nurse (the infant's grandmother, for example—anyone who has previously breastfed can fairly easily relactate) requires the additional complexity that the wet-nurse refrain from any activities that could cause her to become infected while breastfeeding, as newly infected persons are particularly infectious. While adherence to this regimen would provide effective prevention of post-birth transmission of HIV, and while many families might be able to achieve it, the public health community has eschewed it as a prevention message.

Another advantage to putting the decision in the hands of individuals is that it may increase the total number of individuals who adopt any measure. If safe methods are chosen, this could enhance overall prevention effectiveness.

2.2 Disadvantages

Providing multiple options should be done only when research has been conducted on how they will be cognitively processed, particularly when they vary in their effectiveness. This is because a substantial literature from social and cognitive psychology indicates that decision-making is not always straightforward. Rather than doing complex cost-benefit computations, people tend to employ effort-saving "heuristics" that greatly simplify the process of decision-making, but that sometimes lead to poor decisional outcomes. These are described in detail elsewhere (Kahneman, Slovic & Tversky, 1982; Nisbett & Ross, 1980). One example is the "availability" heuristic, in which individuals are more likely to think of solutions whose mental representations are vivid. A woman who has observed her partner engaged in sex with someone else might be particularly likely to choose condom use over negotiated safety. Another heuristic is called "elimination by aspects" (Tversky, 1972). In this process, the decision-maker identifies one value of one dimension that is salient and important, and then subsets to only options in which this condition is met. In the case of purchasing an automobile, for example, the person might subset to convertibles, or high-gas mileage cars. To give an example from HIV prevention: In the hierarchical message situation in which a microbicide is listed as possible option (see chapter by Moore and Rogers, this volume), this might take the form of eliminating all options that require negotiation with a partner (i. e., presently, the known-effective methods) then deciding among the remaining ones. This could result in her using microbicide, even if she would have been able to respond to a condom-only message. For this example, there is evidence to support that this occurs. Miller and colleagues (1998) randomized women either to receive a male-condom message, a hierarchical message, or a no-message control condition. Women receiving the hierarchical message were significantly less likely to perceive male condoms as effective (45%vs. 64%and 70%)and were less willing to consider using male condoms (36% vs. 60%and 52%).

It is also not clear that all individuals, or even most, would prefer to be given multiple options. Again, more research is needed on this issue. It may be that some individuals prefer to simply be given a single recommendation. For example, a study by Eagly and Warren found that complex messages were more likely to change attitudes of more educated people, but that simple messages changed only the attitudes of less-educated people.

3. SHOULD INTERVENTIONS FOCUS ON LIMITED BUT APPROPRIATE OPTIONS?

3.1 Advantages

The most obvious advantage to putting the decision into the hands of intervention designers, who are usually medical or public health experts, is that they generally know more than the layperson about the biological processes involved in the effectiveness of the prevention strategy. For example, community-wide STD treatment, or the use of antidepressant medication to treat sexual compulsivity, are not ideas likely to occur to a lay individual. Some that are likely to occur (or that have occurred) to lay persons, such as avoiding partners who are physically dirty, are not based on sound scientific evidence and are therefore unlikely to be effective. Similarly, the interventionist is likely to know characteristics of target persons or populations that influence the suitability of match with prevention strategy.

Another advantage to expert decision-making is that, for the most part, experts are a credible source of information. One study of attitude change found, for example, that a message advocating a certain number of hours of sleep was more effective when the source was a Nobel-prize winning physicist than when the source was a YMCA director (Petty & Cacioppo, 1981). Indeed, the power of the health care provider to change behavior using brief interventions has been demonstrated many times (see Elder, Ayala, & Harris, 1999, for a review), and has been underutilized in HIV prevention.

One case in which the public health specialist must be a decision-maker is when the good of the individual and the good of the public at large are incompatible. At first blush, one might imagine the optimal public health strategy to be to offer each individual the prevention strategy most likely to prevent that person from contributing to the epidemic (i.e., neither becoming infected nor transmitting the virus to others). However, there are several reasons why this might not always be true. First, any monies spent to prevent HIV infection among those at very low risk may not be cost-effective on a national level. Second, individualizing prevention measures may decrease the cost-effectiveness of our efforts if fewer infections per dollar are averted than would have been the case had a single, moderately effective approach been universally disseminated. Indeed, the process of assessing individuals' relevant lifestyles and characteristics in order to achieve the optimal matching might be prohibitively costly. At a more basic level, we may need to expand our prevention focus from the individual to the population. Some time ago Geoffrey Rose introduced into public health the importance of differences between "sick individuals" and "sick populations" and argued that different prevention strategies may be needed for the control of individual and population level health problems (Rose 1985). Given the clustering of HIV infection and most other sexually transmitted infections in distinct subpopulations, the concept of "sick populations" appears to be particularly relevant to the epidemiology of HIV infection and other STDs. At a minimum, it is important to focus on HIV infection and other STDs as multilevel problems (Padian, 1999). In prevention research and prevention programs, the mechanism of change may be at individual, group or population levels while the target of the intervention may be an individual, group or population. Moreover, the beneficiary of the intervention may be the same or different individual, group or population. For example, peer–led interventions (that employ individuals to implement change) that target groups of sex workers may benefit the clients of sex workers and the wives and other sex partners of the clients to a greater extent than they benefit the sex workers themselves. Ultimately the general population is the beneficiary of such interventions; the benefit to the population may exceed the benefit to individual sex workers (Padian, 1999). To give another example, emphasis on preventing acquisition of infection among all susceptible individuals in the community, and emphasis on preventing transmission of infection from a relatively smaller number of infected individuals, produce different distributions of costs and benefits across the population (Aral, 1996). Focusing prevention efforts on individuals who are already infected may not benefit those individuals at all, but are likely to benefit others.

3.2 Disadvantages

One downside to expert-provided recommendations is that such messages may attract less buy-in on the part of the target audience member. Evidence indicates that directive approaches to behavior change can at times be counterproductive because they foster resistance on the part of the message recipient (see Brehm, 1972). Much of the psychological research that identified effective behavior-change techniques used in public health interventions, such as those of cognitive-behavioral therapy, was conducted with help-seeking clinical populations. Help-seekers are presumably already motivated to change, and are likely to appreciate and welcome the assistance that the therapist can provide. However, many individuals at risk for HIV infection do not perceive HIV as a threat prior to intervention. Thus, interventions must inform and motivate participants in addition to helping them to acquire skills. This is recognized explicitly in the HIV prevention field by Fisher's Information-Motivation-Skill model of HIV-related behavior change (Fisher, Fisher, Williams, and Malloy, 1994). .

Indeed, there is evidence that resistence to limited options is affecting some HIV risk-taking particularly among MSM (Rofes, 1996; 1998). While early efforts to prevent the spread of HIV were firmly lodged within the gay community itself, current efforts appear to be more often located within public health bodies and other outside sources–leading many gay men to resent what they see as a lifetime prescription for abstinence or condom use.

4. COMBINING MEDICAL AND INDIVIDUAL EXPERTISE

How can decisions be based on the scientific expertise and expert power of the public health specialist, while taking into consideration target population characteristics and avoiding resistance? One model would be a process in which the participant retains substantial latitude in the problem-solving process, an approach detailed by Freire in the context of literacy training (Freire, 1983). Indeed, motivational interviewing (Miller, 1998; Miller & Rollnick, 1991) was developed as a strategy for motivating alcoholics non-directively; this approach has recently been adapted for HIV prevention interventions (Belcher et al., 1998; Carey et al., 1997).

However, this relies on one-to-one interactions between the provider and client. Many public health messages are delivered across mass media, within institutions such as schools and workplaces, or through product labeling or other structural/policy interventions affecting large numbers of diverse people. How can these messages be matched to audience member?

One possibility would be to deliver conditional–"if – then"–messages rather than one-size-fits-all ones. For example, a message targeting gay men could be: "If you are in a committed relationship and know that you are both HIV-negative, then discuss monogamy or using condoms with others." Or, "If you haven't had sex yet, consider the reasons to wait". Another would be to target specific audiences via the venues used to deliver messages. For example, sexually compulsive men could be reach through self-help groups or sex-related publications or websites. In fact, the internet may be a particularly effective way to reach specific audiences with tailored public health messages.

5. CONCLUSION

As the chapters in this volume make clear, the job of HIV prevention is becoming increasingly complex. Messages and prevention strategies will need to be tailored to the needs and characteristics of different individuals and populations. We have discussed numerous issues in achieving this matching process, from individual cognitive processing limitations and emotional factors, to public health exigencies that better serve the population than particular individuals. We need more high-quality research into what is effective for whom, and how best to frame messages and deliver interventions so that the reach the appropriate people effectively. Just as condoms are not a magic bullet for HIV prevention, there is no magic bullet for conducting prevention triage.

REFERENCES

Aral SO, Holmes KK, Padian NS, Cates W Jr. Overview: individual and population approaches to the epidemiology and prevention of sexually transmitted diseases an(human immunodeficiency virus infection. *Journal of Infectious Diseases* 1996; 174(Supp 2):S127-133.

Beeker, C., Guenther-Grey, C., & Raj, A. (1998).Community empowerment paradigm drif and the primary prevention of HIV/AIDS. *Social Science & Medicine, 46,* 831-842.

Belcher L, Kalichman S, Topping M, Smith S, Emshoff J, Norris F, & Nurss J. (1998). A randomized trial of a brief HIV risk reduction counseling intervention for women. *Journa of Counsling and Clinical Psychology, 66,* 856-861.

Brehm, J. W. (1972). *Responses to loss of freedom: A theory of psychological reactance* Morristown, NJ: General Learning Press.

Carey, M. P., Maisto, S.A., Kalichman, S. C., Forsyth, A. D., Wright, E. M., & Johnson, B.T (1997). Enhancing motivation to reduce the risk of HIV infection for economicall disadvantaged urban women. *Journal of Counsling and Clinical Psychology, 65,* 531-541.

Celentano DD, Nelson KE, Suprasert S, Eiumtrakul S, Tulvatana S, Kuntolbutra S, Akarasew P, Matanasarawoot A, Wright NH, Sirisopana N et al. Risk factors for HIV-seroconversion among young men in northern Thailand. *JAMA* 1996; 275(2):122-127.

Centers for Disease Control, 1981a. *Pneumocystis* Pneumonia--Los Angeles. MMWI 30:250-252.

Centers for Disease Control, 1981b. Kaposi's sarcoma and *pneumocystis* pneumonia amon homosexual men--New York City and California. MMWR 30305-308.

Centers for Disease Control, 1982a. Persistent, generalized lymphadenopathy amon homosexual males. MMWR 31:249-252.

Centers for Disease Control, 1983. Prevention of acquired immune deficiency syndrom (AIDS): report of inter-agency recommendations. MMWR 32:101-104.

Centers for Disease Control, 1984. Antibodies to a retrovirus etiologically associated wit acquired immunodeficiency syndrome (AIDS) in populations with increased incidences o the syndrome. MMWR 33:377-379.

Centers for Disease Control, 1985. Heterosexual transmission of human T-lymphotropi virus type III/lymphadenopathy-associated virus. MMWR 34:561-563.

Centers for Disease Control, 1986. Additional recommendations to reduce sexual and dru abuse-related transmission of human T-lymphotropic virus type III/lymphadenopathy associated virus. MMWR 35:152-155.

Centers for Disease Control, 1994. Current Trends Heterosexually Acquired AIDS-- Unite States, 1993. MMWR 43:155-160.

Centers for Disease Control, 1995. Update: AIDS Among Women-- United States, 1994 MMWR 44:81-84.

Centers for Disease Control, 1998. Trends in Sexual Risk Behaviors Among High Schoo Students -- United States, 1991-1997. MMWR 47:749-752.

Coutsoudis A, Pillay K, Spooner E, Kuhn L, Coovadia HM. (1999). Influence of infant feeding patterns on early mother-to-child transmission of HIV-1 in Durban, South Africa a prospective cohort study

Eagly, A. H., & Warren, R. (1976). Intelligence, comprehension, and opinion change *Journal of Personality, 44,* 226-242.

Elder, J. P., Ayala, G. X., & Harris, S. (1999). Theories and intervention approaches t health-behavior change in primary care. *American Journal of Preventive Medicine, 17* 275-284.

Fisher, J. D, Fisher, W. A, Williams, S. S, Malloy, T. E. (1994). Empirical tests of an information-motivation-behavioral skills model of AIDS preventive behavior with gay men and heterosexual university students. *Health Psychology, 13*, 238-250.

Freire, P. (1983). *Education for critical consciousness.* New York: Continuum Press.

Kahneman, D., Slovic, P., & Tversky, A. (1982). *Judgement under uncertainty: Heuristics and biases.* Cambridge, UK: Cambridge University Press.

Kegeles, S. M., Hays, R. B., Coates, T. J. (1996). The Mpowerment Project: A community-level HIV prevention intervention for young gay men. *American Journal of Public Health, 86,* 1129-1136.

Kilmarx PH, Limpakarnjanarak K, Uthaivoravit W, St. Louis ME, Young N, Korattana S, Kaewkungwal J, Mastro TD. Declining prevalence of gonorrhoea (GC) and chlamydia (CT)in female sex workers (FSW), Chiang Rai, Thailand, 1991 - 1994. Abstract presented at the XI International Conference on AIDS, Vancouver, July 7-12, 1996; Mo.C.440.

Miller, L., Murphy, S. T., Clarke, L., & Moore, J. (1998). Increasing options or condom substitution? Impact of hierarchical messages on women's evaluations of HIV prevention methods. *International Conference on AIDS,* 12: 684 (abstract no. 33479).

Miller, W. R. (1998). Enhancing motivation for change. W. R. Miller, Heather, N., et al.(Eds). *Treating addictive behaviors (2nd ed.)* (pp. 121-132). New York, NY, USA: Plenum Press.

Miller, W. R., & Rollnick, S. (1991). Motivational interviewing: Preparing people to change addictive behavior. New York, NY, USA: Guilford Press.

Morris M, Podhisita C, Wawer MJ, Handcock MS. (1996). Bridge populations in the spread of HIV/AIDS in Thailand. *AIDS,10,*1265-1271.

Nduati R, John G, Mbori-Ngacha D, Richardson B, Overbaugh J, Mwatha A, Ndinya-Achola J, Bwayo J, Onyango FE, Hughes J, & Kreiss J. (2000). Effect of breastfeeding and formula feeding on transmission of HIV-1: A randomized clinical trial. *Journal of the American Medical Association, 28*, 1167-1174.

Nisbett, R., & Ross, L. (1980). *Human inference: Strategies and shortcomings of social judgment.* Englewood Cliffs, NJ: Prentice-Hall.

O'Leary, A. (1999). Preventing HIV infection in heterosexual women: What do we know? What must we learn? *Applied and Preventive Psychology, 8,* 257-263.

Padian N, Aral SO, Holmes, KK. (1999). Individual, group, and population approaches to STD/HIV prevention. Sexually Transmitted Diseases, Third Edition. King K. Holmes et al (Editors). McGraw-Hill.

Peterson, J. L. & DiClemente, R. J. (Eds), (2000). *Handbook of HIV prevention.* New York: Kluwer/Plenum.

Petty, R. E., & Cacioppo, J. T. (1981). *Attitudes and persuasion: Classic and contemporary approaches.* Dubuque, IO: William C. Brown.

Rofes, E. E. (1998). Context is everything: Thoughts on effective HIV prevention and gay men in the United States. *Journal of Psychology & Human Sexuality, 10*, 133-142.

Rofes, E. E. (1996). *Reviving the tribe: Regenerating gay men's sexuality and culture in the ongoing epidemic.* New York, NY, USA: Harrington Park Press/Haworth Press, Inc.

Rose G: (1985). Sick individuals and sick populations. *International Journal of Epidemiology, 14*, 32-38.

Tversky, A. (1972). Elimination by aspects: A theory of choice. *Psychological Review, 79,* 281-299.

Index

MIX
Papier aus verantwortungsvollen Quellen
Paper from responsible sources
FSC® C105338

If you have any concerns about our products,
you can contact us on
ProductSafety@springernature.com

In case Publisher is established outside the EU,
the EU authorized representative is:
Springer Nature Customer Service Center GmbH
Europaplatz 3, 69115 Heidelberg, Germany

Printed by Libri Plureos GmbH
in Hamburg, Germany